Manual of

Nutrition and Therapeutic Diet

Manual of

Nutrition and Therapeutic Diet

(As per INC Syllabus)

Second Edition

TK Indrani BSc (N)

Ex Assistant Lecturer
College of Nursing
Sri Ramachandra Medical College and Research Institute
Sri Ramachandra Deemed University
Porur, Chennai, India

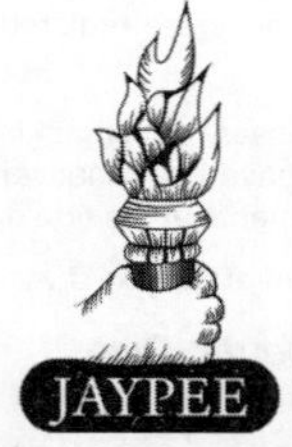

JAYPEE BROTHERS MEDICAL PUBLISHERS
The Health Sciences Publisher
New Delhi | London

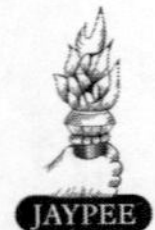

Jaypee Brothers Medical Publishers (P) Ltd

Headquarters
Jaypee Brothers Medical Publishers (P) Ltd
EMCA House, 23/23-B
Ansari Road, Daryaganj
New Delhi 110 002, India
Landline: +91-11-23272143, +91-11-23272703
+91-11-23282021, +91-11-23245672
Email: jaypee@jaypeebrothers.com

Corporate Office
Jaypee Brothers Medical Publishers (P) Ltd
4838/24, Ansari Road, Daryaganj
New Delhi 110 002, India
Phone: +91-11-43574357
Fax: +91-11-43574314
Email: jaypee@jaypeebrothers.com

Overseas Office
JP Medical Ltd.
83, Victoria Street, London
SW1H 0HW (UK)
Phone: +44 20 3170 8910
Fax: +44 (0)20 3008 6180
Email: info@jpmedpub.com

Website: www.jaypeebrothers.com
Website: www.jaypeedigital.com

Inquiries for bulk sales may be solicited at: jaypee@jaypeebrothers.com

Manual of Nutrition and Therapeutic Diet

First Edition: 2001
Reprint: 2005, 2008, 2012
Second Edition: 2017
Reprint: 2023, 2024, **2025**
ISBN: 978-93-86261-60-1

Printed at Rajkamal Electric Press, Kundli, Haryana-131 028.

Dedicated to

Jaypee Brothers Medical Publishers (P) Ltd, for showing keen interest to publish the book.

Preface to the Second Edition

Diet plays an important role not only in the maintenance and development of health conditions of the individuals but also in the early recovery from the illness to the patients.

The purpose to bring out *Manual of Nutrition and Therapeutic Diet* with new INC syllabus is to help undergraduates, graduate nursing students, dietic students, and medical students. The nursing teachers can use this book for preparing lesson plans.

The new syllabus has additional information for agencies who helps in preparing the nuritional programs in India and also to plan menu according to the illness of patients.

The general public can make use of this book for knowledge on diets and menu planning.

TK Indrani

Preface to the First Edition

Diet plays a sine qua non role not only in the maintenance and development of health conditions of individuals but also in the early recovery from the illness to the patients. The purpose of bringing out *Nursing Manual of Nutrition and Therapeutic Diet* is to help graduate, undergraduate and nursing students in planning the diets of the patients according to their disease conditions. This is a reference book prepared especially to help the students to prepare a concise and elaborate teaching notes according to their needs on the subject of nutrition and therapeutic diet. A cursory look of the book can enable them to plan menu for the requirement of individual patient according to the nature of disease. The chapters on Constituents of Food and its Function, Food Requirements, Planning for Nutritional Needs and Diet and the Patient have been dealt exhaustively keeping in mind the above purpose. In addition, chapters on Diet therapy in various health disorders also serve the same purpose. The discussions on nutritions for geriatric people, industrial workers and obese persons deserve special significance.

The book is mainly designed to suit the needs of nursing students. I hope the students will be benefited maximally. Readers comments for further improvement of the text are welcome.

TK Indrani

Acknowledgments

The success of this book was due to the active participation of the publisher. This is to record my appreciation for the support extended by Shri Jitendar P Vij (Group Chairman), Mr Ankit Vij (Group President), Ms Chetna Malhotra Vohra (Associate Director-Content Strategy), Mr Venugopal Vishnumurthy [Associate Director-South (Sales & Marketing)], Bengaluru Production Unit/Bengaluru Branch and their associates of M/s Jaypee Brothers Medical Publishers (P) Ltd, New Delhi, India, for readily conceding my request to publish the book and taking all pains to bring this book to my utmost satisfaction.

INC Syllabus

NUTRITION

Placement: First Year

Time: Theory 60 hours

Course Description: The course is designed to assist the students to acquire knowledge of nutrition for maintenance of optimum health at different stages of life and its application for practice of nursing.

Unit	*Time (Hrs)*		*Learning objectives*	*Content*	*Teaching learning activities*	*Evaluation*	*Chapter*
	Th.	*Pr.*					
I	4		• Describe the relationship between nutrition and health.	**Introduction** • Nutrition: – History – Concepts • Role of nutrition in maintaining health • Nutritional problems in India • National nutritional policy • Factors affecting food and nutrition: Socioeconomic, cultural, tradition, production, system of distribution, lifestyle and food habits, etc. • Role of food and its medicinal value • Classification of foods • Food standards • Elements of nutrition: Macro and micro • Calorie, BMR	• Lecture discussion • Explaining using charts • Panel discussion	• Short answers • Objective type	Section I 1, 2, 3, 4, 5

Unit	*Time (Hrs)*	*Learning objectives*	*Content*	*Teaching learning activities*	*Evaluation*	*Chapter*
II	2	• Describe the classification, functions, sources and recommended daily allowances (RDA) of carbohydrates	**Carbohydrates** • Classification • Caloric value • Recommended daily allowances • Dietary sources • Functions • Digestion, absorption and storage, metabolism of carbohydrates • Malnutrition: Deficiencies and over consumption	• Lecture discussion • Explaining using charts	• Short answers • Objective type	Section II 6, 7, 8, 9
III	2	• Describe the classification, functions, sources and recommended daily allowances (RDA) of fats	**Fats** • Classification • Caloric value • Recommended daily allowances • Dietary sources • Functions • Digestion, absorption and storage, metabolism • Malnutrition: Deficiencies and over consumption	• Lecture discussion • Explaining using charts	• Short answers • Objective type	Section III 10, 11, 12,13

Unit	*Time (Hrs)*	*Learning objectives*	*Content*	*Teaching learning activities*	*Evaluation*	*Chapter*
IV	2	• Describe the classification, functions, sources and recommended daily allowances (RDA) of proteins	**Proteins** • Classification • Caloric value • Recommended daily allowances • Dietary sources • Functions • Digestion, absorption, metabolism and storage • Malnutrition: Deficiencies and over consumption	• Lecture discussion • Explaining using charts	• Short answers • Objective type	Section IV 14, 15, 16, 17
V	3	• Describe the daily calorie requirement for different categories of people	**Energy** • Unit of Energy—Kcal • Energy requirements of different categories of people • Measurements of energy • Body Mass Index (BMI) and basic metabolism • Basal Metabolic Rate (BMR) — determination and factors affecting	• Lecture discussion • Explaining using charts • Exercise • Demonstration	• Short answers • Objective type	Section V 20

Unit	Time (Hrs)	Learning objectives	Content	Teaching learning activities	Evaluation	Chapter
VI	4	• Describe the classification, functions, sources and recommended daily allowances (RDA) of vitamins	**Vitamins** • Classification • Recommended daily allowances • Dietary sources • Functions • Absorptions, synthesis, metabolism storage and excretion • Deficiencies • Hypervitaminosis	• Lecture discussion • Explaining using charts	• Short answers • Objective type	Section V 18
VII	4	• Describe the classification, functions, sources and recommended daily allowances (RDA) of minerals	**Minerals** • Classification • Recommended daily allowances • Dietary sources • Functions • Absorptions, synthesis, metabolism storage and excretion • Deficiencies • Over consumption and toxicity	• Lecture discussion • Explaining using charts	• Short answers • Objective type	Section V 19

Unit	Time (Hrs)		Learning objectives	Content	Teaching learning activities	Evaluation	Chapter
VIII	3		• Describe the sources, functions and requirements of water & electrolyte	**Water and Electrolytes** • Water: Daily requirement, regulation of water metabolism, distribution of body water • Electrolytes: Types, sources, composition of body fluids • Maintenance of fluid and electrolyte balance • Over hydration, dehydration and water intoxication • Electrolyte imbalances	• Lecture discussion • Explaining using charts	• Short answers • Objective type	Section VI 21, 22, 23, 24, 25
IX	5	15	• Describe the cookery rules and preservation of nutrients • Prepare and serve simple beverages and different types of foods	**Cookery rules and preservation of nutrients** • Principles, methods of cooking and serving – Preservation of nutrients • Safe food handling-toxicity • Storage of food • Food preservation, food additives and its principles • Prevention of Food Adulteration Act (PFA) • Food standards • Preparation of simple beverages and different types of food	• Lecture discussion • Demonstration • Practice session	• Short answers • Objective type • Assessment of practice session	Section VIII 37, 38, 39, 40, 41, 42

Unit	*Time (Hrs)*		*Learning objectives*	*Content*	*Teaching learning activities*	*Evaluation*	*Chapter*
X	7	5	• Describe and plan balanced diet for different categories of people	**Balanced Diet** • Elements • Food groups • Recommended daily allowance • Nutritive value of foods • Calculation of balanced diet for different categories of people • Planning menu • Budgeting of food • Introducion to therapeutic diets: Naturopathy—diet	• Lecture discussion • Explaining using charts • Practice session • Meal planning	• Short answers • Objective type • Exercise on menu planning	Section VII 26, 27, 28, 29, 30, 31, 32, 33, 34, 35, 36
XI	4		• Describe various national programmes related to nutrition • Describe the role of nurse in assessment of nutritional status and nutrition education	**Role of Nurse in Nutritional Programmes** • National programmes related to nutrition – Vitamin A deficiency programme – National iodine deficiency disorders (IDD) programme – Mid-day meal programme – Integrated child development scheme (ICDS) • National and international agencies working towards food/nutrition – NIPCCD, CARE, FAO, NIN, CFTRI (Central food technology and research institute), etc. • Assessment of nutritional status • Nutrition education and role of nurse	• Lecture discussion • Explaining with • Slide/Film shows • Demonstration of assessment of nutritional status	• Short answers • Objective type	Section IX 43, 44, 45

Contents

Section I: Nutrition

Section II: Carbohydrates

Section III: Fats

Section IV: Proteins

Section V: Vitamins, Minerals and Energy

Section VI: Water and Electrolytes

Section VII: Balanced Diet

Section VIII: Food Preservation and Hospital Diets

Section IX: Nutritional Programs/ Education and Role of Nurse

Section I

Nutrition

1. History of Nutrition
2. Introduction to Nutrition
3. Medicinal Benefits of Whole Foods
4. Food Classification/Standards and Elements of Nutrition
5. Measurements of Energy

Chapter 1

History of Nutrition

Nutritional discoveries from the earliest days of history have had a positive effect on health and well-being. The word nutrition itself means "the process of nourishing or being nourished, especially the process by which a living organism assimilates food and uses it for growth and replacement of tissues". Nutrients are substances that are essential to life, which must be supplied by food.

Today more than ever, obtaining nutritional knowledge can make a big difference in lives. Air, soil and water pollution in addition to modern farming techniques, have depleted soils of vital minerals. The widespread use of food additives, chemicals, sugar and unhealthy fats in diets contributes to many of the degenerative diseases of the day such as cancer, heart disease, arthritis and osteoporosis. Here is a brief history of the science that offers the hope of improving health naturally.

400 BC: Hippocrates, the 'Father of Medicine', said to his students, "let thy food be thy medicine and thy medicine be thy food". He also said "a wise man should consider that health is the greatest of human blessings."

400 BC: Foods were often used as cosmetics or as medicines in the treatment of wounds. In some of the early far-Eastern biblical writings, there were references to food and health. One story describes the treatment of eye disease, now known to be due to a vitamin A deficiency, by squeezing the juice of liver onto the eye. Vitamin A is stored in large amounts in the liver.

1500s: Scientist and artist Leonardo da Vinci compared the process of metabolism in the body to the burning of a candle.

1747: James Lind, a physician in the British Navy, performed the first scientific experiment in nutrition. At that time, sailors were sent on long voyages for years and they developed scurvy (a painful, deadly, bleeding disorder). Only non-perishable foods such as dried meat and breads were taken on the voyages, as fresh foods would not last. In his experiment, Lind gave some of the sailors sea water, others vinegar and the rest limes. Those given the limes were saved from scurvy. As Vitamin C was not discovered until the 1930s, Lind did not know it was the vital nutrient. As a note, British sailors became known 'Limeys'.

1770: Antoine Lavoisier, the 'Father of Nutrition and Chemistry' discovered the actual process by which food is metabolized. He also demonstrated where animal heat comes from. In his equation, he describes the combination of food and oxygen in the body, and the resulting byproduct giving off heat and water.

Early 1800s: It was discovered that foods are composed primarily of four elements—carbon, nitrogen, hydrogen and oxygen, and methods were developed for determining the amounts of these elements.

1840: Justus Liebig of Germany, a pioneer in early plant growth studies, was the first to point out the chemical makeup of carbohydrates, fats and proteins. Carbohydrates were made of sugars, fats were made up of fatty acids and proteins were made up of amino acids.

1897: Christiaan Eijkman, a Dutchman working with natives in Java, observed that some of the natives developed a disease called beriberi, which caused heart problems and paralysis. He observed that when chickens were fed the native diet of white rice, they developed the symptoms of beriberi. When he fed the chickens unprocessed brown rice (with the outer bran intact), they did not develop the disease. Eijkman then fed brown rice to his patients and they were cured. He discovered that food could cure disease. Nutritionists later learned that the outer rice bran contains vitamin B1, also known as thiamine.

1912: McCollum EV, while working for the US Department of Agriculture at the University of Wisconsin, developed an approach that opened the way to the widespread discovery of nutrients. He decided to work with rats rather than large farm animals such as cows and sheep. Using this procedure, he discovered the first fat-soluble vitamin, i.e. vitamin A. He found that rats fed butter were healthier than those fed lard, as butter contains more vitamin A.

1912: Casimir Funk was the first to coin the term 'vitamins' as vital factors in the diet. He wrote about these unidentified substances present in food, which could prevent the diseases of scurvy, beriberi and pellagra (a disease caused by a deficiency of niacin, vitamin B_3). The term vitamin is derived from the words 'vital' and 'amine', because vitamins are required for life and they were originally thought to be amines—compounds derived from ammonia.

1930s: William Rose discovered the essential amino acids, the building blocks of protein.

1940s: The water-soluble B and C vitamins were identified.

1940s: Russell Marker perfected a method of synthesizing the female hormone progesterone from a component of wild yams called diosgenin.

1950s to the present: The roles of essential nutrients as part of bodily processes have been brought to light. For example, more became known about the role of vitamins and minerals as components of enzymes and hormones that work within the body.

1968: Linus Pauling, a Nobel Prize winner in chemistry, created the term orthomolecular nutrition. Orthomolecular is, literally, 'pertaining to the right molecule'. Pauling proposed that by giving the body the right molecules in the right concentration (optimum nutrition), nutrients could be used by people to achieve better health and prolong life. Studies in the 1970s and 1980s conducted by Pauling and colleagues suggested that very large doses of vitamin C given intravenously could be helpful in increasing the survival time and improving the quality of life of terminal cancer patients.

1994–2000: Have you ever wondered why vitamin bottle labels and nutritional websites include a phrase saying that their products and information are not intended to diagnose, cure or prevent any disease? These also usually state that their health claims have not been evaluated by the food and drug administration (FDA). Here is why—the Dietary and Supplement Health and Education Act was approved by Congress in October 1994 and updated in January 2000. It sets forth what can and cannot be said about nutritional supplements without prior FDA review.

While this law limits what vitamin manufacturers can claim about preventing or curing diseases; its passage has been a major milestone in the natural health field. It acknowledges millions of people who believe dietary supplements can improve their diets and bestow good health. It opens the way for people to obtain the information they need to make the best nutritional choices for themselves. In January 2000, the FDA clarified that supplement makers will state that their products can improve the structure or function of the body or improve common or minor symptoms. Allowable statements include things such as 'maintains a healthy heart', 'helps you relax', 'is good for symptoms of premenstrual syndrome (PMS)', 'strengthens joint structure', etc. Overall, due to this law, vitamins, herbs and nutrient manufacturers have greater freedom to say what their products can do to improve the health.

Chapter 2

Introduction to Nutrition

NUTRITIONAL BASIC CONCEPTS

The science of human nutrition is mainly concerned with defining the nutritional requirement for the promotion, protection and maintenance of health in all groups of population. In this context, variety of terms have been used to define the amount of nutrients needed by the body such as:

1. Optimum requirements.
2. Minimum requirements.
3. Recommended intake or allowances.
4. Safe level intake.

Of those, the term recommended daily allowance (RDA) or intake has been widely accepted.

Recommended Daily Allowance

The term recommended daily allowance is defined as the amount of nutrients sufficient for the maintenance of health in nearly all people. They are reference standards of nutritional intakes. This value will meet the requirement of 97.5% of the population. In fact for many individuals, this level will be in excess of their needs. The recommendation is estimated to meet the requirements of practically all the healthy people. They are reference standards of nutritional intakes for all nutrients; except energy, estimates of allowances are based on the defined 'minimum requirement' plus a safety margin are often generous.

Nutrition

Nutrition signifies a dynamic process in which the food that is consumed is utilized for nourishing the body. The word nutrition is derived from 'nutricus' meaning 'to suckle'; no clear distinction is made between food and nutrients.

Nutrition may be defined as the science of food and its relationship to health. Nutrition plays an important role in the promotion and maintenance of health, and in the prevention of human diseases. Malnutrition and undernutrition are the greatest international health problems of present day.

Food

Food is a composite mixture of various substances; the quantity of which may vary from a fraction of a grams in certain cases to hundreds of grams in others.

Foodstuff

The term foodstuff is defined as "anything, which can be used as food."

Malnutrition

Malnutrition has been defined as "a pathological state resulting from a relative or absolute deficiency, or excess of one or more essential nutrients"; it comprises of four forms as follows:

- Undernutrition
- Overnutrition
- Imbalance
- Specific deficiency.

Undernutrition

Undernutrition is the condition, which results when insufficient food is eaten over an extended period of time. In extreme cases, it is called starvation.

Overnutrition

Overnutrition is the pathological state resulting from the consumption of excessive quantity of food over an extended period of time. The high incidence of obesity atheroma and diabetes in western societies is attributed to overnutrition.

Imbalance

Imbalance is the pathological state resulting from a disproportion among essential nutrients without the absolute deficiency of any nutrients.

Specific Deficiency

Specific deficiency is the pathological state resulting from a relative or absolute lack of an individual nutrient.

Ecology of Malnutrition

Malnutrition is a man-made disease. It is a disease of human societies. It begins quite commonly in the womb and ends in the grave. The great advantage of looking at malnutrition as a problem in human ecology is that it allows for variety of approaches towards prevention. Ecological factors related to malnutrition are as follows:

- Conducting influences
- Cultural influences
- Socioeconomic factors
- Food production
- Health and other services.

A sound knowledge of nutrition is therefore essential for a nurse. In the global campaign of health for all, promotion of proper nutrition is one of the eight elements of primary health care. Greater emphasis is now placed on integrating nutrition into primary healthcare systems whenever goals to promote health and nutritional status of families and communities.

Definition of Terms

Nutrient

Food factor used for specific dietary constituents such as proteins, vitamins and minerals.

Dietetics

It is the practical application of the principles of nutrition. It includes the planning of meals for the well and the sick.

Role of Nutrition in Maintaining Health

1. Good nutrition is a basic component of health. The role of nutrition in health may be seen from the following viewpoints:
   a. Good nutrition is essential for the attainment of normal growth and development; not only for physical growth and development but also for the intellectual development; learning and behavior is affected by malnutrition:
      i. Malnutrition during pregnancy may affect the fetus resulting in stillbirth, premature birth and small-for-date babies.
      ii. Malnutrition during early childhood delays physical and mental growth. Such children are slow in passing their milestones and are slow learners in school.

iii. Good nutrition is essential for adult to maintain optimum health and efficiency. In short, nutrition affects human health from birth till death.

2. Malnutrition is directly responsible for certain specific nutritional deficiency diseases. The commonly reported ones in India are:
   a. Kwashiorkor
   b. Marasmus
   c. Blindness due to vitamins deficiency
   d. Anemia
   e. Beriberi
   f. Goiter

   Good nutrition therefore is essential for the prevention of specific nutritional deficiency disease and promotion to health.
3. To give resistance against infection—malnutrition predisposes to infection such as tuberculosis. Infection in turn may aggravate malnutrition by affecting food intake, absorption and metabolism.
4. Nutrition helps to reduce morbidity (death due to disease) and mortality (death). Indirect effects of malnutrition are:
   a. High general death rate.
   b. High infant mortality rate.
   c. High sickness rate or morbidity rate.
   d. Lower expectation of life.
   e. Overnutrition, which is another form of malnutrition. It is responsible for:
      i. Obesity
      ii. Diabetes
      iii. Hypertension
      iv. Cardiovascular diseases
      v. Renal diseases
      vi. Disorder of the liver and gallbladder.

NUTRITIONAL PROBLEMS IN INDIA

A number of factors influence the food habits. These include educational and economic level of the community, availability and cost of foods, and social and cultural practice, etc. Once the food habits are established, they are handed down from generation to generation.

The other factors that influence food habits are:

- Cultural influences
- Geographic locations
- Religious beliefs
- Traditional beliefs
- Food fads and cults
- Changing food habits.

People choose diets because of cultural influences, which vary widely from country to country and from region to region. These may be stated as follows:

- Food habits, customs, beliefs, traditions and attitudes
- Religion
- Food fads
- Cooking practices
- Child-rearing practices
- Miscellaneous.

Food Habits, Customs, Beliefs, Traditions and Attitudes

Food habits are among the oldest and most deeply entrenched aspects of any culture. They have deep psychological roots and are associated with love, affection, warmth, self-image and social prestige. The family play an important role in shaping the food habits and these habits are passed from one generation to another.

Rice is the staple cereal in the Eastern and Southern states of India and wheat is the staple cereal in the Northern states. During the Second World War, when wheat was made available in place of rice in South India, people refused to buy wheat because it was not their staple cereal. The crux of the problem is that many customs and beliefs apply most often to vulnerable groups, i.e. infants, toddlers, expectant and lactating women. For example:

1. Papaya is avoided during pregnancy because it is believed to cause abortion.
2. In Gujarat, valuable goods such as pulses, green leaves, rice and fruits are avoided by the nursing mother.
3. These is a widespread belief that if a pregnant women eats more, her baby will be healthy and delivery gets difficult.
4. Certain 'foods are forbidden,' as being harmful for the child.
5. Then there are certain beliefs about hot and cold foods, and also light and heavy foods.

Religion

Religion has a powerful influence on the food habits of the people. Hindus do not eat beef; Muslims do not prefer pork. Some orthodox Hindus and Jains do not eat meat, fish, eggs and certain vegetables such as onion and garlic. These are known as 'food taboos', which prevent people from consuming nutritious foods even when these are easily available.

Food Fads

In the selection of foods, personal likes and dislikes play an important part. These are called 'food fads'. The food fads may stand in the way of correcting nutritional deficiencies.

Cooking Practices

Draining away the rice water at the end of cooking, prolonged boiling in open pans, peeling of vegetables, etc. all influence the nutritive value of foods.

Child-rearing Practices

The practices vary widely from region to region and influence the nutritional status of infants and children. Examples of this situation are premature curtailment of breastfeeding, the adoption of bottle feeding and commercially produced refined foods.

Miscellaneous

In some communities, men eat first and women eat last and poorly. Consequently, the health of women in these societies may be adversely affected.

Production

Consumption of diets based predominantly on these foods has given rice to large scale incidence of protein-calorie malnutrition among preschool children in these regions. This may also explain the large scale cultivation of certain roots and tubers, viz. cassava, yam, sweet potato and maize (corn) in many countries of Africa, Central and South America over the past several centuries. For example, pellagra was also widely prevalent among poor maize eaters.

Rice is the main food crop in the tropical countries where rainfall is high and water is available for irrigation, while millets are cultivated in areas of low rainfall. Wheat is mainly cultivated in temperate regions. Incidence of beriberi was high among the population consuming highly milled raw rice.

NATIONAL NUTRITIONAL POLICY

The Government of India has initiated several programs in nutrition on a national scale to control/prevent major nutritional problems; these programs may be classified as:

1. **Programs designed to improve the overall nutritional status:**
   a. Applied Nutrition Program.
   b. Supplementary Feeding Programs.
   c. Mid-day Meal Program for school children.
2. **Programs aimed at overcoming specific deficiency diseases:**
   a. National Goiter Control Program.
   b. Vitamin A Prophylaxis Program.
   c. Iron and Folate Distribution Program.
3. **Others:**
   a. Integrated Child Development Scheme (ICDS).
   b. India Population Project.

Applied Nutrition Program

The Applied Nutrition Program was launched by the Government of India in 1963 with aid from United Nations Children's Fund (UNICEF), Food and Agriculture Organization (FAO), and World Health Organization (WHO) for improving the nutrition of the nursing and expectant mothers and children.

The chief aim of the program is to stimulate the production of protective foods such as eggs, fish, milk, vegetables and fruits, and by means of health education to promote their consumption by mothers and children who are the vulnerable group from the nutrition standpoint. Health education is an important component of the program, in fact the program has been developed to teach the village people how they can increase and improve their food supply through their own efforts. An important aspect of the programs is to train various categories of personnel such as rural health workers, teachers, doctors, youth and women leaders.

The Applied Nutrition Program is one of the longest single programs assisted by UNICEF in many countries. In India, it now covers 1,375 community development blocks and serves 1.7 million women and children. It is connected with the program that has not made the expected impact in terms of stated aims and objectives. Its demonstration effect has not been felt in most areas.

Supplementary Feeding Programs

The Special Nutritional Program (SNP) was started in 1970 for the nutritional benefit of preschool children (6 month to 6 year), pregnant women and nursing mothers, under the overall charge of the Ministry of Social Welfare, Government of India. Beneficiaries are selected from the weaker section of the population. In the initial stages, children in tribal areas and urban slums were covered. Later it was extended to selected backward areas and demoniacally drought affected areas. The supplementary food supplies 300 cal and 10–12 g of protein per child per day. The mothers receive daily 500 cal and 25 g of protein. This supplement is provided to them for about 300 days in a year.

The Balwadi Nutrition Program (BNP), which was started in 1970–71 is also under the overall charge of the department of social welfare. Balwadis were established in rural areas for providing preparatory education to children in the age group of 3–6 years. The supplement provided to the beneficiaries supplies 300 cal and 10 g of protein per child per day.

Mid-day Meal Program

The Mid-day Meal Program has been in operation in many parts of the country since 1962–1963, after it was first organized successfully in Tamil Nadu in 1957. Nearly 12 million children were covered by the program in 1974. The two basic objectives of the program are improvement in the nutritional status of children and importing nutrition education. The Tamil Nadu Government introduced in 1982, a new nutrition meal program for children aged 2–10 years. The Andhra Pradesh Government has also launched an ambitious school meal program.

The National Institute of Nutrition, Hyderabad has prepared model recipes for the preparation of school meals, suitable for North and South Indians. The National Institute of Nutrition is of the view that the number of feeding days in a year should be at least 250 to have the desired impact on the children. The important goals to be accomplished are reorientation of eating habits, incorporation of nutrition education into the curriculum; encouraging the use of local commodities; improving school attendance as well as educational performance of the pupils.

National Goiter Control Program

The National Goiter Control Program is in operation since 1962. Iodized salt is sold at the same price as common salt in goiter-endemic areas. Government aims to reduce prevalence of goiter endemic areas. Government aims to reduce prevalence of goiter under the program of 'Health for All by 2000'. Reduction of 50% of cases by 1985, and 95% by 2000 is planned. As a result, a major national program—the iodine deficiency disorder (IDD) control program was mounted to 1986 with the objective to replace the entire edible salt by iodine salt, in a phased manner.

Vitamin A Prophylaxis Program

One of the components of the national program for control of blindness is to administer a single massive dose oily preparation of vitamin A containing 200,000 IU (110 mg). of retinol palmitate orally to all preschool children in the community every 6 months through peripheral health workers. The program was launched by the Ministry of Health and Family Welfare in 1970 on the basis of technology developed at the National Institute of Nutrition at Hyderabad. An evaluation of the program has revealed a significant reduction in vitamin A deficiency in children.

Prophylaxis Against Nutritional Anemia

In view of its public health importance, a national program for the prevention of nutritional anemia has been launched by the Government of India during the fourth Five-year Plan. The program consist of distribution of iron and folic acid tablets for pregnant women and young children (1–12 year).

Mother and child health (MCH) centers in urban areas, primary health centers in rural areas and ICDS projects are engaged in the implementation of this program. The technology for the control of anemia through iron fortification of common salt has also been developed at the National Institute of Nutrition at Hyderabad.

Integrated Child Development Service Program

The ICDS program was started in 1975 in pursuance of the national policy for children. There is a strong nutrition component in this program in the form of supplementary nutrition, vitamin A prophylaxis and iron and folic acid distribution. The beneficiaries are preschool children below 6 years, pregnant and lactating mothers. The states and union territories are encouraged to undertake additional ICDS projects on the central pattern to cover more beneficiaries.

The workers at the village level who deliver the services are called anganwadi workers. Each anganwadi worker covers a population of about 1,000. A network of mahila mandals has been built up in ICDS project areas to help anganwadi workers in providing health and nutrition services. The work of anganwadis if supervised by mukhya sevikas. Field supervision is done by the child development project officer (CDPO).

Monitoring and Evaluation of Nutrition Programs

Since, health and nutrition of the young child is indivisible from the health and nutrition of the family as a whole. In the long new, one can hope to improve the nutritional status of the children only through improvement in the economic conditions of the community to a level at which families can afford balanced diets; organized state-sponsored feeding program cannot be the permanent answer to the problem. Factors affecting food and nutrition are:

- Socioeconomic, cultural and traditional beliefs
- Production
- System of distribution
- Lifestyle
- Food habits.

Traditional Beliefs

Traditional beliefs in food habits are still prevalent with a large majority of the population who are illiterate or ignorant regarding the nutritive value of foods. These beliefs influence profoundly the pattern of food eaten. For example:

1. In South Pacific Islands, it is believed that certain shell fish eaten during pregnancy will cause the child to be born with scales on its head.
2. In Ethiopia, a pregnant woman must avoid roasted meat, as it is believed to induce abortion. Eggs are thought to cause baldness or sterility and hence not consumed by pregnant women.
3. In India, consumption of papaya fruit by pregnant women is believed to lead abortion.
4. Milk, which is an essential protective food in Western countries, is disliked in many Asian and African countries and not even fed to weaned infants and preschool children.

5. In some parts of India (West Bengal), it was believed that consumption of milk and fish at the same meal will lead to the development of leprosy and leukoderma. Other similar beliefs include the following:
   a. Consumption of animal's brain will lead to premature graying of hair and baldness of head.
   b. Consumption of tongue of goat by children will make them talkative.
   c. Eating goat's leg by children will lead to improper development of knees and ankle joints.
   d. Consumption of pig's stomach by girls and young women will darken their complexion.
   e. Consumption of meat from the underside of an animal by young married women will prevent childbearing.
   f. In some parts of Africa, it is believed that eggs, if given to children before the teeth have erupted, will lead to stupidity; such will produce skin rashes and heat that will make a child greedy.

Hot and Cold Foods

Foods are classified as 'hot' and 'cold' by different cultures in many countries. 'Hot' foods are believed to produce more heat in the body and lead to the development of boils. 'Cold' foods are supposed to lower the heat production and lead to the development of cold, sore throat, etc. Meat, eggs, legumes, nuts and oilseeds supposed to be 'hot' foods, while fruits, vegetables and milk are supposed to be 'cold' foods.

Pica

Pica is a common practice among pregnant women and children in many countries. Pica is the habit of eating dirt, clay, chalk, limestones, plaster, ashes, starch, etc.

Socioeconomic Factors

Malnutrition is largely the byproduct of poverty, ignorance, insufficient education, lack of knowledge regarding the nutritive value of foods, etc. These factors bear most directly as the quality of life and are the true determinants of malnutrition in society.

Food Production

Increased food production should lead to increased food consumption. But increased food production will not cure the basic problem of hunger and malnutrition in much of the developing world. Scarcity of food, as a factor responsible for malnutrition, may be true at the family level; but it is not true on global basis nor it is true for most of the countries, where malnutrition is still a serious problem. It is said that there will be very little malnutrition in India today if all the food available can be equitably distributed in accordance with physiological needs.

Chapter 3

Medicinal Benefits of Whole Foods

HEALTH BENEFITS OF FOODS

For the first 5,000 years of civilization, humans relied on foods and herbs for medicine. Only in the past 50 years we have forgotten the medicinal 'roots' in favor of patent medicines. While pharmaceuticals have their value, we should not forget the well-documented, non-toxic and inexpensive healing properties of whole foods. The following list is about a sampling of the health benefits from whole foods.

Apple

Apples are very good to eat in their raw state, including the skin. They are a wonderful health builder and can help to alleviate constipation. Apples are an excellent blood purifier and they help to lower cholesterol and relieve liver congestion. They are anti-inflammatory fruit, and also useful for lung health.

Artichoke

Artichoke helps to detoxify the liver by facilitating the elimination of waste material. It is liver protective and good for the kidneys, especially in cases of fluid retention. Artichokes are helpful with digestive problems and are very good for diabetes and blood sugar issues. They are high in inulin and should be included in any diet of those needing to regulate blood sugar. Artichokes are also excellent for the skin.

Asparagus

Asparagus stimulates kidney function. It promotes the flow of urine by eliminating fluids that are stored in the tissues. Asparagus contains potassium, phosphorus, iron, magnesium and is one of the vegetables that are highest in protein, but low in calories. It is a great food for weight loss and also heart and bone health. Asparagus is also a good blood purifier.

Avocado

Avocado is a very nourishing food and an excellent body builder. Avocados are rich in vitamin B and dietary fiber. They are very high in potassium, which makes them excellent for the cardiovascular system. Potassium is a wonderful mineral for regulating blood pressure. Avocados are also good for anemia and nervous disorders and excellent for maintaining a healthy blood sugar level. The avocado is also the most protein-rich fruit, containing all of the essential amino acids.

Banana

Bananas are another food that are very high in potassium, making them a good medicinal food. They are a great energy food. Bananas help to alkalize the blood and eliminate excessive uric acid, which make them a very good food for those suffering from arthritis and gout. Two bananas a day provide 1,000 mg of potassium, excellent for maintaining a healthy heart.

Barley

Barley was long known as 'heart medicine' in the Middle East. It reduces cholesterol; has antiviral and anticancer activity; contains potent antioxidants, including tocotrienols.

Beans (Legumes)

Legumes (including navy, black, kidney, pinto, soy and lentils) are very rich in protein and fiber. They are excellent for constipation. Black beans may be the easiest to digest. Legumes are another food that is very rich in potassium, making them an excellent food for hypertension. They are beneficial for hair follicles and have been recommended for hair loss. Legumes contain more amino acids than any other plant food. They are a great meat substitute and should be eaten by those who are undernourished.

Beans (String)

String beans can be more nourishing than leafy vegetables and help to invigorate the body. String beans are very good for constipation, rheumatism, bladder and kidney issues. They are a good diuretic and help to reduce blood glucose levels. String beans are anti-inflammatory and also low in calories, so they are very good for maintaining a healthy weight.

Beets

Beets are one of the best foods for constipation. Beets fight inflammation, have anticancer properties (especially colon cancer), and help to detoxify the liver and the blood. They can be eaten raw or cooked. Grate them into the salads. Do not throw away the greens, as they are excellent in salads or lightly steamed and very healthy for the large intestine.

Bell Pepper

Bell peppers are rich in antioxidant vitamin C. It helps to fight off cold, asthma, bronchitis, respiratory infections, cataracts, macular degeneration, angina, atherosclerosis and cancer.

Blueberry

Blueberries are a wonderful blood purifiers and improve blood circulation. They are good for anemia, constipation, poor complexion, and obesity. Blueberries help to improve vision. They aid in cancer prevention and are very high in antioxidants that provide powerful protection against many degenerative diseases.

Broccoli

Broccoli is very rich in the mineral potassium. It is excellent for the circulatory system and the heart. Broccoli is a very powerful anticarcinogenic food and is great cancer preventative. Because broccoli is low in calories and sugars, it is a great food for diabetics and is a wonderful source of dietary fiber.

Brussel Sprouts

Cruciferous family possesses some of the same powers as broccoli and cabbage. Definitely anticancerous, estrogenic and packed with various antioxidants and indoles.

Cabbage (Including Bok Choy)

Cabbages are an excellent healing food. The juice will help to heal ulcers. Cabbages are especially helpful for lowering the risk of stomach and colon cancer. They are also high in calcium and potassium, which makes them valuable for the heart, helping to reduce fluid retention and blood pressure.

Carrot

Carrots are very rich in vitamin A and beta carotene. Carrots are a great medicine for the eyes, particularly night vision. They help to regulate elimination and are soothing to the intestinal tract. Carrots help to strengthen the liver, immunity and improve the blood. They are the beneficial food for cancer prevention. Carrot's health benefits improve when cooked, but carrot juice is especially beautifying for the skin.

Cauliflower

Cauliflower is an excellent source of fiber. It protects the body against various cancers, such as breast and colon cancer. Cauliflower stimulates the immune system. It is rich in potassium and calcium and is more digestible than other cruciferous vegetables. Cauliflower helps to regulate the transit time in the colon. It has diuretic properties and is helpful for the cardiovascular system.

Celery

Celery is one of the oldest remedies for controlling high blood pressure. It cleanses the blood. It is good for fluid retention and gout. Celery makes a wonderful juice and is also good blended in smoothies with apples. It has an astringent quality and helps with digestion and weight loss. Celery juice can help to lower cholesterol.

Chili Pepper

Chili pepper helps to dissolve blood clots, opens up sinuses and air passages, breaks up mucus in the lungs, acts as an expectorant or decongestant, helps prevent bronchitis, emphysema and stomach ulcers. Most of of chili pepper's pharmacological activity is credited to capsaicin (from the Latin 'to bite'), the compound that makes the pepper taste hot. Also a potent painkiller, alleviating headaches when inhaled and joint pain when injected. Hot paprika made from hot chili peppers is high in natural aspirin, antibacterial and antioxidant activity. Putting hot chili sauce on food also speeds up metabolism, burning off calories. Chili peppers do not harm the stomach lining or promote ulcers.

Cinnamon

A strong stimulator of insulin activity, thus potentially helpful for those with type 2 diabetes; mild anticoagulant activity.

Clove

Used to kill the pain of toothache and acts as an anti-inflammatory against rheumatic diseases; has anticoagulant effects (antiplatelet aggregation) and its main ingredient, eugenol, is anti-inflammatory.

Coffee

Most, but not all of coffee's pharmacological impact, comes from its high concentration of caffeine—a psychoactive drug. Caffeine, depending on an individual's biological makeup and peculiar sensitivity, can be a mood elevator and mental energizer. Improves mental performance in some. An emergency remedy for asthma; dilates bronchial passages; mildly addictive; triggers headaches, anxiety and panic attacks in some. In excess, may cause psychiatric disturbances. Promotes insomnia; it stimulates stomach acid secretions (both caffeinated and decaf) can aggravate heartburn. Promotes bowel movements in many, causes diarrhea in others. Caffeine may promote fibrocystic breast disease in some women.

Collard Greens

Collard greens are very high in calcium and promote good bone health. They help with vision health and offer antioxidant protection. Collards are cancer protective. They are good food for weight control, due to low-calorie and high-fiber count. Collards are rich in vitamin C and folate, and promote healthy liver function. The health benefits of collard greens are better when the leaves are steamed. They make a great addition to soups.

Corn

Anticancer and antiviral activity are possibly induced by corn's content of protease inhibitors. Corn has estrogen-boosting capabilities. A very common cause of food intolerance linked to symptoms of rheumatoid arthritis, irritable bowel syndrome, headaches and migraine-related epilepsy in children. Be sure to use only non-genetically modified organic (GMO) corn.

Cranberry

Strong antibiotic properties with unusual abilities to prevent infectious bacteria from sticking to the cells lining the bladder and urinary tract. Thus, it helps prevent recurring urinary tract (bladder) infections; also has antiviral activity.

Cucumbers

Cucumbers are high in silica and are a good food for the complexion and nails. They cool the body temperature. Cucumbers are excellent for obesity, skin eruptions, fevers, heart health and constipation. They hydrate the body and are rich in many alkalizing minerals. Cucumber juice is great to drink in the summer time.

Dates

High in natural aspirin; has laxative effect. Dried fruits, including dates, are linked to lower rates of certain cancers, especially pancreatic cancer. Contains compounds that may cause headaches in susceptible individuals.

Eggplant

Eggplant substances, called glycoalkaloids, made into a topical cream medication that have been used to treat skin cancers such as basal cell carcinoma, according to Australian researchers. Also, eating eggplant may lower blood cholesterol and help counteract some detrimental blood effects of fatty foods. Eggplant also has antibacterial and diuretic properties.

Fenugreek Seed

A spice common in the Middle East and available in many US food markets. Fenugreek has antidiabetic powers. Helps control surges of blood sugar and insulin. Also antidiarrheal, antiulcer, antidiabetic, anticancer, tends to lower blood pressure, helps prevent intestinal gas.

Flax Seeds and Oil

Used primarily for constipation; in cases of gastritis, colitis or other inflammations of the digestive tract. Lowers blood fat levels; often associated with heart attacks and strokes. Reduces harmful blood cholesterol levels with its soluble fibers. Prevents colon and breast cancer through its rich source of lignins, a documented anticancer agent. Improves moods, diminishes allergies and produces healthier skin.

Fig

Fig helps to prevent cancer. Both extract of figs and the fig compound, benzaldehyde, have helped shrink tumors in humans according to Japanese tests. Also possess laxative, antiulcer, antibacterial and antiparasitic powers. Triggers headaches in some people.

Fish and Fish Oil

An ounce a day has been shown to cut risk of heart attacks by 50%. The omega-3 oil in fish can relieve symptoms of rheumatoid arthritis, osteoarthritis, asthma, psoriasis, high blood pressure, Raynaud's disease, migraine headaches, ulcerative colitis and possibly, multiple sclerosis. May help ward off strokes. A known anti-inflammatory agent and anticoagulant. Raises good type [high density lipoprotein (HDL)] cholesterol. Lowers triglycerides; guards against glucose intolerance and type 2 diabetes. Some fish are high in antioxidants, such as selenium and coenzyme Q10. Exhibits anticancer activity, especially in blocking development of colon cancer and spread of breast cancer. Fish highest in omega-3 fatty acids include sardines, mackerel, herring, salmon and tuna.

Garlic

Garlic is a natural antibiotic and it stimulates immune system and digestive system. It helps to lower blood pressure. Garlic helps to reduce inflammation in the body and increase blood fluidity. It is excellent for respiratory problems. If raw garlic is eaten twice a week, it can lower the risk for lung cancer by 44%. The use of garlic as a medicine goes back to the time of Hippocrates.

Ginger

Used to treat nausea, vomiting, headaches, chest congestion, cholera, colds, diarrhea, stomachache, rheumatism and nervous diseases. Ginger is a proven antinausea antimotion sickness remedy that matches or surpasses drugs such as Dramamine. Helps thwart and prevent migraine headaches and osteoarthritis. Relieves symptoms of rheumatoid arthritis. Acts as an antithrombotic and anti-inflammatory agent in humans; is an antibiotic in test tubes (kills *Salmonella* and *Staphylococcus* bacteria), and an antiulcer agent in animals. Also, has antidepressant, antidiarrheal and strong antioxidant activity; high in anticancer activity.

Grapes

Grapes are rich in antioxidant compounds. Red grapes (but not white or green grapes) are high in the antioxidant 'quercetin'. Grape skins contain resveratrol, is shown to inhibit blood-platelet clumping (and consequently, blood clot formation) and boost good type HDL cholesterol. Red grapes are antibacterial and antiviral in test tubes. Grape seed oil also raises good type cholesterol.

Grapefruit

The pulp contains a unique pectin (in membranes and juice sacs—not in juice) that lowers blood cholesterol and reverses atherosclerosis (clogged arteries) in animals. It has anticancer activity and appears particularly protective against stomach and pancreatic cancer. The juice is antiviral and high in various antioxidants, especially vitamin C.

Honey

Honey has strong antibiotic properties. It has sleep-inducing, sedative and tranquilizing properties; use sparingly, as it is high in sugar.

Kale

Kale is one of the healthiest foods and is particularly protective against at least five different types of cancer. It has detoxification properties that make it very good food for liver function. Kale is high in bone-building calcium and is one of the vegetables whose health benefits improve when steamed.

Kiwi Fruit

Kiwi is commonly prescribed in Chinese traditional medicine to treat stomach and breast cancer. It is high in vitamin C.

Lecithin

Lecithin protects the nerves, improves memory and may help thyroid and adrenal hypertension. It protects cells against damage by oxidation. It emulsifies fat in the blood.

Lemon

Lemon is generally a good blood and body purifier and a mild diuretic. It works as an antiseptic for external use. Lemons improve blood fluidity, circulation and help with removal of toxins from the body. Lemons help strengthen the capillary walls and lower blood pressure. They alkalize the blood and are helpful with arthritic conditions and digestive disorders. Squeeze the juice of a half lemon into water and drink several times a day. It is helpful for weight loss and also helps to correct liver function.

Licorice

Licorice has strong anticancer powers, possibly because of a high concentration of glycyrrhizin. Mice drinking glycyrrhizin dissolved in water have fewer skin cancers. Also kills bacteria, fights ulcers and diarrhea; may act as a diuretic. Too much licorice can raise blood pressure; also it is not advised for pregnant women. Only real licorice has these powers. Licorice 'candy' sold in the US is made with anise instead of real licorice. Real licorice is called 'licorice mass'. Imitation licorice is labeled as 'artificial licorice' or 'anise'.

Melon

Melon—green and yellow, such as cantaloupe and honeydew does anticoagulant (blood-thinning) activity; contains the antioxidant beta-carotene.

Milk

Milk fat promotes cancer and heart disease. Milk has also an unappreciated terror in triggering 'allergic' reactions that induce joint pain and symptoms of rheumatoid arthritis, asthma, irritable bowel syndrome and diarrhea. In children and infants, milk is suspected to cause or contribute to colic and respiratory problems, sleeplessness, itchy rashes, migraines, epileptic seizures, ear infections and even diabetes. It may retard healing of ulcers.

Mushroom (Asian, Including Shiitake)

A longevity tonic, heart medicine and cancer remedy in Asia. Current tests show that mushrooms such as maitake, help prevent and/ or treat cancer and viral diseases such as influenza and polio, high blood cholesterol, sticky blood platelets and high blood pressure. If eaten daily, maitake or shiitake, fresh (3 ounce) or dried (1-3 ounce), cut cholesterol by 7–12% respectively. A shiitake compound, lentinan, is a broad-spectrum antiviral agent that potentiates immune functioning. It is used to treat leukemia in China and breast cancer in Japan. Eating black ('tree ear') mushroom thins the blood. No therapeutic effects are known for the common US button mushroom. Some claim that this species has cancer-causing potential (hydrazides) if not cooked.

Mustard (Including Horseradish)

Recognized for centuries as a decongestant and expectorant. Helps break-up mucus in air passages. A good remedy for congestion caused by colds and sinus problems; also antibacterial. Increases metabolism, burning off extra calories. In one British test, about three fifths of a teaspoon of ordinary yellow mustard increased metabolic rate by about 25%, burning 45 extra calories in 3 hours.

Nuts and Seeds

Nuts and seeds are foods that deeply nourish the body. They are good for nervous system and brain function, and also help in the prevention of cardiovascular disease. They are high in calcium, potassium, magnesium and phosphorus. They have a higher concentration of protein than other plants. Nuts and seeds are best in their raw state and not roasted. If roasted or heated, they may become toxic. Walnuts and flax seeds are high in omega-3s. Sesame seeds are high in calcium. Almonds are rich in magnesium, which is beneficial to the muscles, teeth and bones. Pumpkin seeds are high in zinc and beneficial for immunity. Cashews are high in magnesium and helps to promote relaxation and prevent osteoporosis. If weight is an issue, eat in a smaller amounts, such as small handful for an energetic snack and healthy blood sugar regulation.

Nutritional Yeast

Nutritional yeast contains a high quality protein that is easily digested and tastes delicious, sprinkled on vegetables or organic non-GMO popcorn. It adds nutritional value and flavor to soups. Nutritional yeast is a great alternative to animal protein. It is rich in B complex, especially vitamins B_{12}, so is very good for vegetarians and is mineral rich. Nutritional yeast is truly on the list of great superfoods.

Oats

Oats can depress cholesterol 10% or more, depending on individual responses. Oats help stabilize blood sugar, have estrogenic and antioxidant activity. They also contain psychoactive compounds that may combat nicotine cravings and have antidepressant powers. High doses can cause gas, abdominal bloating and pain in some.

Olive Oil

Lowers bad, low-density lipoprotein (LDL) cholesterol without lowering good HDL cholesterol. It helps keep bad cholesterol from being converted to a toxic or 'oxidized' form. Thus, helps protect arteries from plaque. Reduces blood pressure; helps regulate blood sugar. It has potent antioxidant activity. Best oil for kitchen cooking and salads.

Onion

Onions (including chives, shallots, scallions and leeks) were reputed in ancient Mesopotamia to cure virtually everything. An exceptionally strong antioxidant. It is full of numerous anticancer agents. Blocks cancer dramatically in animals. The onion is the richest dietary source of quercetin, a potent antioxidant (in shallots, yellow and red onions only, not in white onions). Specifically linked to inhibiting human stomach cancer. Thins the blood, lowers cholesterol, raises good type HDL cholesterol (preferred dose—half a raw onion a day), wards off blood clots, fights asthma, chronic bronchitis, hay fever, diabetes, atherosclerosis and infections. Anti-inflammatory, antibiotic, antiviral, thought to have diverse anticancer powers. Quercetin is also a sedative. Onions aggravate heartburn and may promote gas.

Orange

Natural cancer inhibitor, includes carotenoids, terpenes and flavonoids. Also rich in antioxidant vitamin C and beta carotene. Specifically tied to lower the rates of pancreatic cancer. In a test orange juice protected mice sperm from radiation damage. Because of its high vitamin C, oranges may help ward off asthma attacks, bronchitis, breast cancer, stomach cancer, atherosclerosis, gum disease and boost fertility and healthy sperm in some men. May aggravate heartburn.

Parsley

Parsley is anticancerous because of its high concentrations of antioxidants, such as monoterpenes, phthalides, polyacetylenes. It helps in detoxifying carcinogens and neutralize certain carcinogens in tobacco smoke. Also, it has diuretic activity.

Pineapple

Pineapple, if eaten fresh contains bromelain, which helps to prevent indigestion. It is also highly anti-inflammatory, and is good for arthritis, sore throat and cold symptoms. Pineapple is a good complement to weight loss diets. It is protective against stomach cancer. Pineapple/Parsley juice made in a blender is great for weight loss.

Plum

Plum is antibacterial and antiviral; it also acts as laxative.

Potato (White)

Patato contains anticancer protease inhibitors. It is high in potassium, thus may help prevent high blood pressure and strokes, and it has some estrogenic activity.

Prune

A well-known laxative, high in fiber, sorbitol and natural aspirin.

Pumpkin

Extremely high in beta carotene, the antioxidant reputed to help ward off numerous health problems, including heart attacks, cancer and cataracts.

Raspberry and Strawberry

Raspberry and strawberry are both good for digestion and urinary tract infections. Both berries are cleansing and detoxifying, and both are antiaging. They are a good remedy for constipation, are high in fiber and have the ability to prohibit cancer cells from growing. Berries are high in potassium and good for high blood pressure prevention. They are good for liver disorders. Use only organic berries, due to high pesticide use.

Rice

As other seeds, rice has antidiarrheal and anticancer properties, contains anticancer protease inhibitors. Of all grains and cereals, it is least likely to provoke intestinal gas or adverse reactions (intolerances) causing bowel distress such as spastic colon. Rice bran is excellent against constipation, lowers cholesterol and tends to block development of kidney stones.

Seaweed and Kelp

Seaweed and kelp (brown or laminaria type seaweed) are the best foods that one can eat in cases of hypothyroid. It is rich in many important minerals. The antibacterial and antiviral activity in brown laminaria type seaweed known as kelp helps kill herpes virus. For example, kelp may also lower blood pressure and cholesterol. Wakame boosts immune functioning. Nori kills bacteria and seems to help heal ulcers. A chemical from wakame seaweed is a clot buster, in a test conducted which was twice as powerful as the common drug heparin. Most types of seaweed have anticancer activity. Might aggravate acne flare-ups.

Soybean

Soybean is rich in hormones, it boosts estrogen levels in postmenopausal women. It has anticancer activity and is thought to be especially antagonistic to breast cancer, possibly one reason rates of breast and prostate cancers are low among the Japanese. Soybeans are the richest source of potent protease inhibitors, which are anticancer and antiviral agents. Soybeans lower blood cholesterol substantially. In animals, soybeans seem to deter and help dissolve kidney stones.

Spinach

Spinach provides strength to the muscles and protects the retina of the eye. It is very low in calories and contains great nutritive power from its richness in minerals and vitamins. Spinach is good for anemia and helps to prevent macular degeneration. It helps with the production of red blood cells and is protective against prostate cancer. Spinach is an excellent food for constipation. Raw spinach can be blended into a smoothie.

Spirulina

Spirulina helps to strengthen the immune system and is cancer protective. It is low in calories and helps with weight loss, curbs hunger and helps decrease inflammation. It is helpful in the treatment of allergies. Spirulina has a balance of all nine essential amino acids and is considered a complete protein. It is high in chlorophyll, easy to digest, and gives the body abundant energy on a cellular level.

Sugar

Sugar helps to heal wounds when applied externally. Similar to other carbohydrates, sugar helps to induce cavities. Also may be related to

Crohn's disease. Triggers rise in blood sugar and stimulates insulin production. One teaspoon of sugar is said to set the immune system back to 3½ hours. Causes fatigue and adrenal weakness.

Sweet Potato (Yams)

A source of the antioxidant beta carotene, linked to preventing heart disease, cataracts strokes and numerous cancers. One-half cup of mashed sweet potatoes contains about 23,000 international units (IUs) of beta carotene, according to Department of Agriculture estimates.

Swiss Chard

Swiss chard is a blood purifier. It helps with digestion and is good for constipation. Similar to spinach, it is good for anemia and weight loss.

Tea

Tea (including black, oolong and green tea, not herbal teas) has an amazing and diverse pharmacological activity, mainly due to catechins. Tea acts as an anticoagulant, artery protector, antibiotic, antiulcer agent, cavity-fighter, antidiarrheal agent, antiviral agent, diuretic (caffeine), analgesic (caffeine) and mild sedative (decaffeinated). In animals, tea and tea compounds are potent blockers of various cancers. Tea drinkers appear to have less atherosclerosis (damaged, clogged arteries) and fewer strokes. Excessive tea drinking because of its caffeine could aggravate anxiety, insomnia and symptoms of premenstrual syndrome (PMS). Tea may also promote kidney stones because of its high oxalate content. Green tea, popular in Asian countries, is highest in catechins, followed by oolong and ordinary black tea, common in the US. Green tea is considered most potent. One human study, however, found no difference in benefits to arteries from green or black tea.

Tomato

A major source of lycopene, an antioxidant and anticancer agent that intervenes in devastating chain reactions of free radical molecules of oxygen. Tomatoes are linked in particular to lower rates of pancreatic and cervical cancer.

Turmeric

Turmeric is truly one of the marvelous medicinal spices of the world. Its main active ingredient is curcumin, which gives turmeric its intense cadmium yellow color. Curcumin studies show that it is an anti-inflammatory agent on a par with cortisone and has reduced inflammation in animals and symptoms of rheumatoid arthritis in humans. In other tests, it lowered cholesterol, hindered platelet aggregation (blood clotting), protected the liver from toxins, boosted stomach defenses against acid, lowered blood sugar in diabetics and was a powerful antagonist of numerous cancer-causing agents and is anticancerous.

Watermelon

Watermelon has high amounts of lycopene and glutathione, antioxidant and anticancer compounds; also mild antibacterial and does anticoagulant activity.

Wheat

High-fiber whole wheat and particularly wheat bran, ranks as the world's greatest preventives of constipation. The bran is potently anticancerous. Remarkably, in humans, wheat bran can suppress the disorder, which can develop into colon cancer and is antiparasitic. Ranks exceedingly high as a trigger of food intolerances and allergies, resulting in symptoms of rheumatoid arthritis, irritable bowel syndrome and neurological illnesses.

Yogurt

Goat yogurt is preferred most. An ancient wonder food, strongly antibacterial and anticancerous. A cup or two of yogurt a day boosts immune functioning by stimulating production of gamma interferon. Also spurs activity of natural killer cells that attack viruses and tumors. A daily cup of yogurt reduces colds and other upper respiratory infections in humans. Helps to prevent and cure diarrhea. Daily a cup of yogurt with acidophilus cultures prevents vaginitis (yeast infections) in women. Helps fight bone problems, such as osteoporosis, because of high available calcium content. Acidophilus yogurt cultures neutralize cancer-causing agents in the intestinal tract. Yogurts with *Lactobacillus bulgaricus* and *Streptococcus thermophilus* cultures, both live and dead, blocks lung cancers in animals. Yogurt with live cultures is safe for people with lactose intolerance.

Zucchini

Zucchini is a great food to eat freely in the summer time. It is good for constipation, high blood pressure, kidney and bladder health, as well as weight loss. Zucchini is soothing to the intestinal tract and easy to digest. It is very good for heart health. Refer the highly nourishing Bieler's broth recipe in this publication.

Chapter 4

Food Classification/ Standards and Elements of Nutrition

There are many ways to classify foods:

1. **Classification by origin:**
   a. Foods of animal origin
   b. Foods of vegetable origin.
2. **Classification by chemical compositions:**
   a. Proteins
   b. Fats
   c. Carbohydrates
   d. Vitamins
   e. Minerals.
3. **Classification by predominant functions:**
   a. Body-building foods, for example milk, meat, poultry, fish, eggs, pulses, peas, nuts, etc.
   b. Energy-giving foods, for example cereals, sugars, roots and tubers, fats and oils.
   c. Protective foods, for example vegetables, fruits and milk.
4. **Classification by nutritive value:**
   a. Cereals and millets
   b. Pulses (legumes)
   c. Vegetables
   d. Nuts and oil seeds
   e. Fruits
   f. Animal foods
   g. Fats and oils
   h. Sugar and jaggery
   i. Condiments and spices
   j. Miscellaneous foods.

DEFINITION OF NUTRITION

Nutrients are organic and inorganic complexes contained in food. These are about 50 different nutrients, which are normally supplied through the foods we eat. Each nutrient has specific functions in the body. Most of the natural foods contain more than one nutrient. These may be divided into:

1. Macronutrients.
2. Micronutrients.

Macronutrients

Macronutrients are proteins, fats and carbohydrates, which are often called 'proximate principles', because they form the main bulk of food in the Indian diet. They contribute to the total energy intake in the following proportions:

- Proteins: 1–15%
- Fats: 10–30%
- Carbohydrates: 65–80%.

Micronutrients

Micronutrients are vitamins and minerals. They are called so because they are required in small amounts, which may vary from a fraction of a milligram to several grams.

FOOD STANDARDS

Food and Agriculture Organization (FAO)/World Health Organization (WHO) formulates food standards for international market. Codex Alimentarius Commission is the principal organ of the joint FAO/WHO food standards program. The standards in India are based on the standards of the Codex Alimentarius.

Any food that does not confirm to the minimum standard is said to be of adulterated standards. Provisions have been laid down under this act for various foods. In 1954, the Government of India enacted a central prevention of food adulteration act. The act has been amended several times; the latest amendment is that of 1976 and in lately in 1986 to make the act more stringent. Although it is central act; its implementation is largely carried out by the local bodies and state governments.

Prevention of Food Adulteration Standards

Under the Prevention of Food Adulteration (PFA) Act, 1954, standards have been established, which are revised from time to time by the 'control committee for food standards'. The purpose of PFA standards is to obtain a minimum level of quality of foodstuffs attainable under Indian conditions.

Agmark Standards

The Agmark standards are set by the Directorate of marketing and inspection of the Government of India. The Agmark gives the consumer an assurance of quality in accordance with the standards prescribed by the Bureau of Indian Standards (BIS) for that commodity.

Bureau of Indian Standards

The Indian Standards Institute (ISI) mark on any article of food is a guarantee of food quality in accordance with the standards prescribed by the BIS for that commodity. The Agmark and ISI standards are not mandatory; they are purely voluntary. They express degree of excellence above PFA standards.

Chapter 5

Measurements of Energy

CALORIE

The energy value of foods has long been expressed in terms of the kilocalories (kcal). The kcal or the large calorie used in nutrition work is defined as the heat required to raise the temperature of 1 kilogram of water by 1°C and is 1,000 times the calorie usually referred to in physics. This has been replaced by the 'Joule', which has been accepted internationally. The conversion factors are as follows:

- 1 kcal : 184 kJ
- 1,000 kcal : 4.184 kJ
- 1,000 kcal : 40184 MJ
- 1 kJ : 0.239 kcal
- 1,000 kJ : 239 kcal
- 1 MJ : 239 kcal.

The dietary sources of energy are protein, fat and carbohydrate. They supply energy at the following rates:

- Protein : 4 kcal/g or 17 kJ
- Fat : 9 kcal/g or 37 kJ
- Carbohydrate : 4 kcal/g or 17 kJ.

BASAL METABOLIC RATE

Basal metabolic rate (BMR) is the amount of energy required by a person who is awake, but he/she is nearly as possible as at complete mental and physical rest, and has had no food for 12–14 hours.

Factors Affecting the Basal Metabolic Rate

There are many factors, which affect the BMR; the most important of which are:

1. **Surface area of the body:** Larger the surface area of the body in relation to bulk, greater is the heat lost by radiation. For example, tall man will have greater surface area of the body than a short

fat man; therefore he will lose more heat by radiation and his BMR will be higher. This may explain, at least in part, why a thin man often eats more than a fat man of the same weight.

2. **Sex:** The BMR is higher per square meter of body surface area in man than in women. According to Western Standards, the requirements are:
   - About 40 cal/hr/m^2 for man
   - About 30 cal/hr/m^2 for woman.
3. **Age:** Growing children and adolescents have higher BMRs in relation to their weight than adults.
4. **Diseases:** Some diseases, especially of the thyroid gland, may raise or lower the BMR. A rise in the body temperature of 1°F is found to increase BMR by about 7%. This is important to remember during fever.
5. **Nutrition:** Under prolonged or chronic undernutrition, the BMR is decreased.
6. **Stress:** Psychological tension caused by worry or stress will increase the BMR.

Section II

Carbohydrates

Chapter 6

Classification and Functions

The third major component of food is carbohydrate, which is the main source of energy, providing 4 kcal/1 g of carbon. There are three main sources of carbohydrates, which are as follows:

1. **Starch:** It is basic to the human diet. It is found in abundance in cereals, roots and tubers.
2. **Sugars:** Free sugars along with starches constitute a key source of energy.
3. **Cellulose:** It is the indigestible component of carbohydrate with scarcely any nutritive value that contributes to dietary fiber.

The carbohydrate reserve (glycogen) of a human adult is about 500 g. This reserve is rapidly saturated where man is fasting. If the dietary carbohydrate do not meet the energy needs of the body, protein and glycerol from dietary and endogenous sources are used by the body to maintain glucose (homeostasis).

CLASSIFICATION OF CARBOHYDRATES

The carbohydrates are classified into three groups:

1. **Monosaccharides or simple sugars:** It includes glucose, fructose and galactose, which are detailed as follows:
   a. Glucose: It is also called dextrose, grape sugar or corn sugar. It is found in fruits such as grapes, sweet corn and certain roots.
   b. Fructose: It is known as levulose or fruit sugar. It is the sweetest of all sugar, e.g. honey, ripen fruits and vegetables.
   c. Galactose: It is the result of the hydrolysis of lactose or milk sugar. It does not occur in the free state in nature.
2. **Disaccharides or compound sugars:** It includes sucrose, lactose and maltose, which are detailed as follows:
   a. Sucrose: Sugarcane juice, sugar beet, sorghum cane, fruits and vegetables.

b. Lactose: Also known as milk sugar; it is produced only by mammals.
c. Maltose: Also known as malt sugar and found in malted products such as cereals.

3. **Polysaccharides:** It includes starch, glycogen, cellulose, which are detailed as follows:
   a. Starch: The sources include cereals, grains, seeds, roots, potatoes and green banana.
   b. Glycogen: Animal starch is the form in which the animal stores carbohydrates in liver.
   c. Cellulose: It is non-digestible dietary constituent. They are composed of more than two sugars. They contain pentose and hexose. They are present in all vegetables and bran of cereals.

Carbohydrates that are utilized by the body are starch, dextrin and glycogen. Carbohydrates, which are not utilized by the body are cellulose, hemicellulose, starch, etc. These are not acted upon by digestive juices and hence are voided or excreted in the feces.

FUNCTIONS OF CARBOHYDRATES

1. They are the main source of energy.
2. They are also essential for the oxidation of fats and for the synthesis of certain non-essential amino acids.
3. When consumed in excess, they may be converted into fats and stored in the body.

SOURCES OF CARBOHYDRATES (DIETARY SOURCES)

The main sources of carbohydrates are:

1. **Starches:** Cereals, rice, wheat, roots, tubers, potatoes, jowar, sweet potatoes and tapioca.
2. **Sugar:** Glucose and fructose.
3. **Cellulose:** Fruits and cereals.

DAILY REQUIREMENT OF CARBOHYDRATES

About 50–60% of total calories are from carbohydrates or 500 calories as minimum dietary level. It is increased in case of pregnancy and lactation.

DEFICIENCY OF CARBOHYDRATES

Reduction in carbohydrate intake causes marasmus and protein energy malnutrition in children, and malnutrition in adults.

CALORIC REQUIREMENT (TABLE 6.1)

Table 6.1: Calories required for human body

Category	Man (53 kg)	Woman (45 kg)
Sedentary worker	2,400 kcal	2,000 kcal
Heavy worker	2,800 kcal	2,300 kcal
Pregnancy	–	2,300 kcal
Lactation	–	2,700 kcal

FIBERS

Fiber or roughage consists of cellulose and hemicellulose. This part of carbohydrates are not digested by the digestive juices. They are left unchanged after digestion.

Functions of Fibers

1. The fiber absorbs water and this increases the bulk of stool and helps to reduce the tendency of constipation by encouraging bowel movements.
2. The cholesterol-lowering effect of certain types of dietary fiber appears firmly established.
3. Fiber may also have a role in weight reduction, people who eat well-balanced diet obtain enough roughage.

Chapter 7

Digestion, Absorption and Storage

DIGESTION

Digestion of food takes place through two processes, i.e. mechanical and chemical. The enzymes present in the digestive system plays a major role in the digestion process (Table 7.1).

Table 7.1: Digestion of carbohydrates

Site	Substrate	Enzyme	Digestion Product
Mouth	Starch	Ptyalin	Dextrin
Stomach	Sucrose	Pancreatic amylase	Maltose
Small intestine	Starch and dextrin	–	–
	Maltose	Maltase	Glucose
	Sucrose	Sucrase	Glucose and fructose
	Sucrose	Lactase	Glucose and galactose

Digestion in Mouth

In mouth, salivary digestion takes place. While the digestion of all types of foods (proteins, fats and carbohydrates) begins in the mouth with the mechanical process of mastication. Food is chewed in the mouth, where it mixes with saliva. Carbohydrates are broken down by mastication and the saliva prepares the broken pieces of food for swallowing. Salivary amylase—ptyalin, the enzyme secreted by the parotid glands is mixed with the food during the chewing process, and begins the conversion of glycogen, starch and dextrin into the disaccharide maltose.

Digestion in Stomach

In stomach, muscular contractions churn the food, break it up and mix it with the gastric juices secreted by gastric glands in the stomach wall. The gastric juices contain a lot of water, hydrochloric acid (HCl) and enzyme amylases. The acid enhances hydrolysis and food breaks down into microfragments. Before the complete mixing of food with gastric secretions, about 30% of the starche may have been changed into maltose.

While digestive action continues in the stomach, the food is prevented from moving on through the alimentary canal by a muscular valve called pylorus. From time to time, the pylorus relaxes, allowing some of the chyme to pass into the small intestine.

Digestion in Small Intestine

The food moves through the gastrointestinal tract (GIT) by the regular contractions of the smooth muscles of the system. These movements are wave-like and called peristaltic movements, and the process is called peristalsis. Peristalsis aids by mixing and moving the chyme. Chemical digestion is completed in the small intestine by two enzymes, viz. pancreatic amylase and intestinal secretions. Amylase of the pancreatic juice hydrolyzes the remaining starch into maltose.

At this stage in the digestive process, polysaccharides (starch, dextrin and glycogen) have been converted into disaccharides (maltose, sucrose and lactose) and then converted into monosaccharides. The intestinal mucosa contains sucrase, maltase and lactase enzymes. These enzymes convert sucrose into glucose and fructose, maltose into glucose, and lactose into glucose and galactose. These amylases are secreted by the wall of the small intestinal part called villi. The end products of carbohydrates digestion are glucose, galactose and fructose, and are absorbed in the intestine:

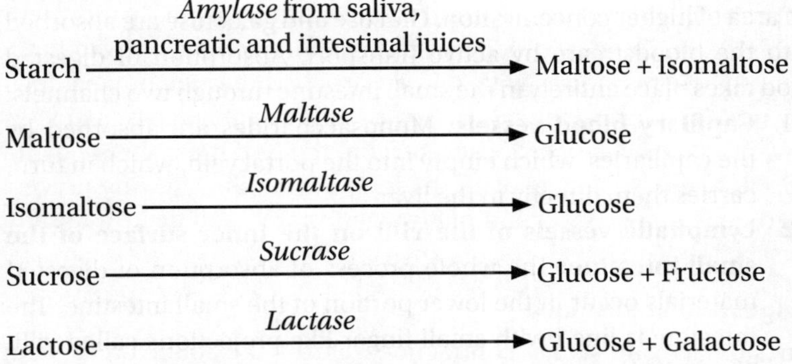

The non-digestible carbohydrates present in the food such as cellulose, hemicelluloses, pentosans, galactans, fructosans, etc. are not acted upon by the digestive juices. They add bulk to the contents of large intestines and are excreted in the feces. Some of these are fermented by bacteria present in the large intestine.

Digestion in Large Intestine

All carbohydrates that reach the large intestine may be fermented by the colonic microflora with the production of short-chain fatty acids and gas.

ABSORPTION

The absorption of carbohydrates from the intestine is controlled by certain factors such as condition of the intestinal tract, muscle tone, endocrine glands (anterior pituitary, thyroid and adrenal cortex) and their functions, and vitamin B complex content in the diet. Substances or nutrients pass through the intestinal membrane through the process of osmosis in one of the following two ways:

- Diffusion
- Active transport.

Diffusion

Nutrients in the intestinal tract that are in higher concentration across the membrane in the blood and lymph pass through by diffusion. Fructose is absorbed by diffusion.

Active Transport

Active transport is the osmotic pressure used when nutrients are absorbed from an area of low concentration across a membrane to an area of higher concentration. Glucose and galactose are absorbed into the bloodstream by active transport. Absorption of digested food takes place entirely in the small intestine through two channels:

1. **Capillary blood vessels:** Monosaccharides are absorbed by the capillaries, which empty into the portal vein, which in turn, carries them directly to the liver.
2. **Lymphatic vessels of the villi on the inner surface of the small intestine:** The whole process of absorption of digested materials occur in the lower portion of the small intestine. The intestine is lined with small finger-like projections called villi. Through these, simple sugars diffuse from the intestines into the blood.

STORAGE

Carbohydrates are stored either as glycogen or fat. Glycogen is a large polymer of glucose. The process of glycogen formation is called glycogenesis. A small part of glucose is stored in liver and muscle as glycogen and some portion of glucose is converted into fat and stored in adipose tissue.

Chapter 8

Metabolism and Synthesis

METABOLISM (TABLE 8.1)

Once absorbed, the nutrients enter the bloodstream, which distributes them to all cells of the body where they undergo metabolism. Metabolism is the chemical phenomenon containing of two processes:

1. **Anabolism:** The process in which absorbed food is converted to body tissue.
2. **Catabolism:** The breaking down of the body tissue and production of energy required for various vital processes.

Table 8.1: Enzyme's action on disaccharides

Disaccharides	Enzymes	Monosaccharides
Sucrose	Sucrase	Fructose
Lactose	Lactase	Galactose
Maltose	Maltase	Glucose

Process of Metabolism

Carbohydrates in the form of starch and sugar are acted upon by the enzymes of the saliva, pancreatic and intestinal juices, and converted into simple sugars such as glucose, galactose and fructose. This simple sugar absorbed by the villi of the small intestine passes into the blood capillaries and is carried by the portal vein to the liver.

Glucose, galactose and fructose absorbed in the intestines pass through the portal circulation of the liver. In the liver, apart from glucose, the entire galactose and fructose are converted into glycogen. A part of the glucose passes into the general circulation and to the various tissues for being oxidized and used as energy. A small part of glucose is sorted in liver and muscle as glycogen, and some portion of the glucose is converted into fat and stored in adipose tissue. The oxidation of glucose in the tissues occurs in two stages as indicated below:

1. Glycogen $\rightleftharpoons$ Glucose $\rightarrow$ Pyruvic acid $\rightleftharpoons$ Lactic acid

2. Pyruvic acid $\xrightarrow{\text{Oxidation}}$ $CO_2 + H_2O$

The first stage is called 'glycolysis'. The oxidation of pyruvic acid takes place through a series of reactions known as tricarboxylic acid cycle (Krebs cycle). The use of glucose is to serve as the main body fuel for production of energy for work and heat. The glucose required for immediate use is carried straight through the liver into hepatic veins and inferior vena cava, and enters the circulation. Any excess not required for the body's immediate need is converted into glycogen by the liver cells, which is insoluble and is stored in the liver until required for use.

When sugar is needed by the body, the glycogen is converted back into glucose, which the body fluids dissolve, so that it passes into bloodstream. Both the formation of glycogen from glucose and the forming of glucose from glycogen are the work of enzymes produced by liver cells. Glucose is specially required by the most active tissues of the body—the muscles and glands, but all tissues need it to some extent. The muscles, e.g. the liver, are able to store it to a slight extent in the form of glycogen. Glucose is burnt to produce energy for muscle contraction, but more energy is released by complete combustion that is required for the work of muscles and the excess energy is used to build up glycogen again.

Actually, it is estimated that only about one fifth of the fuel is completely burnt down into the waste products (i.e. CO_2 and H_2O). The remaining four fifth after partial combustion, is built up again into glycogen, ready for use, when the muscles require it. The energy for this building up work is obtained from the complete combustion of the other one fifth of the fuel. The waste products of the combustion of carbohydrates are CO_2 and H_2O, which are carried away by the bloodstream and excreted from the body. The end product CO_2 and H_2O are also got rid off by the skin and kidneys. The metabolism of carbohydrate is controlled by insulin—the internal secretion of the pancreas. Without insulin, the tissues are not able to burn neither glucose nor the liver to store it as glycogen. If the insulin supply is normal, the amount of glucose in the blood varies very slightly.

If there is deficiency of insulin, the blood sugar raises too high; liver and muscles store glucose to the normal extent. Too much insulin in the blood causes excess glucose to be stored in liver and leaves it insufficient in the bloodstream. This is very serious and may cause coma and death.

SYNTHESIS

The carbohydrates are not synthesized in the body, but are taken from the food such as starch and sugar. The various forms of synthesis are as follows:

1. **Glucose formation from non-carbohydrate sources:** The glucose can be formed from the metabolism of proteins and glycerol of fat. It has been estimated that the glycerol present in 100 g of fat can give rise to 12 g glucose that can be reconverted into glucose in the liver.
2. **Formation of carbohydrates from proteins:** Carbohydrates can be formed from proteins. This happens during starvation, when carbohydrates are formed from the tissue proteins, which are broken down to meet energy needs. Glucose is also formed from proteins in the disease, i.e. diabetes mellitus.
3. **Carbohydrates from fats:** Carbohydrates can be formed from the entire glycerol present in fats. Fatty acids with even number of carbon atoms cannot be readily converted into glucose, as the body cannot convert acetyl-CoA derived from oxidation of fatty acids to pyruvic acid, which is key material for the synthesis of carbohydrates.

Chapter 9

Malnutrition and Overconsumption

Carbohydrates are main sources of energy. These are an important dietary nutrient and the key source of caloric energy. Foods containing carbohydrates provide with vitamins and minerals. A variety of foods, including fruits, vegetables and whole grains supply carbohydrates. Within these foods, there are different types of carbohydrates that absorb gradually or quickly during digestion, depending on the molecular structure. A carbohydrate deficiency can occur when one restricts the diet of carbohydrate-containing foods, thus limiting the primary source of energy from glucose.

DEFICIENCIES

Hypoglycemia

Hypoglycemia is also known as low blood sugar or low blood glucose, occurs when glucose levels in the blood drop below normal. While hypoglycemia is often associated with diabetes, it can be caused by lack of carbohydrates in healthy people. Symptoms of tiredness, weakness, lightheadedness, confusion and hunger. Carbohydrates are the main source of glucose because they are broken down into simple sugars during digestion and enter the cells with the help of insulin, providing energy. Eating a small amount of carbohydrates will quickly treat hypoglycemia.

Blood Glucose/Blood Sugar Tests

Glucose, a simple sugar is the major source of energy for all cells. The three most frequently prescribed blood sugar tests to determine the glucose level in the blood are described below.

Fasting blood sugar: The blood test has to be performed after 12 hours of fasting. That means the person must refrain from eating approximately 12 hours prior to this blood test. Normal range of fasting blood sugar (FBS) is 70–115 mg/dL.

Postprandial blood sugar: Prior to this test, the person fasts overnight and then consumes a carbohydrate meal. Approximately between 1½ and 2 hours after eating, a blood sample from vein is drawn for testing. Normal range of postprandial blood sugar (PPBS) is 70–140 mg/dL.

Glucose tolerance test (GTT): The test is performed after consuming a concentrated amount of glucose dissolved in water. The normal range of fasting sugar level should be 80–120 mg; after 2 hours (food taken), it should be 120–150 mg.

Random blood sugar test: It is also common to monitor blood glucose levels. In this case, the blood sample can be taken at any time irrespective of the consumption of food. Normal range of random blood sugar test (RBS) is 70–130 mg/dL.

Glycosuria

Glycosuria is the presence of sugar in the urine. Less than 0.1% of glucose normally filtered by the glomeruli, appears in the urine and less than 130 mg should appear in the urine over a 24-hour period. It most commonly results from diabetes mellitus, but may occur from a lowered renal threshold (renal glycosuria) in pregnancy, organic renal disease and patients taking adrenocorticosteroids.

Galactosemia

Galactose is a sugar that is present in milk, and in some fruits and vegetables. A deficient enzyme or liver dysfunction can alter the metabolism, which can lead to high levels of galactose in the blood causing galactosemia. Symptoms include vomiting, jaundice, diarrhea and abnormal growth. The diagnosis is based on a blood test. Even with adequate treatment, affected children still develop mental and physical problems.

Newborns with galactosemia seem normal at first, but within a few days or weeks, lose their appetite, vomit, become jaundiced, have diarrhea and stop growing normally. White blood cell function is affected and serious infections can develop. If treatment is delayed, affected children remain short and become intellectually disabled or may die. Galactosemia is treated by completely eliminating milk and milk products—the source of galactose from an affected child's diet. Galactose is also present in some fruits, vegetables and sea products such as seaweed. Doctors are not sure whether the small amounts in these foods cause problems for the long term. People who have the disorder must restrict galactose intake throughout their life.

Pentosuria

Pentosuria is a condition where the sugar xylitol pentose present in the urine is in unusually high concentrations. It was characterized as an inborn error of carbohydrate metabolism and is excretion of 1–4 g of the pentose L-xylulose in the urine per day. Those diagnosed with pentosuria are predominantly of Jewish root. However, it is a harmless defect and no cure is needed.

Ketosis

When body does not have enough carbohydrates to produce energy from glucose, it begins to burn fat for energy instead. Ketones are acids in the blood that form when fat is used as an energy source. Over time, the accumulation of acidic ketones causes to lose minerals vital to normal health functions such as fluid balance, nerve transmission and muscle contraction. Dangerously high levels of ketones in bloodstream increase the risk of electrolyte imbalance, dehydration, fatigue and digestive disturbance. In diabetics, this deficiency can lead to ketoacidosis, a life-threatening condition. Mild ketosis can cause mental fatigue, bad breath, nausea and headache, but severe ketosis can lead to painful swelling of the joints and kidney stones. Aim for 225–325 g of carbohydrates a day to prevent ketosis and other health problems.

MALNUTRITION

Malnutrition/Undernutrition may be defined as a state of partial starvation. Inadequate nutrition resulting from lack of food or failure of the body to absorb or assimilate nutrients properly.

Types

Undernutrition is of two types, i.e. primary and secondary.

Primary Undernutrition

Primary undernutrition is one of the most basic types of malnutrition and occurs in people who do not have enough nutrients in their diet, i.e. progressive loss of body energy.

Causes

- Lack of energy (fats and carbohydrates)
- Lack of foodstuffs
- Scarcity of certain foodstuffs.

Secondary Undernutrition

Steady state at which a person is in an energy balance, although at cost either in terms of increased risk to health or as an impairment of functions and health.

Causes

- Failure of absorption
- Increased nutritional requirements (growth, injuries, burns, surgical procedures, pregnancy, lactation and fever)
- Excessive excretion (diarrhea).

Signs and Symptoms

- Feeling tired all the time and lacking energy
- Delayed wound healing
- Poor concentration
- Diarrhea
- Taking a long time to recover from infection
- Irritability
- Depression.

Diagnosis

- Comparing a patient's weight to standardized charts
- Calculating body mass index (BMI) according to formula that divides height and weight
- Physical examination.

Prevention

- Supplements of carbohydrates are often advised
- Intake of carbohydrates need to be gradually increased by the patients with malnutrition
- To provide health education to the people.

Treatment

1. Regularly consuming fruits, which contain carbohydrates and starchy vegetables. Fiber is an essential component in the diet for cancer prevention and healthy digestion.
2. Without some whole grains, one would need to consume a large amount of fruits, vegetables and legumes to meet daily fiber requirements (35 g/day for men and 30 g/day for women).

OVERCONSUMPTION

1. Excessive consumption of refined sugars could be one of the causes of dental carries or tooth decay.
2. Excessive sugar depresses the appetite, provides hollow calories and could result in malnutrition.
3. High intake of sugar and refined carbohydrates increases the blood triglyceride levels leading to heart diseases.
4. When excessive carbohydrates are consumed, they are converted into fat and deposited in the adipose tissue, which could lead to obesity.
5. Excessive fiber could irritate the intestinal lining causing cramps or bloating due to gas formation.
6. Excessive fiber interferes with the absorption and availability of mineral elements such as iron and calcium.
7. Excessive consumption of carbohydrates may lead to overweight.

Symptoms

1. **Hypertension:** High blood pressure (BP) defined as a repeatedly elevated BP exceeding 140 over 90 mm Hg—a systolic pressure above 140 or a diastolic pressure above 90.
2. **Hyperlipidemia:** Elevated lipid (fat) levels in the blood. Hyperlipidemia can be inherited and increases the risk of disease of the blood vessels leading to stroke and heart disease.
3. **Asthma:** A respiratory condition marked by attacks of spasm in the bronchi of the lungs, causing difficulty in breathing. It is usually connected to allergic reaction or other forms of hypersensitivity.
4. **Sleep apnea:** It is a type of sleep disorder characterized by pauses in breathing or instances of shallow or infrequent breathing during sleep.
5. **Metabolic syndrome:** A cluster of biochemical and physiological abnormalities associated with the development of cardiovascular disease and type 2 diabetes.
6. **Low back pain:** It is a common disorder involving the muscles and bones of the back. It affects about 40% of people at some point in their lives.
7. **Depression:** It is a common mental disorder characterized by sadness, loss of interest or pleasure, feeling of guilt or low self-

worth, disturbed sleep or appetite, feeling of tiredness and poor concentration.

8. **Low self-esteem:** It is a debilitating condition that keeps individuals from realizing their full potential. A person with low self-esteem feels unworthy, incapable and incompetent. In fact, the person with low self-esteem feels so poorly about himself/herself.

Prevention

1. Daily diet should be a balance of carbohydrates and protein. A plate should contain twice as many carbohydrates as proteins.
2. Base each of the meals on a complex carbohydrate such as potato, wholemeal bread for the toast.
3. Cut down the amount of refined white flour products in the diet such as white bread, pizza and white pasta and rice. The refining process produces simple carbohydrates where many vitamins and minerals are lost.
4. Fruit is naturally high in sugar, so are fruit juices and smoothies. In liquid form, these sugars can damage teeth, but these drinks count towards our 'five-a-day' (consumption of at least five portions of fruit or vegetables each day) and contain fiber, vitamins and minerals. To avoid tooth decay, it is best to drink them with a meal.

Treatment

To decrease obesity by the exercises. Maintain healthy diet and prescribed medicines for this complication of overconsumption of carbohydrates.

Section III

Fats

10. Classification, Requirements and Functions
11. Digestion, Absorption and Storage
12. Metabolism and Synthesis
13. Malnutrition and Overconsumption

Chapter 10

Classification, Requirements and Functions

Fats and oils are important items in the diet of people. They contain carbon, hydrogen and oxygen. Fats and oils are concentrated sources of energy.

CLASSIFICATION OF LIPIDS

Simple Lipids

'Oils and fats' are called simple lipids These are esters of fatty acids and glycerol. Oils are liquids at 20°C, while fats are solids at 20°C. Simple lipids that consist of fats and oils are triglycerides.

Compound Lipids

The compound lipids contain, in addition to fatty acids and glycerol, some other organic compounds:

1. **Phospholipids (phosphatides):** These contain phosphoric acid and a nitrogenous base in addition to fatty acids and glycerol, e.g. lecithin and cephalin.
2. **Glycolipids:** Complex lipids containing carbohydrates in combination with fatty acids and glycerol (e.g. cerebrosides).
3. **Waxes:** These are esters of fatty acids and long aliphatic alcohol.
4. **Derived lipids:** These include sterols, fatty acids and alcohols.

CLASSIFICATION OF FATTY ACIDS (CHEMISTRY)

Fatty acids are divided into two main groups:

1. Saturated fatty acids.
2. Unsaturated fatty acids (one or double unsaturated bonds).

Common Saturated Fatty Acids

- N-butyric
- Caproic
- Caprylic

- Capric
- Lauric
- Myristic
- Palmitic
- Stearic
- Arachidonic.

Common Unsaturated Fatty Acids

- Oleic
- Linoleic
- Linolenic
- γ-linolenic
- Eleostearic.

The polyunsaturated fatty acids are mostly found in vegetable oils and the saturated fatty acids mainly in animal fats. Coconut and palm oils, although vegetable oils, have an extremely high percentage of saturated fatty acids. On the other hand fish oils, although they are not vegetable oils, contain poly- and mono-unsaturated fatty acids.

Essential Fatty Acids (Table 10.1)

Essential fatty acids are those that cannot be synthesized by humans. They can be derived only from food. The most important essential fatty acids (EFA) are linoleic acid and arachidonic acids, which

Table 10.1: Dietary sources of essential fatty acids

Essential fatty acids	Dietary sources	Content (%)
Linoleic	Safflower oil	73
	Corn oil	57
	Sunflower oil	56
	Soybean oil	51
	Sesame oil	40
	Groundnut oil	39
	Mustard oil	15
	Palm oil	9
	Coconut oil	2
Arachidonic acid	Meat, eggs, milk (fat)	0.5–0.3 0.4–0.6
Eicosapentaenoic	Fish oil	10

serves as a basis for the production of other essential fatty acids. Not all polyunsaturated fatty acids are essential fatty acids. Linoleic acid is abundantly found in vegetable oils. The dietary sources of EFA are detailed below.

CHEMICAL PROPERTIES OF FAT

Hydrogenation

The hydrogenated fat is known as 'vanaspati' or vegetable ghee, which is a popular cooking medium in India. When vegetable oils are hydrogenated under conditions of optimum temperature and pressure in the presence of a catalyst, and liquid oils are converted into semisolid and solid-fat, it is known as vanaspati or vegetable ghee. During the process of hydrogenation, unsaturated fatty acids are converted into saturated acids and the essential fatty acid content is drastically reduced. The main advantage of vanaspati is its ghee-like consistency and its keeping quality even in hot humid climates. Vanaspati is lacking in fat-soluble vitamins. It is fortified with vitamins A and D.

Refined Oils

Refining oil is usually done by treatment with steam, alkaline, etc. Refining and deodorization of raw oil is done mainly to remove the free fatty acids and rancid materials. Refining the oil improves only the quality and taste of oils. Refined oils are costly.

FAT REQUIREMENTS

In developed countries, dietary fats provide 30–40% of total energy intake. The World Health Organization (WHO) Expert Committee on prevention of coronary heart disease has recommended only 20–30% of total dietary energy to be provided by fats. The Indian Council of Medical Research (1981) has recommended a daily intake of not more than 20% of total energy intake. At least 50% of fat intake should consist of vegetable oils rich in essential fatty acids.

VISIBLE AND INVISIBLE FATS

Nutrition scientists have classified fats into two types:

1. **Visible fats:** Those that are used during cooking or that are separated from their natural source, e.g. ghee, butter from milk, cooking oils from oil-bearing seeds and nuts.

2. **Invisible fats:** Those which we generally do not take notice or which are not visible to the naked eye. They are present in almost every particle of food such as cereals, pulses, nuts, milk, eggs and meat.

CALORIC VALUE AND RECOMMENDED DAILY ALLOWANCES

Caloric Value

A calorie is the unit used to measure the energy-producing value of food. Technically, a calorie is defined as the amount of heat necessary to raise the temperature of 1 g of water by 1°C. When burned (metabolized), they provide energy. About 1 g of fat yields 9 kcal or 38 Joules of energy.

Recommended Daily Allowances

- Depending upon the level of calories consumed, i.e. 20% of the total energy (ICMR, 1976):
  - Normal adults, expectants and nursing mothers: 10–20 g of fat/day
  - Children and adolescents (2–8 year): 15–20 g of fat/day
  - Infants: 25–30 g of the fat/day.
- Caloric value of fats:
  - In bomb calorimeter: 9 kcal
  - In human body: 9 kcal or 38 kJ.
- The WHO Expert Committee on prevention of the coronary heart disease has recommended only 20–30% of total dietary energy to be provided by fats

Table 10.2: Recommended daily allowances of fats for different age groups according to ICMR, 2010

Category	Daily values
Men	20 g/day
Women	20 g/day
Pregnant	30 g/day
Lactation	30 g/day
Infants	45 g/day
Children	25 g/day
Adolescents	22 g/day

- The Indian Council of Medical Research (1981) has recommended a daily intake of not more than 20% of total energy intake (Table 10.2)
- At least 50% of fat intake should consist of vegetable oils rich in essential fatty acids
- In developed countries, dietary fats provide 30–40% of total energy intake.

DIETARY SOURCES

The dietary source of fats may be classified as animal fats, vegetable fats and other sources:

1. **Animal fats:** These are ghee, butter milk, cheese, eggs, fish oils, fat of meat and fish. Animal fats are poor sources of EFA with exception of marine fish oil such as cod liver oil and sardine oil, but they are good source of retinol and cholecalciferol, which all lack in vegetable oils.
2. **Vegetable fats:** They include various edible oils such as groundnut oil, gingelly, mustard oil, sesame oil, palm oil, coconut oil and sunflower oil. Mostly all vegetable oils (except coconut oil) are rich sources of EFA.
3. **Other sources**: Small quantities of invisible fat are found in most other foods such as cereals, pulses, nuts and vegetables:
   - Rice : 3%
   - Wheat: 3%
   - Jowar : 4%
   - Bajra : 6.5%.

Large cereal consumption as in India provides considerable amounts of invisible fat. Moreover, the body can convert carbohydrate into fat.

FUNCTIONS OF FATS

Fats have always been elevated with calories. They are high-energy foods, providing as much as 6 kcal for every gram. Fat is much more concentrated source of energy:

1. Fats are essential for the transportation and absorption of fat-soluble vitamins such as A,D, E and K.
2. Fats are sources of essential fatty acids.
3. Excess fat is stored as fat depot in the body. Fat not used by the body is stored by adipose tissue (or fats are stored in the form of adipose tissue) in various parts of the body.

4. Fats supply fatty acids.
5. Fats beneath the skin, provide insulation against cold or the adipose tissue under the skin acts as an insulating material against cold.
6. Fats add taste to the foods.
7. Some of the animal fats such as fish, liver oils, butter and ghee supply vitamin A.
8. Food fats supply the EFA, i.e. linolenic acid, linoleic acid and arachidonic acid, which are needed for the growth and maintenance of the body. Linoleic acid, one of the EFA, prevents scaly skin formation.
9. Fat in the diet adds flavor and taste to foods and gives a feeling of fullness in the stomach.
10. Compound lipids such as phospholipids are essential constituents of nervous tissue.
11. At the time of starvation, stored fat will be used for energy. Padding of the fatty tissue supports and protects vital organs such as heart and kidney.
12. The fat layer below the skin plays an important role in maintaining body temperature.

'Non-calorie' Roles of Fat

Vegetable fats are rich sources of essential fatty acids, which are needed by the body for growth, structural integrity of the cell membrane and decreased platelets adhesiveness. Diets rich in essential fatty acids reported to reduce serum cholesterol and low density such as proteins. Polyunsaturated fatty acids are precursors of prostaglandins—now recognized as 'local hormones'; they play a major role in controlling many of the physiological functions of the body such as:

- Vascular homeostasis
- Kidney function
- Acid secretion in stomach
- Gastrointestinal motility
- Lung physiology and reproduction.

Cholesterol is essential as a component of membranes and nervous tissue, and is a precursor for the synthesis of steroid hormones and bile acids.

Chapter 11

Digestion, Absorption and Storage

DIGESTION AND ABSORPTION

Fats arenot digested in the stomach. The presence of fats in the diet delays the emptying of the food from the stomach. Fats are hydrolyzed by the pancreatic and intestinal lipases in the intestines into a mixture of digestion and absorption, as it helps to emulsify the fats before digestion. The products of digestion pass into the cells of the intestinal wall, where synthesis of new glycerides and characteristic of the animal species takes place. The resynthesized lipids pass through the lacteals of the small intestines to the thoracic duct and then to the bloodstream in the form of fine particles known as chylomicrons. A greater part of the cholesterol present in vegetable fats and oils are not absorbed.

When a person takes food, it enters the stomach where gastric lipase produces slight hydrolysis of fat (hydrolysis means the process of splitting into smaller molecules by inciting with water). Then the food enters duodenum, where bile secretion emulsifies fats. Pancreatic and intestinal lipase breakdown the fats in the small intestine; glycerine and fatty acids are absorbed by the lacteals, and pass into the thoracic duct, which enter the bloodstream. In the blood, fat is carried to every cell of the body.

The liver assists in the oxidation of fats and prepares fats for deposition in the tissues. In the tissues, some of the fat is oxidized (in the presence of CHOs) to give heat and energy. Some of the fat is stored in the fat depots. This stored fat contains vitamin A and D. The waste products, which result from the combustion of fat in tissues are excreted by the lungs as water and CO_2, by the skin as sweats and by the kidneys as urine (water):

$$\text{Fat} \xrightarrow{\textit{Pancreatic and intestinal lipase}} \text{Diglyceride + Monoglyceride + Fatty acid}$$

STORAGE

Fat is stored in our body. Excessive fat storage leads to obesity and coronary heart diseases.

Adipose Tissue

Adipose tissue is of two types. White adipose tissue is found all over the body. Brown adipose tissue is found in small amounts in newborn animals as well as human infants, and in large amounts in hibernating animals.

White Adipose Tissue

1. Human adipose tissue usually contains about 85% of fat (triglycerides) as well as 15% of cell material and supporting tissue.
2. The protein content is about 2% and water content is about 10%. A healthy adult male weighing 70 kg will have about 10–15 kg of adipose tissue and a healthy woman of 60 kg will have about 12–20 kg of adipose tissue.
3. About 50–60% of the extra body weight of obese subjects consist of adipose tissue.

Brown Adipose Tissue

1. Brown adipose tissue is present in small amounts in newborn animals and human infants, around the neck and between the shoulder blades.
2. Adult human beings and animals contain very little brown adipose tissue.
3. Brown adipose tissue has rich blood and nerve supply, and contains cells with round nuclei, granular cytoplasm and numerous fat droplets. The granularity of the cytoplasm is due to the high concentration of cytochrome pigments.
4. This tissue has a large capacity for generating energy in the form of heat and thus protects the newborn animals against exposure to cold.

Chapter 12

Metabolism and Synthesis

FAT METABOLISM

Fat is emulsified by alkalis and split up into fatty acids and glycerol by the lipase of the pancreatic juice. These substances are absorbed by the lacteals and pass through the lymphatic circulation up the thoracic duct into the bloodstream. The use of fat is to serve as fuel for the production of heat and energy in the tissues. Fat is a better fuel than glucose; in that, it produces twice as much heat and energy per gram of fuel used compared to glucose. On the other hand, it is less easy to digest and absorb, and less satisfactory to burn; provided, it is burnt with sufficient sugar, it is completely burnt and converted into carbon dioxide and water.

If there is little or no sugar to burn with it, combustion is incomplete and ketone bodies are formed (acetone and diacetic acid), which in small quantity, produce a sense of fatigue and in large quantity, after the reaction of the blood, reducing its alkalinity and causing the condition known as acidosis that results in drowsiness, coma and finally death—if the condition is not corrected by providing the tissues with glucose. This acidosis occurs in starvation and in diabetes; and in the second condition, insulin must be provided as well as glucose to enable the tissues to make use of this fuel. Fats, before they can be used as body fuel, must be prepared for combustion in the tissues by the liver. This is again a chemical process carried out by the liver cells and is known as the desaturation of fats. Fat is also required for the building of various tissues, e.g. nerve tissue, fatty tissue and marrow; fat derivatives are found in the secretions of certain glands.

Fat is not required for immediate use, as fuel can be stored as fatty tissue. This is found particularly in the subcutaneous tissue and in the body cavities, but whereas sugar can only be stored in very limited quantities; the total being about 225 g in liver and muscles. Fat can be stored in very large quantities and may be found in large amounts even in the muscles themselves. This is however, undesirable, as it causes increase in weight. Putting on fat does not necessarily mean that too much fat is being eaten, as the body can convert excess glucose into fat for storage and excess protein not required for body building into glucose. The metabolism of the three foodstuffs (carbohydrate, fat and protein) is therefore closely linked up and the taking the food of any kind in excess of the needs of the tissues will lead to an increase in weight. The waste products of fat metabolism are carbon dioxide and water; if combustion is complete, they are excreted by the lungs, skin and kidneys. If the combustion is incomplete, the acetone bodies formed, also leave the body by the same routes. The volatile acetone can be smelt in the 'sweet' breath, and acetone and diacetic acid can be found in the urine.

Summary of Fat Metabolism

1. Short chain fatty acids enter the circulation directly, but most of the fatty acids are re-esterified with glycerol in the intestines to form triglycerides that enter into the blood as lipoprotein particles called chylomicrons.
2. Lipoprotein lipase acts on these chylomicrons to form fatty acids. These may be stored as fat in adipose tissue, used for energy in any tissue with mitochondria, using oxygen and re-esterified to triglycerides in the liver and exported as lipoproteins called very-low-density lipoproteins (VLDL).
3. The VLDL has a similar outcome as chylomicrons and eventually is converted to low-density lipoproteins (LDL). Insulin stimulates lipoprotein lipase.
4. During starvation for long periods of time, the fatty acids can also be converted to ketone bodies in the liver. These ketone bodies can be used as an energy source by most cells that have mitochondria:

$$\underset{(1)}{\text{Palmitic acid}} \longrightarrow \underset{\text{oxidation (8)}}{\text{Acetic acid}} \longrightarrow \underset{(16)}{CO_2} + \underset{(16)}{H_2O}$$

Role of Liver in Lipid Metabolism

1. A greater part of the lipid metabolism in the body was formerly thought to take place in the liver.
2. Most tissues have the ability to oxidize fatty acids completely and that the adipose tissue has all the enzymes for the synthesis of fatty acids and triglycerides, and for the hydrolysis of fat, have helped to modify to some extent, the emphasis on the role of liver in fat metabolism.
3. The important roles of liver in lipid metabolism are the following:
   a. Liver is an important site for the synthesis of fatty acids and triglycerides from acetyl coenzyme A (acetyl-CoA) obtained from the oxidation of glucose.
   b. It is an important site for the synthesis of cholesterol from acetyl-CoA obtained from the oxidation of carbohydrates, fatty acids and some amino acids.
   c. Liver is a major site for the oxidation of fatty acids.
   d. Liver is the most important site for the for the formation of ketone bodies.

FAT SYNTHESIS

Fat is not synthesized in our body. But it is taken from the foods such as oils, cheese, butter, fish, liver oils, etc. Fat is synthesized from fatty acids. Fatty acids are synthesized by three methods, as detailed below.

Cytoplasmic De Novo Fatty Acid Synthesis

1. This is the most important system for synthesis of fatty acids from acetyl-CoA obtained from the oxidation of glucose.
2. The steps involved are:
   - Conversion of acetyl-CoA to malonyl-CoA
   - Reaction of malonyl-CoA with acetyl-CoA to yield fatty acids:

     Acetyl-CoA (1 mol) C_2 + Malonyl-CoA (1 mol) C_2 ⟶ Butyric acid

     Acetyl-CoA (1 mol) C_2 + Malonyl-CoA (8 mol) ⟶ Stearic acid (C_{16})
3. In the above manner, fatty acids ranging from butyric (C_4) acid can be synthesized.

Mitochondrial System for the Elongation of Fatty Acids

Starting from fatty acids C_{10}–C_{16}, the next higher fatty acid can be synthesized by this system:

Myristic acid		Acetyl-CoA		Palmitic acid
C_{14}	+	C_2	→	C_{16}
Palmitic acid		Acetyl-CoA		Stearic acid
C_{16}	+	C_2	→	C_{18}

Microsomal System for Elongation of Fatty Acids

Microsomal system can synthesize higher fatty acids starting from lower fatty acids by adding 1 mol of malonyl-CoA to a fatty acid:

Myristic acid		Malonyl-CoA		Palmitic acid
C_2	+	C_2	→	C_{16}

Chapter 13

Malnutrition and Overconsumption

Malnutrition is a condition that results from eating a diet in which nutrients are not enough or are too much such that it causes health problems. Malnutrition occurs among the people who are either undernourished or overnourished. Malnutrition may range from mild to severe and life-threatening.

DEFICIENCIES

Phrynoderma

1. Deficiency of essential fatty acids in the diet associated with a condition is known as phrynoderma/toad skin.
2. It is characterized by horny papular eruptions on the posterior and lateral aspects of thighs, and on the back and buttocks. It is associated with rough and dry skin. The skin is lusterless.
3. Phrynoderma can be cured rapidly by the administration of sunflower oil, which is rich in essential fatty acids along with vitamins of the B-complex group.

Gaucher's Disease

1. In this condition, glucocerebrosides accumulate in the cells of the reticuloendothelial system.
2. The cerebroside-laden cells are large. Their cytoplasm appears as crumpled silk (Gaucher's cells).
3. Children who have the infantile form usually die within a year, but children and adults who develop the disease later in life, may survive for many years.
4. In Gaucher's disease, glucocerebrosides, which are a product of fat metabolism, accumulate in tissues. Gaucher's disease is the most common lipidosis. The disease is most common among Ashkenazi (Eastern European) Jews. Gaucher's disease leads to

an enlarged liver and spleen, and a brownish pigmentation of the skin. Accumulation in the bone marrow can cause pain and destroy bone.

5. Many people with Gaucher's disease can be treated with enzyme replacement therapy in which enzymes are given by vein, usually every 2 weeks.
6. Enzyme replacement therapy is most effective for people who do not have nervous system complications.

Tay-Sachs Disease

Tay-Sachs disease is caused by a build-up of gangliosides in the tissue. This disease results in early death. In Tay-Sachs disease, gangliosides, which are products of fat metabolism, accumulate in tissues. The disease is most common among families of Eastern Jewish origin. At a very early age, children with this disease become progressively intellectually disabled and appear to have floppy muscle tone. Spasticity develops and is followed by paralysis, dementia and blindness. These children usually die by age 3–4. The disease cannot be treated or cured. Before conception, parents can find out whether they carry the gene that causes the disease. During pregnancy, Tay-Sachs disease can be identified in the fetus by chorionic villus sampling or amniocentesis.

Niemann-Pick Disease

1. Niemann-Pick disease is caused by a buildup of sphingomyelin or cholesterol in the tissues. This disease causes many neurologic problems.
2. In Niemann-Pick disease, the deficiency of a specific enzyme results in the accumulation of sphingomyelin (a product of fat metabolism) or cholesterol.
3. Some forms of Niemann-Pick disease can be diagnosed in the fetus by chorionic villus sampling or amniocentesis. Afterbirth, the diagnosis can be made by a liver biopsy (removal of a tissue specimen for examination under a microscope). Niemann-Pick disease can be cured and children tend to die of infection or progressive dysfunction of the central nervous system.

Fabry's Disease

1. Fabry's disease is caused by a build-up of glycolipid in tissues. This disease causes skin growth, pain in the extremities, poor vision, recurrent episodes of fever and kidney or heart failure.

2. In Fabry's disease, glycolipid, which is a product of fat metabolism, accumulates in tissues. Because the defective gene for this rare disorder is carried on the X chromosome, the full-blown disease occurs only in males (refer X-Linked inheritance).
3. The accumulation of glycolipid causes non-cancerous (benign) skin growths (angiokeratomas) to form on the lower part of the trunk. The corneas become cloudy, resulting in poor vision. A burning pain may develop in the arms and legs, and children may have episodes of fever.
4. Children with Fabry's disease eventually develop kidney failure and heart disease, although most often, they live into adulthood. Kidney failure may lead to high blood pressure, which may result in stroke.
5. Fabry's disease can be diagnosed in the fetus by chorionic villus sampling or amniocentesis. The disease cannot be cured or even treated directly, but researchers are investigating a treatment in which the deficient enzyme is replaced by transfusion.
6. Treatment consists of taking analgesics to help relieve pain and fever or anticonvulsants.
7. People with kidney failure may need a kidney transplant.

OVERCONSUMPTION

Excessive consumption of fats causes obesity, coronary heart disease, cancer and others.

Obesity

Excessive consumption of fats lead to obesity (i.e. overweight). In fat people, adipose tissue may increase up to 3%. Most of the body fat (99%) in the adipose tissue is in the form of triglycerides. The human body can synthesize triglycerides and cholesterol. In the normal human beings, adipose tissue constitute between 10 and 15% of body weight. The accumulation of 1 kg of adipose tissue corresponds to 7,700 kcal of energy.

Causes

- An inactive lifestyle
- Genes and family history
- Medicines
- Smoking

- Pregnancy
- Environment
- Health conditions
- Emotional factors
- Age
- Lack of sleep.

Signs and Symptoms

- Osteoarthritis
- Stroke
- Sleep apnea (when you periodically stop breathing during sleep)
- Heart disease
- Diabetes.

Diagnosis

Diagnostic tests may include:

- Taking the health history
- Calculating the body mass index (BMI)
- A general physical examination
- Checking for other health problems
- Measuring the waist circumference
- Blood tests.

Prevention

- Obesity is managed and treated to decrease the health risks caused by it and to improve quality of life
- An appropriate weight management program usually combines physical activity, healthy diet and change in daily habits
- Other programs may also involve psychological counseling and in some cases, drug therapy is also indicated
- People who are medically obese, should consult a doctor or dietitian for a safe and personalized weight loss program.

Treatment

1. The body needs a minimum amount of energy from food to function normally. No daily diet with less than 1,000–1,200 calories should be used without medical supervision.
2. To lose weight successfully and to maintain a healthy weight, it requires lifelong changes in eating and exercise habits.

3. Regular physical activity is an important part of weight management. In addition to managing weight, exercise also improves overall health and can help reduce the risk of diseases such as certain cancers, heart disease and osteoporosis.
4. Medications may be part of a weight management program. Medications are not 'magic cures' leading to permanent weight loss. They are generally used in combination with a proper diet and exercise program.

Coronary Heart Disease

High-fat intake, i.e. dietary fat representing 40% or over the energy supply and containing a high proportion of saturated fats has been identified as a major risk factor for coronary heart disease (CHD) (atherosclerosis). Excessive fatty acids in the body lead to increased blood cholesterol levels associated with atherosclerosis and cardiovascular stroke. There is high blood cholesterol, which is deposited as plaques in the arterial walls. This predisposes to coronary artery disease.

Causes

1. Fatty material and other substances form a plaque buildup on the walls of coronary arteries. The coronary arteries bring blood and oxygen to the heart.
2. This build-up causes the arteries to get narrow.
3. As a result, blood flow to the heart can slow down or stop.

Symptoms

- Early stages of heart disease
- Chest pain or discomfort (angina)
- It may feel heavy or as someone is squeezing one's heart; may feel it under the breast bone (sternum) and also in neck, arms, stomach or upper back
- Emotion
- Shortness of breath and fatigue with activity (exertion)
- General weakness.

Diagnosis

Diagnostic tests may include:

- Coronary angiography—an invasive test that evaluates the heart arteries under X-ray

- Echocardiogram (ECG)
- Electron-beam computed tomography (EBCT)—to look for calcium in the lining of the arteries; the more calcium, higher the chance for CHD
- Exercise stress test
- Heart computed tomography (CT)
- Nuclear stress test.

Prevention

- Stop smoking/using tobacco
- Exercise for 30 minutes on most days of the week
- Eat a heart-healthy diet.

Treatment

To take one or more medicines to treat blood pressure, diabetes or high cholesterol levels. Follow the doctor's directions closely to help prevent coronary artery disease from getting worse.

Cancer

In recent years, there has been some evidence that diets high in fat increase the risk of colon cancer and breast cancer.

Causes

- Genetics
- Diet and physical activity
- Radiation exposure and cancer risk
- Uses tobacco
- Sun and ultraviolet (UV) exposure
- Other carcinogens.

Signs and Symptoms

- Fatigue
- Lump or area of thickening that can be felt under the skin
- Weight changes, including unintended loss or gain
- Skin changes, such as yellowing, darkening or redness of the skin, sores that will not heal or changes to existing moles
- Changes in bowel or bladder habits
- Persistent cough
- Difficulty swallowing
- Hoarseness

- Persistent indigestion or discomfort after eating
- Persistent unexplained muscle or joint pain
- Persistent unexplained fevers or night sweats.

Diagnosis

- Blood tests
- Bone marrow biopsy (most often for lymphoma or leukemia)
- Chest X-ray
- Complete blood count (CBC)
- Liver function tests.

Prevention

- Do not use tobacco
- Eat plenty of fruits and vegetable
- Stop drinking alcohol regularly
- Eat a healthy diet
- Limit fat consumption
- Maintain a healthy weight and be physically active.

Treatment

- Chemotherapy
- Surgery
- Radiation
- Medications.

Others

The skin lesions of kwashiorkor and those induced by essential fatty acid deficiency are similar.

Section IV

Proteins

Chapter 14

Classification, Requirement and Functions

The word protein means, which is of first importance. Indeed they are of the greatest importance in human nutrition. Proteins are complex organic nitrogenous compounds. They are composed of carbon, hydrogen, oxygen, nitrogen and sulfur in varying amounts. Some proteins also contain phosphorus and iron, and occasionally other elements. Proteins contribute about 20% of the body weight in adults. The quality of dietary protein is closely related to its pattern of amino acids. From the nutritional standpoint, animal proteins are rated superior to vegetable proteins because they are 'biologically complete', e.g. milk and egg proteins have a pattern of amino acids considered most suitable for humans.

CLASSIFICATION OF PROTEINS (BASED ON AMINO ACID)

Both essential and non-essential amino acids are needed for synthesis of tissue proteins.

Essential Amino Acid

Proteins are made up of smaller units, called amino acids. Some 24 amino acids are stated to be needed by the human body of which 9 are called 'essential', because the body cannot synthesize them. They must be obtained from dietary proteins. The 9 essential amino acids are as follows:

- Leucine
- Isoleucine
- Lysine
- Methionine
- Phenylalanine
- Threonine
- Valine

- Tryptophan
- Histidine.

Some of the essential amino acids have important biological functions, for example, formation of niacin from tryptophan, the action of methionine as a donor of methyl group for the synthesis of choline, folates and nucleic acids. New tissues cannot be formed unless all the essential amino acids (EAA) are present in the diet. A protein is said to be 'biologically complete,' if it contains all the EAA in essential amounts corresponding to human needs. When one or more of the EAA are lacking, the protein is said to be 'biologically incomplete.'

Non-essential Amino Acids

- Arginine
- Asparaginic acid
- Serine
- Glutamic acid
- Proline
- Glycine.

Non-essential amino acids are needed for synthesis of tissue proteins. It can be synthesized by the body, provided, other building blocks are present.

SUPPLEMENTARY ACTION OF PROTEINS

Cereal proteins are deficient in lysine and threonine and pulse proteins in methionine. These are known as 'limiting amino acids.' Thus with proper planning, it is possible for a vegetarian to obtain a high-grade protein, from mixed diets of cereals, pulses and vegetables. This is known as supplementary action of proteins.

ASSESSMENT OF PROTEIN NUTRITION STATUS

At the present time, the best measure of the state of protein nutrition is probably serum albumin concentration. It should be more than 3.5 g/dL. A level of 3.5 g/dL is considered as mild degree of malnutrition and a level of 3.0 g/dL as severe malnutrition.

Biological Value

A method for determining biological value of proteins was developed by Mitchell in 1925. It measures the quantity of dietary protein utilized by the body for meeting its protein needs for maintenance and growth:

$$\text{Biological value} = \frac{\text{Nitrogen digested} - \text{Nitrogen lost in metabolism}}{\text{Nitrogen digested}} \times 100$$

Protein Efficiency Ratio

The method is developed by Osborne Mendel and Ferry in 1919 to use the evaluation of protein quality:

$$\text{Protein efficiency ratio} = \frac{\text{Gain in body weight (kg)}}{\text{Protein intake (g)}}$$

Net Protein Utilization

Mitchell in 1922 introduced the term net protein utilization (NPU), which is a product of digestibility coefficient and biological value divided by 100:

$$\text{Net protein utilization} = \frac{\text{Digestibility coefficient} \times \text{Biological value}}{100}$$

Caloric Value

A calorie is the unit used to measure the energy-producing value of food. Technically, a calorie is defined as the amount of heat necessary to raise the temperature of 1 g of water to 1°C. When burned (metabolized), they provide energy; 1 g of protein yields:

- 4.1 kcal in bomb calorimeter
- 4.1 kcal or 17 kJ in human body.

RECOMMENDED DAILY ALLOWANCES (TABLE 14.1)

The daily protein requirement depends upon the age, sex, physical, physiological, psychological and certain other factors. Indian Council of Medical Research (1981) recommended 1 g of protein/kg of bodyweight/day, for an Indian adult, assuming a NPU of 65 g for the dietary pattern (Table 14.2). An extra amount is to be provided for heavy workers and also should be provided in ailments involving either loss, destruction or degeneration of body tissues, e.g. blood loss, surgery, etc.

Table 14.1: Recommended protein allowances

Group	Particulars	Protein allowance	
		(g/kg/day)	(g/day)
Men	Sedentary work	1	55.0
	Moderate work	–	–
	Heavy work	–	–
Women	Sedentary work	1	45.0
	Moderate work	–	–
	Heavy work	–	–
	Pregnancy	1	+14.0
	Lactation (0–6 month)	1	+ 25.0
Infants	0–3 month	2.3*	–
	3–6 month	1.8*	–
	6–9 month	1.8†	–
	9–12 month	1.5†	–
Children	1–3 year	1.83	22.0
	4–6 year	1.56	29.0
	7–9 year	1.35	36.0
Adolescents	Males		
	10–12 year	1.24	43.0
	13–15 year	1.10	52.0
	16–18 year	0.94	53.0
	Females		

*In terms of milk protein alone; †In terms of mixed protein of NPU-65 relative to egg.

Table 14.2: RDA* of proteins for different age groups according to ICMR† 2010

Group	Category	Body weight (kg)	Protein (g/day)
		Revised	Revised
Infants	0–6 month	5.4	1.16/kg
	6–12 month	8.4	1.69/kg
Children	1–3 year	12.9	1.67
	4–6 year	18.0	20.1
	7–9 year	25.1	29.5
Boys	10–12 year	34.3	39.9
Girls	10–12 year	35.3	40.4
Boys	13–15 year	47.6	54.3
Girls	13–15 year	46.6	51.9
Boys	16–17 year	55.4	61.5
Girls	16–17 year	52.1	55.5
Men	Sedentary	–	–
	Moderate	60	60
	Heavy	–	–
Women	Sedentary	–	–
	Moderate	–	55
	Heavy	55	–
	Pregnant	–	78
	Lactation < 6 month	–	74

*RDA, recommended dietary allowance; †ICMR, Indian Council of Medical Research.

DIETARY SOURCES

There are two main sources of proteins (Table 14.3), i.e. animal and vegetable sources.

Animal Sources

Proteins are found in animal origin, e.g. meat, egg, fish, milk, cheese and liver. Animal proteins contain all the essential amino acid in

Table 14.3: Food source of proteins

Foods	Proteins in g/100 g of food
Animal foods	
Milk	3.2–4.3
Cow's milk	3.5
Buffalo's milk	4.3
Meat	18–26
Egg	13
Fish	15–23
Plant foods	
Cereals	6–13
Bajra or pearl millet	11.6
Jowar or sorghum	10.4
Maize	11.1
Ragi	7.1
Milled rice	7.0
Whole wheat	11.8
Pulses	21–28
Bengal gram dal	22.5
Black gram dal	24.0
Green gram dal	24.0
Red gram dal	22.3
Vegetables	1–4
Leafy vegetables	
Amaranth, tender (Amaranthus tricolor)	4.9
Agathi (Sesbania grandiflora)	8.4
Cabbage	1.8
Coriander	3.3
Curry leaves	6.1
Drumstick leaves	6.7
Ipomoea leaves	2.9
Mint	4.8
Spinach	1.9
Others vegetables	
Broad beans	4.5
Cauliflower	3.5
Cluster beans	3.7

adequate amounts. It is called First class protein/superior proteins, as they are more easily digestible and contain more of amino acids of different types. The essential amino acids are to be derived from the food we eat. Egg proteins are considered to be the best among good proteins because of their high biological value and digestibility. They are used in nutrition studies as a reference protein.

Vegetable Sources

Proteins are found in pulses, beans, nuts, oil seed, cereals, etc. They are poor in EAA. In developing countries such as India, cereals and pulses are the main sources of dietary protein, because they are cheap, easily available and consumed in bulk:

1. **Pulses:** Red gram, Bengal gram, black gram, soybeans (are also called poor man's meat).
2. **Nuts:** Peanuts.
3. **Cereals:** Wheat and parboiled rice.

Pulses are poor in essential amino acids. Pulses contain about 25% of proteins and they are cheap. By proper combination of two or more vegetable foods (cereals, pulses and vegetables), it is possible to produce a mixture containing all the essential amino acids cheaper than animal proteins. In developing countries such as India, cereals and pulses are the main sources of dietary protein because they are cheap, easily available and consumed in bulk.

FUNCTIONS (TABLE 14.4)

1. **Proteinhelpsforthebodybuilding:** Themostimportantfunction of protein is to supply amino acids to cells for the continuous replacement of cells throughout the life, i.e. from consumption to growth at various levels, e.g. fetus, infant, child, pregnancy and lactation. Sometimes, tissue proteins are broken down and new substances are continuously synthesized in body. Muscles and other tissues, bones and cartilage contains fairly high amount of proteins. Our hair, nails and skin also contain proteins.
2. **Protein helps for the growth and development of body tissues:** Through the digestion of proteins, amino acids will be absorbed by small intestine and they go to liver or tissues to maintain their growth and development.

Table 14.4: Role of proteins

Functions	How it works?
Structural, mechanical support and maintenance	Proteins are body's building materials, providing strength and flexibility to tissues, tendons, ligaments, muscles, organs, bones, nails, hairs and skin. Protein are also needed for the ongoing maintenance of the body
Enzymes and hormones	Proteins are needed to make most enzymes that speed up reactions in the body and many hormones that direct specific activities, such as regulating blood glucose levels
Fluid balance	Proteins play a major role in ensuring that body fluids are evenly dispersed in the blood inside and outside cells
Acid-base balance	Proteins act as buffers to help keep the pH of body fluids within a tight range. A drop in pH will cause body fluids to become too acidic, whereas a rise in pH can make them too basic
Transport	Proteins shuttle substances such as oxygen, waste products and nutrients (such as sodium and potassium) through the blood into and out of cells
Antibodies and the immune response	Proteins creates specialized antibodies that attack pathogens that may cause illness
Energy	Proteins provide 4 cal/g of energy, they can be used as fuel

3. **Protein is a source of energy:** Proteins enable the blood to maintain their slight alkalinity, thus helping various sites of chemical reaction to maintain its pH:
   a. Oxyhemoglobin and their alkaline salts makes oxygen to enter into the tissues and receive carbonic acid from the cells. This process helps the removal of 92–97% of all CO_2 from the tissue.
   b. Plasma proteins, especially albumin and globulin play an important role in regulating osmotic pressure and water balance within the body. When plasma proteins are decreased, the water balance gets upset and accumulation of fluids in the body takes place.

c. Protein is generally considered the building material of the body. But, when diet contains insufficient carbohydrates and fats for fuel, proteins are used as a fuel by the body. Each gram of protein yields 4 calories. But it is not a wide contribution, because the nitrogen (N_2) excretion increases along with the cost of food.

4. **Protein forms hormones and enzymes:** Protein, supply raw materials for the body to synthesize enzymes such as trypsin and pepsin; hormones such as insulin and thyroxin are proteins in nature. Digestive juices contain proteins. Antibodies, which give resistance power to the body are proteins in nature. They are known as immune proteins.
5. **Protein forms a part of vital compounds in body:** Nitrogenous compounds are present in certain substances of immunological and antigenic reactions, e.g. globulin of blood serum and chromatin in nucleus, methionine or amino acids provide methyl group for the formation of creatinine and choline.
6. **Protein help the transport of drug:** They also help the transport of drugs by binding them into protein molecules. Contractile protein molecules (myosin, actin) regulate muscle contraction.
7. **Proteins are needed by the body for:**
   a. Body building.
   b. Repair and maintenance of body tissues.
   c. Maintenance of osmotic pressure.
   d. Synthesis of certain substances such as:
      - Antibodies
      - Plasma proteins
      - Hemoglobin
      - Enzymes
      - Hormones
      - Coagulation factors.
8. **Proteins are connected with the immune mechanism of the body:** The cell-mediated immune response and the bactericidal activity of leukocytes have been found to be lowered in severe forms of protein-energy malnutrition.
9. **Protein supply energy:** They can also supply energy (4 kcal/g) when the calorie intake is inadequate, but this is not their primary function. It is considered wasteful, if proteins were used for such a purpose.

Chapter 15

Digestion, Absorption and Storage

DIGESTION

Digestion of proteins takes place in the stomach and intestines. As a result of this, the proteins are broken down to amino acids and absorbed.

Sites of Protein Digestion

1. **Gastric digestion:** The proteolytic enzyme present in gastric juice is called pepsin. It acts on proteins in an acid medium and hydrolyzes them to simpler compounds as polypeptide.
2. **Intestinal digestion:** The digestion of proteins is further carried on in the intestine by the action of proteolytic enzymes (trypsin, chymotrypsin and peptidases) present in the pancreatic and intestinal juices. The polypeptides produced by gastric digestion are hydrolyzed to free amino acids by the above enzymes. The amino acids are absorbed in the small intestines and enter the blood circulation through the portal vein.

Mechanism of Proteins Digestion

- Proteins are first acted upon by the enzyme pepsin present in the stomach
- Pepsin converts protein into peptones
- Renin converts caseinogen to casein
- Pepsin converts casein to peptones:

$$\text{Protein} \xrightarrow{\textit{Pepsin}} \text{Peptones}$$

$$\text{Caseinogen} \xrightarrow{\textit{Renin}} \text{Casein}$$

$$\text{Casein} \xrightarrow{\textit{Pepsin}} \text{Peptones}$$

- When the food enters into duodenum, it mixes with pancreatic fluid, which contains an enzyme called trypsin that reduces proteins and peptones into polypeptides and amino acids:

$$\text{Protein} \xrightarrow{\textit{Trypsin}} \text{Polypeptides + Amino acids}$$

$$\text{Peptones} \xrightarrow{\textit{Trypsin}} \text{Polypeptides + Amino acids}$$

ABSORPTION

The absorption of digested food takes place entirely in the small intestine through two channels or ways:

1. The capillary blood vessels.
2. The lymphatics of villi on the inner surface of small intestines.

The amino acids are absorbed in the blood through the capillary blood vessels and then carried through the portal vein to the liver.

Formation of Urea

The liver receives amino acids, which have been absorbed by the blood. In the liver cells, deamination takes place, which means (that the nitrogen is separated from the amino acid part and the ammonia is converted into urea) urea is removed by the liver. It is taken to the kidneys and excreted in the urine. The remaining part is used by the tissue for repair and body build.

STORAGE

The proteins are stored in every part of the body except in adipose tissue. When a high-dietary protein intake is consumed, there is an increase in urea excretion, which suggests that amino acid oxidation is increased. High levels of protein intake increase the activity of branched-chain ketoacid dehydrogenase. As a result, oxidation is facilitated and the amino group of the amino acid is excreted to the liver. This process suggests that excess protein consumption results in protein oxidation and that the protein is excreted. The body is unable to store excess protein. Protein is digested into amino acids, which enter the bloodstream.

Excess amino acids are converted to other usable molecules by the liver in a process called deamination. Deamination converts nitrogen from the amino acid into ammonia, which is converted by the liver into urea in the urea cycle. Excretion of urea is performed by the kidneys. These organs can normally cope with any extra workload; but, if kidney disease occurs, a decrease in protein will often be prescribed. When there is excess protein intake, amino acids can be converted to glucose or ketones, in addition to being oxidized for fuel.

When food protein intake is periodically high or low, the body tries to keep protein levels at an equilibrium by using the 'labile protein reserve,' which serves as a short-term protein store to be used for emergencies or daily variations in protein intake. However, the reserve is not utilized as long-term storage for future needs.

Chapter 16

Metabolism and Synthesis

METABOLISM

The metabolism of proteins may be discussed under the following headings:

- Breakdown and synthesis of tissue proteins
- Nitrogen balance
- Oxidation of amino acid.

Breakdown and Synthesis of Tissue Proteins

1. Recent studies have shown that breakdown and synthesis of tissue proteins proceed simultaneously.
2. A part of the tissue proteins is broken down continuously and is replaced by the formation of new tissue protein from the amino acids supplied by the diet.
3. The breakdown of tissue proteins is called catabolism and the formation of new tissue proteins is called anabolism.

Nitrogen Balance

1. The primary function of dietary proteins are to make up the endogenous losses of nitrogen from the body and to meet the protein needs for growth, convalescence, pregnancy, lactation, etc. Nitrogen balance is calculated by subtracting the nitrogen lost in urine, feces and sweat from nitrogen intake, i.e.:

   Nitrogen balance = Nitrogen intake
   – Nitrogen loss (in urine, feces and sweat)

2. The nitrogen balance can be positive, zero or negative depending on the protein intake from the diet. Data on the effect of varying protein intake on nitrogen balance in a boy are given in Table 16.1:

Table 16.1: Nitrogen balance in a boy aged 15 years on different proteins intake (mean values per day)

Protein intake (g)	Nitrogen intake from diet (g)	Nitrogen losses			Nitrogen balance (g)
		Urine (g)	Feces (g)	Total (g)	
50.0	8.0	5.0	1.8	6.8	+ 1.2 (positive nitrogen balance)
37.5	6.0	4.3	1.7	6.0	0 (nitrogen equilibrium)
25.0	4.0	3.6	1.6	5.2	- 1.2 (negative nitrogen balance)

a. Positive nitrogen balance: If the nitrogen lost from the body in urine, feces and sweat is less than the nitrogen intake, the body is in positive nitrogen balance.
b. Nitrogen equilibrium: When the nitrogen intake equals the nitrogen lost in urine, feces and sweat in the body, it is in a state of nitrogen equilibrium.
c. Negative nitrogen balance: If the nitrogen lost from the body in urine, feces and sweat is greater than nitrogen intake, the body is in negative nitrogen balance. Negative nitrogen balances are observed in persons suffering from under-nutrition, burns, fever, injury, after surgery and in starvation, and also inadequate protein intake.

Oxidation of Amino Acids

The amino acids are not utilized for the formation of tissue proteins and are oxidized by enzymes:

$$\text{Amino acid} \xrightarrow{\text{Oxidation}} \text{Ketoacids} + NH_3$$

The ammonia thus formed is converted into urea in this level and excreted in the urine. The ketoacids are oxidized to yield energy. Proteins are converted into amino acids by enzymes of the gastric pancreatic and intestinal juices. These are absorbed by the villi of the small intestine and carried by the portal vein to the liver.

The chief use of protein is to provide material for body building. The new tissue required for the purpose of growth and repair can only be made from this foodstuff, since no other foodstuff contains the nitrogen essential for the making of a living cell. The amino acids required for tissue building pass through the liver and are carried by the bloodstream to all parts of the body for this purpose. Protein can also be used as body fuel. Excess protein and protein unsuitable for body building, such as the second class proteins obtained from plant foods are split up in the liver into two forms:

- Body fuel in the form of glucose (containing carbon, hydrogen and oxygen)
- Urea or nitrogenous waste matter (containing nitrogen, which is incombustible and hydrogen).

This process is termed as deamination of the amino acids. The nitrogenous content of the amino acids are not required for the body building and converted first into ammonia, which is combined with carbonic acid and water in the liver. The glucose is either burnt or stored as required. The urea is readily soluble and being useless for fuel, is carried away by the bloodstream and excreted from the blood by the kidneys. Protein will also serve as fuel in conditions of starvation. Combustion must go on continuously to maintain life.

The waste products of protein metabolism are urea, uric acid and creatinine. Uric acid is less soluble than urea and comes particularly from the nuclear material in the food. Creatinine is the waste product of the breaking down of our own body protein. All these protein wastes are excreted by the kidneys in the urine. About 30 g of urine leave the body each day.

SYNTHESIS

1. Several studies using amino acids containing radioactive isotopes have been carried out to assess the rate of protein synthesis and breakdown in human and different animals.
2. The rates of protein synthesis and breakdown is expressed as grams of proteins per kilogram body weight per day, which was found to be 4–6 g in man.
3. Thus, a 70 kg adult man synthesizes and degrades about 280–420 g of proteins daily, as compared with daily intake of 50–100 g of protein from the diet.
4. The total amount of free amino acids in the body (in body fluids and tissues) in an adult man weighing 70 kg is of the order of 20–30 g.
5. The whole body of a 70 kg adult man will contain about 12 kg proteins. if we assume the half-life of total body proteins to be 80 days, then one eightieth of the total proteins, i.e. 12 × 1,000/80 = 150 g proteins will be synthesized and breakdown daily.

Chapter 17

Malnutrition and Overconsumption

The term malnutrition generally refers both to undernutrition and overnutrition; but in this guide, we use the term to refer solely to a deficiency of nutrition. Many factors can cause malnutrition, most of which relate to poor diet or severe and repeated infection, particularly in underprivileged populations. Inadequate diet and disease, in turn, are closely linked to the general standard of living the environmental conditions, and whether a population is able to meet its basic needs such as food, housing and health care. Malnutrition is thus a health outcome as well as a risk factor for disease and exacerbated malnutrition and it can increase the risk, both of morbidity and mortality. Although it is rarely the direct cause of death (except in extreme situations such as famine), child malnutrition was associated with 54% of child deaths (10.8 million children) in developing countries in 2001. Malnutrition that is the direct cause of death is referred to as 'protein-energy malnutrition (PEM)' in this guide.

DEFICIENCIES

1. **In adults:** Protein deficiency in adults leads to loss of body weight. Reduced subcutaneous fat, anemia, susceptibility to infection, frequent loose stools, general lethargy, delay in wound healing, nutritional edema, cirrhosis of liver, underweight and incapacity to sustained work.
2. **In pregnancy:** Premature birth, still birth, low-birth-weight babies (weight < 2,500 g).
3. **In infancy and early childhood:** Mental retardation, stunted growth and development.
4. **In children:** Protein deficiency in children is a grave concern, as it may lead to PEM. This is one of the major nutritional problems in India. It is more prevalent in preschool children in the age group of 2–5 years.

PROTEIN-ENERGY MALNUTRITION

Protein-energy malnutrition (kwashiorkor and marasmus) is widely prevalent among weaned infants and preschool children in India, and other developing countries. The diets consumed by weaned infants and preschool children in these countries lack in proteins, calories, certain, vitamins and minerals. PEM is one of the nutrition problems in the country. It affects mainly the child population, especially in the age group of 0–5 years. It is very common condition among children under 5 years of age in poor communities.

Causes

The main cause for the wide prevalence of PEM among children in the developing countries such as India are:

1. Failure of breastfeeding due to death of mother or chronic disease of the mother.
2. Late introduction of supplementary foods.
3. Inappropriate choice of supplementary foods due to ignorance or traditional beliefs.
4. Poverty and inability to buy foods due to high cost.
5. Poor care of children by their siblings, when their mother goes for work.
6. Neglecting smaller children in large families, where the mother has to do too much work.
7. Stoppage of breastfeeding for the first child due to short interval between the two children.
8. Twins receiving only half as much milk and attention from the mother than as a single baby.
9. Economic and cultural factors, i.e. nonavailability of protein-rich and protective foods due to inadequate production, lack of knowledge about the process and preservation of foods, and lack of quick distribution wherever necessary and lack of financial sources, etc.
10. Poverty, illiteracy, less income, unemployment, food fads, customs, superstitions, etc. are the causes of PEM.
11. The environmental factors include infestations and infection due to parasites, bacteria, chemicals, hook worms and round worms, etc.

Signs

The signs of PEM in children are:

- Edema
- Dyspigmentation of the hair
- Thin sparse hair and dull hair
- Straight hair, easily plucked
- Muscle wasting
- Dyspigmentation of the skin
- Moon face
- Flaky paint dermatosis (scaly skin)
- Poor wound healing
- Irritability
- Poor liver protein production, transport and release
- Inadequate fuel supply to the brain
- Amino acid and electrolyte imbalance
- Inadequate protein for new tissue growth
- Hepatomegaly (enlargement of liver).

Classification

Protein-energy malnutrition has been classified in many ways. Two of the important types are mentioned below:

1. **Gomez classification:**
   - Grade 1: 90–75% of expected weight
   - Grade 2: 75–60% of expected weight
   - Grade 3: < 60% of expected weight.
2. **Clinical classification:**
   - Kwashiorkor
   - Marasmus
   - Marasmic Kwashiorkor.

Kwashiorkor

Kwashiorkor comes from an African word meaning 'displaced child' referring to the illness of the older infant who is denied of breast milk, when the new baby is born. Kwashiorkor is common in children between 1 and 5 years. It is due to a protein deficiency, which occurs after protein-rich foods are discontinued during weaning and the child is given food, which is low in proteins and calories.

Definition: A severe malnutrition of infants and young children, primarily in tropical and subtropical regions, caused by deficiency in the quality and quantity of protein in the diet.

Signs and symptoms: The important clinical signs and symptoms of kwashiorkor are as follows:

1. **Growth failure:** This is manifested by decreased body length and low body weight in spite of retention of water in the body (edema) and presence of subcutaneous fat in some children. This growth retardation is primarily due to the general quantitative lack of proteins.
2. **Mental changes:** Several workers have stressed on the constant findings of mental changes described as apathy and peevishness. In advanced cases, children tend to live in inert listless condition and show no interest, in the surrounding.
3. **Edema:** It occurs at first in the feet and lower legs, and then may involve the hands, the thighs and face. The edema is mainly due to lowered serum albumin and probably also due to high-sodium and low-potassium levels in serum. There is also some evidence that the normal diuretic and antidiuretic hormonal control of urine secretion is upset.
4. **Muscle wasting:** It is a constant feature of kwashiorkor and a reduction in the circumference of the upper arm is usually evident. It is less affected by edema than in the forearm or leg.
5. **Moon face:** The full well-rounded face, known as moon face and infiltration of liver is usually present.
6. **Gastrointestinal tract:** Loss of appetite and vomiting are common. Diarrhea is present in most cases.
7. **Skin and hair changes:** The characteristic skin changes of kwashiorkor are known as the 'crazy pavement' dermatosis. This is most marked on the buttocks, back of thighs and axilla. These lesions consist of dark hyperpigmented brownish black areas of skin.
8. **Anemia:** It is invariably present. It is due to the deficiency of iron and folic acid. Anemia may be aggravated by parasitic infection, which prevents the absorption of nutrients.
9. **Vitamin deficiency:** Signs and symptoms of vitamin A deficiency such as xerophthalmia and keratomalacia are widely prevalent. Angular stomatitis and glossitis due to deficiency of riboflavin may be present.

Marasmus

Marasmus is the second clinical form of severe PEM caused by inadequate dietary protein as well as carbohydrate (CHO) called balanced starvation. It is generally seen in children of below 1 year of age, who are bottlefed with diluted milk and prolonged breast feeding not supplemented with other foods for older children.

Definition: Undernourishment causing a child's weight to be significantly low for their age. Marasmus is characterized by growth retardation, muscle wasting, skin changes, vitamin A deficiency and anemia.

Symptoms: The two constant features of nutritional marasmus are growth retardation and severe wasting of muscles, and subcutaneous fat. The similar changes are detailed below:

1. **Growth retardation:** This is usually very severe. Loss of weight is much more marked than decrease in height. The child is usually below 60% of the standard weight.
2. **Wasting of muscles and of subcutaneous fat:** The subject is severely emaciated. The muscles are wasted. The arms are thin and the skin is loose. Subcutaneous fat is practically absent.
3. **Other changes:** The skin is dry and atrophic. The subject shows sign of dehydration. Eye lesions due to vitamin A deficiency and anemia may be present.
4. **Biochemical changes:** There is slight lowering of serum albumin. Vitamin A content of serum is low, the important difference is the clinical and biochemical features between marasmus and kwashiorkor.

Marasmic Kwashiorkor

Marasmic kwashiorkor includes symptoms of both marasmus and kwashiorkor, which represents the gravest form of PEM (Table 17.1). A child with early kwashiorkor can develop nutritional marasmus by severe infective diarrhea and ill-advised prolonged underfeeding. Conversely, an infant with nutritional marasmus may develop kwashiorkor, if it is fed on protein-deficient carbohydrate-rich foods along with adequate common slat.

Definition: The most severe form of PEM characterized by extreme weight loss, weakness edema and features of kwashiorkor.

Table 17.1: Clinical features of kwashiorkor and marasmus

Clinical features	Kwashiorkor	Marasmus
Weight	Below normal, may be marked	Very much below normal
Muscles	Thin upper arms can be marked by edema	Very thin upper arms
Edema of feet and legs	Yes	No
Hair, color and texture	Brighter than in others or reddish and brittle	Normal color/lighter, but softer than others
Skin	Stretched and pale patches	Shriveled and wrinkles
Stools	Often loose	Sometimes loose motion, may also be constipated
Diarrhea	Often	Sometimes
Anemia	Sometimes	Sometimes
Vitamin deficiencies	Usually found	Sometimes found

Investigations

A child suspected of malnutrition needs to be assessed properly, along with a monitoring of the calorie intake. If a child has starved for many days, his/her body cannot handle too much food at once and in all likelihood, the child will vomit or get diarrhea:

1. **Nutritional assessment:** The calorie requirement is calculated as per height and age. The discrepancy between the requirement and actual calorie intake is measured.
2. **Assessment of growth:** The weight and height of the child are calculated and if it is less than the weight of a normal child, it is an indicator of PEM. Also, mid-arm circumference and skin fold thickness is measured as an indicator of PEM.
3. **Blood tests:** For growth hormone, serum albumin (a form of protein), vitamin B_{12} levels and complete blood count (CBC) are important. Routine urine and stool tests are important to check for infection and diabetes.

Treatment

1. Once diagnosed, treatment for a child suffering from PEM need to begin immediately, and in a slow and sustainable manner. The diet in the treatment of marasmic kwashiorkor is the same as that used in the treatment of kwashiorkor.
2. Initially, when the child is admitted to the hospital, intravenous fluids are given to correct dehydration and electrolyte imbalance. Slowly, liquids, semisolids and then solid foods are given over a period of days. If a child is on breast milk, it should be continued in hospital. Vitamin, calcium and iron deficiencies are corrected. Iron and calcium can be given orally, while vitamin A, D and K are given in injectable form.
3. Diet should be charted by a dietician to give calorie dense and nutritious food to accelerate growth and development. Eggs, milk and fruits should be a part of the daily meal.
4. Any infection such as gastroenteritis, worm infestation or tuberculosis should be treated and followed-up.
5. Immunization should be given, if not been given before. The main principles of treatment are to ensure:
   a. An acceptable and readily digestible diet (liquid diet initially for a week) rich in proteins, calories and supplying all other dietary essentials in required amounts.
   b. Treatment of any bacterial and parasitic infections are present.

The diet usually consists of skimmed milk powder (reconstituted), sugar, cooked cereals and banana. Fat is introduced in the diet from the 2nd week of treatment. The daily calorie intake should be 140–150 kcal/kg and protein intake 3–5 g/kg body weight. Vitamin A deficiency is corrected by the administration of the required amounts of synthetic vitamin A.

OVERCONSUMPTION

Protein is not particularly dangerous, but an overconsumption of protein may be associated with the following:

1. **Weight gain:** Excess calories from excess protein may be stored as body fat.
2. **Intestinal irritation:** Too much protein has been linked to constipation, diarrhea and/or excessive gas.
3. **Dehydration:** Experts advise drinking a half gallon of water per 100 g of protein.

4. **Seizures:** These have been linked with excess protein intake, but insufficient amount of water is consumed.
5. **Nutritional deficiencies:** Just focusing on protein intake causes some high-protein dieters to overlook other nutrients. Ensure that the diet is balanced and nutritious.
6. **Risk of heart disease:** This is a bit misleading. A healthy high-protein diet is not associated with heart disease, but if one is getting all of the protein from unhealthy sources that are loaded with unhealthy fats, obviously the risk for heart disease will increase.
7. **Kidney problems:** Some believe that high-protein and low-carbohydrate diets, when taken for long term, can possibly cause kidney issues, but more research needs to be done.

While this list may seem alarming, it is important to remember that many of these side effects are only associated with highly excessive protein diets coupled with unbalanced nutrition and/or dehydration. And this list pales in comparison to the side effects of protein deficiency, which includes general illness, loss of hair, loss of sleep, poor coordination, vision problems, etc.

4. **Seizures:** These have been linked with excess protein intake but insufficient amount of water is consumed.
5. **Nutritional deficiencies:** Just focusing on protein alone causes some high-protein dieters to overlook other nutrients. Ensure that the diet is balanced and nutritious.
6. **Risk of heart disease:** This is a bit misleading. A need for high protein diet is not associated with heart disease, but if one is getting all of the protein from unhealthy sources that are loaded with [illegible] fatty foods, obviously the risk for heart disease will increase.
7. **Kidney problems:** Some believe that high-protein and low-carbohydrate diets, when taken for long term, can possibly cause kidney issues, but more research needs to be done.

While this list may seem alarming, it is important to remember that many of these side effects are only associated with highly excessive protein diets coupled with unbalanced nutrition and/or dehydration. And this list pales in comparison to the side effects of protein deficiency which includes general illness, loss of hair, loss of sleep, poor coordination, vision problems etc.

Section V

Vitamins, Minerals and Energy

Vitamins, Minerals and Energy

Chapter 18

Vitamins

Vitamins are a class of organic compounds categorized as essential nutrients. They are required by the body in a very small amounts, so they fall in the category of micronutrients (Table 18.1). Vitamins do not yield energy, but enable the body to use the other nutrients. Since the body is generally unable to synthesize them (at least in sufficient amounts), they must be provided by food. A well-balanced diet supplies the vitamin needs of a healthy person.

CLASSIFICATION OF VITAMINS (TABLE 18.2)

Vitamins are divided into two groups:

1. **Fat-soluble vitamins:** Vitamins A, D, E and K.
2. **Water-soluble vitamins:** B-group vitamins and vitamin C.

Each vitamin has a specific function to perform and deficiency of any particular vitamin may lead to specific deficiency diseases.

Vitamin A

Vitamin A covers both preformed vitamin—retinal and provitamin—beta carotene, some of which are converted to retinol in the intestinal mucosa. The international units (IU) originally established for vitamin A and provitamin is equivalent to 0.3 microgram (μg) of retinol (or 0.55 μg of retinol palmitate).

Some food composition tables give separate values for retinol and beta carotene. To convert these into a single value, the term 'retinol equivalent' (RE) has been conventionally adopted. The conversion can be done in the following way:

- 1 mg of retinal = 1 μg of RE
- 1 μg of beta carotene = 0.167 μg of RE
- 1 μg of other carotenoids = 0.084 μg of RE.

Table 18.1: Recommended daily intake of vitamins

Age year	Retinol (g)	Vitamin D (g)	Thiamine (mg/1,000 kcal)	Riboflavin (mg/1,000 kcal)	Niacin (mg/1,000 kcal)	Folate (g)	Vitamin B (g)	Vitamin C (mg)
Infancy								
0.0–0.5	400	5	0.5	0.6	6.6	100	0.2	20
0.5–1.0	300	5	0.5	0.6	6.6	100	0.2–1.0	40
Children								
1–3	250	5	0.5	0.6	6.6	100	0.2–1.0	40
4–6	300	5	0.5	0.6	6.6	100	0.2–1.0	40
7–9	400	5	0.5	0.6	6.6	100	0.2–1.0	40
Adolescents								
10–12	600	5	0.5	0.6	6.6	100	0.2–1.0	40
13–12	750	5	0.5	0.6	6.6	100	0.2–1.0	40
16–18	750	5	0.5	0.6	6.6	100	0.2–1.0	40
Adults								
Males	750	5	0.5	0.6	6.6	100	1.0	40
Females	750	5	0.5	0.6	6.6	100	1.0	40
Pregnancy	750	10	0.5	0.6	6.6	300	1.5	40
Lactation	1,150	10	0.5	0.6	6.6	150	1.5	40

Table 18.2: Vitamins essential to human nutrition

Sl No.	Vitamins	Chemical composition	Daily requirements	Sources	Functions/ Actions	Deficiency symptoms	Prevention and control of deficiency
1.	Vitamin A	Retinol, retinal, various retinoids and carotenoids	Infants: 300–400 µg of retinol equivalent Adults: 750 µg Children: 400–600 µg Pregnancy: 750 + 400 µg Lactation: 750 + 400 µg (1 IU of vitamin A = 0.3 µg of retinol)	Yellow vegetables and fruits (carrots, pumpkin, mangoes, papaya, bananas), liver, egg yolk, ghee, cheese, milk and its products eggs, fish, fish liver oil, etc.	Constituents of visual pigment, which helps in normal vision Maintains epithelial cells of skin and mucous membrane Associated with growth, especially regulates skeletal growth Protects body against infections Cornea becomes dry,	Resistance to infection decreases Night blindness, i.e. inability to see in dim light Xerophthalmia (dry eye) characterized by dry conjunctiva, Bitot's spots (grayish, rough and raised patches on conjunctiva)	Diet improvement, regular intake of green leafy vegetables Oral administration of 200,000 IU of vitamin A drops every 6 months to preschool children

Contd...

Contd...

Sl No.	Vitamins	Chemical composition	Daily requirements	Sources	Functions/ Actions	Deficiency symptoms	Prevention and control of deficiency
					hazy as ground glass with ulceration Keratomalacia (softening of a part or whole of the cornea)		
2.	Vitamin D	Cholecalciferol and antirachitic vitamin	Infants and children: 10 µg Adults: 7.50 µg Lactation: 15 µg (1 µg of cholecalciferol = 40 IU of vitamin D)	Fish, liver, fish liver oils, eggs, butter, milk and its products; generated in the skin by action of ultraviolet rays of sunlight	Increases intestinal absorption of calcium and phosphate Mineralization of bones and teeth	Rickets in children and osteomalacia in adults Rickets is characterized by bony deformities in growing children Osteomalacia is characterized	Infants and children are exposed to the sun under appropriate conditions Prophylaxis vitamin D supplements during first 2 years of life

Contd...

Contd...

Sl No.	Vitamins	Chemical composition	Daily requirements	Sources	Functions/ Actions	Deficiency symptoms	Prevention and control of deficiency
						by generalized body pain, especially over bones	
3.	Vitamin E	Tocopherols, tocotrienols	15 IU (10 mg) for normal adults	Milk, oils, eggs, meat, leafy vegetables	Antioxidant Cofactors in electron transport in cytochrome chain	Sterility, muscles wasting and ataxia, fetal death, testicular degeneration and hemolysis of red blood cells in animals	Widely distributed in foods, therefore no deficiency symptoms are produced in humans
4.	Vitamin D	Antihemorrhagic vitamin and phylloquinone, menaquinones	Average diet combined with that formed by intestinal bacteria (approximately 30 μg)	Green leafy vegetables, cereals, fruits; synthesized by bacteria in gastrointestinal tract (GIT)	Catalyzes γ-carboxylation of glutamic acid to activate clotting factors, especially prothrombin	Marked prolongation in blood clotting time leading to generalized bleeding tendencies	Administration of single oral dose of vitamin K to premature infants

Contd...

Contd...

SI No.	Vitamins	Chemical composition	Daily requirements	Sources	Functions/ Actions	Deficiency symptoms	Prevention and control of deficiency
5.	Vitamin B_1	Thiamine	Children: 0.5–1.0 mg Adults: 1.0–1.5 mg Pregnancy and lactation: 1.5–2 mg	Meat, fish liver, eggs, milk, cereals, pulses, grains, nuts, fruits, yeast, vegetables	Cofactor in decarboxylation of acids, thus helps in carbohydrate utilization and maintenance of good appetite and digestion (nervous tissue uses glucose as their primary source of energy)	Beriberi, neurological and mental disturbances, e.g. anesthesia loss of reflexes, paralysis in legs, insomnia, anxiety, depression, cardiomegaly, signs of cardiac failure	Use of parboiled or undermilled rice Addition of thiamine-rich food to the diet
6.	Vitamin B_2	Riboflavin	2 mg	Liver, milk, meat, beer, green leafy vegetables, pulses,	Constituent of 'flavoprotein', which helps in tissue oxidation and respiration	Glossitis, cheilosis, soreness of the tongue, redness and burning	Adequate intake of riboflavin-rich foods

Contd...

Contd...

Sl No.	Vitamins	Chemical composition	Daily requirements	Sources	Functions/ Actions	Deficiency symptoms	Prevention and control of deficiency
				germinating cereals; also synthesized by bacteria in large intestine	Helps in protein, fat and carbohydrate metabolism	sensation in the eyes, dermatitis	
7.	Vitamin B_3	Niacin, niacinamide	10–15 mg	Yeast, meat, kidney, liver, cereals, pulses, germinating seeds, green vegetables; also synthesized in the body	Constituent of coenzyme NAD^+, $NADP^+$ and thus concerned with many of the important enzyme-producing reactions of metabolism This helps in normal functioning of	Pellagra: Characterized by 3Ds, i.e. dermatitis, diarrhea, dementia (memory loss); glossitis, mental disorders with polyneuropathy	Adequate intake of niacin-rich foods

Contd...

Contd...

Sl No.	Vitamins	Chemical composition	Daily requirements	Sources	Functions/ Actions	Deficiency symptoms	Prevention and control of deficiency
					skin, intestinal tract and nervous system		
8.	Vitamin B_5	Pantothenic acid	10 mg for normal adults	Eggs, liver, yeast and many vegetables	Constituent of coenzyme A (CoA)	Dermatitis, enteritis, alopecia (hair loss), adrenal insufficiency	Widely distributed in food and deficiency symptoms, rarely seen
9.	Vitamin B_6	Pantothenic acid	1.5 mg for normal adults	Yeast, wheat, corn, liver, cereals and legumes	Forms prosthetic groups of decarboxylases and transaminases Converted in the body into pyridoxal phosphate	Convulsions, hyperirritability, dizziness and vomiting	Administration of drugs (INH, oral contraceptives) produces vitamin B_6 deficiency These drugs must be

Contd...

Contd...

Sl No.	Vitamins	Chemical composition	Daily requirements	Sources	Functions/ Actions	Deficiency symptoms	Prevention and control of deficiency
					These help in metabolism of amino acids, fats and carbohydrates		supplemented with vitamin B_6
10.	Vitamin B_7	Biotin	In traces	Egg yolk, liver, tomatoes	Catalyzes CO_2 'fixation' (in fatty acid synthesis)	Dermatitis, enteritis	Widely distributed in food and deficiency symptoms rarely seen
11.	Vitamin B_9	Folic acid	Adults and children: 100 µg Lactation: 150 µg	Liver, eggs, green leafy vegetables	Coenzymes for '1 carbon' Involved in methylation reaction (1 and 2) helps in DNA synthesis	Sprue (malabsorption) megaloblastic anemia, sterility, low-birth-weight babies	Avoid overcooking of food, since it destroys folates Demand increases during

Contd...

Contd...

Sl No.	Vitamins	Chemical composition	Daily requirements	Sources	Functions/ Actions	Deficiency symptoms	Prevention and control of deficiency
							pregnancy and in growing children, therefore they must be given extra supplements of folic acid
12.	Vitamin B_{12}	Cyanocobalamin	Children: 0.2–1.0 µg	Liver, meat, eggs, milk, synthesized by bacteria in the colon	Coenzyme in amino acid metabolism Stimulates RBCs production from bone marrow Necessary for DNA synthesis	Pernicious anemia, infertility, neurological and mental disturbances	Prophylactic administration in purely vegetarians, since it is not found in foods of vegetable origin

Contd...

Contd...

Sl No.	Vitamins	Chemical composition	Daily requirements	Sources	Functions/ Actions	Deficiency symptoms	Prevention and control of deficiency
13.	Vitamin C	Ascorbic acid	Infants: 20 mg Children: 40 mg Adults: 40 mg Pregnancy and lactation: 80 mg	Citrus fruits (amla, lemon, orange, guava, tomato); green leafy vegetables; germinating pulses; small amounts in meat and milk	Necessary for hydroxylation of proline and lysine in collagen (connective tissue) synthesis Helps in wound healing prevents bleeding from small blood vessels	Scurvy, which is characterized by painful swelling of gums and joints Multiple hemorrhages, anemia	Milk-fed children should be given supplements of vitamin C

Functions of Vitamin A

1. Vitamin A is essential for normal vision. It contributes to the production of retinal pigments, which are needed for vision in dim light. It supports growth, especially skeletal growth.
2. It is necessary for maintaining integrity and normal functioning of glandular and epithelial tissue, which lines intestinal, respiratory and urinary tracts as well as the skin and eyes.
3. It is anti-infective. There is increased susceptibility to infection and lowered immune response in vitamin A deficiency.
4. It may protect against some epithelial cancers such as bronchial cancers.

Sources of Vitamin A (Table 18.3)

Vitamin A is widely distributed in animal and plant foods—in animal foods as preformed vitamin A (retinol) and in plant foods as provitamins (carotenes).

Table 18.3: Important sources of vitamin A

Sources	Vitamin A content (mg/100 g)
Rich sources	
Fish liver oils	6,660–1,000,000
Cod liver oil	10,000–100,000
Cod liver oil (BP)	18,000
Shark liver oil	9,000–16,000
Shark liver oil (IP)	6,660
Liver (sheep, goat, ox or pig)	6,000–10,000
Good sources	
Butter	720–1,200
Ghee (clarified butter fat)	600–700
Egg (hen—whole)	300–400
Egg yolk	600–800
Milk powder, full cream	400–450
Fair sources	
Milk cow's or buffalo's (whole)	50–60
Fatty fish	30–40

Animal foods: The foods rich in retinol are:

- Liver
- Eggs
- Butter
- Cheese
- Whole milk
- Fish and fish liver oil
- Meat.

Fish liver oils are the richest natural sources of retinol, but they are generally used as nutritional supplements rather than as food sources.

Plant foods: The cheapest source of vitamin A is green leafy vegetables such as spinach and amaranth, which are found in abundance in nature throughout the year. The darker the green leaves, the higher is its carotene content.

Vitamin 'A' also occurs in yellow fruits and vegetables, e.g. papaya, mango, pumpkin and in some roots, e.g. carrots. The most important carotenoid is beta carotene, which has the highest vitamin A activity. Carotenes are converted to vitamin A in the small intestine. This action is poorly accomplished in malnourished children and those suffering from diarrhea.

Fortified foods: The foods fortified with vitamin A, e.g. vanaspati, margarine, milk can be an important source.

Effects of Vitamin A Deficiency

The signs of vitamin A deficiency are predominantly ocular. They include night blindness, conjunctival xerosis, Bitot's spots, corneal xerosis and keratomalacia. The term 'xerophthalmia' (dry eye) comprises all the ocular manifestations of vitamin A deficiency from night blindness to keratomalacia.

Ocular manifestations

Given below is a short description of the ocular manifestations.

Night blindness

Lack of vitamin A first causes night blindness or inability to see in dim light. The mother herself can detect this condition when her child cannot see in late evenings or find her in darkened room. Night blindness is due to impairment in dark adaptation. Unless vitamin A intake is increased, the condition may get worse, especially when children also suffer from diarrhea and other infections.

Conjunctival xerosis

The condition is the first clinical sign of vitamin A deficiency. The conjunctiva becomes dry and nonwettable. Instead of looking smooth and shiny, it appears muddy and wrinkles.

Bitot's spot

Bitot's spots are triangular, 1–2 cm diameter size, pearly white or yellowish, foamy spots on the sclera or white part of the eyeball on either side of cornea. They are frequently bilateral. Bitot's spots in young children usually indicate severe vitamin A deficiency. In older individuals, these spots are often inactive sequelae of earlier disease.

Corneal xerosis

Corneal xerosis stage is particularly serious. The cornea appears dull, dry and nonwettable, and eventually opaque and does not have a moist appearance. In more severe deficiency, there may be corneal ulceration. The ulcer may heal leaving a corneal scar, which can affect vision.

Keratomalacia

Keratomalacia or liquefaction of the cornea is a grave medical emergency. The cornea (a part or whole) become soft and may burst open. The process is rapid one. If the eye collapses, vision is lost. Keratomalacia is one of the major causes of blindness is India and is frequently with protein-energy malnutrition (PEM).

Extraocular manifestations

1. These comprise follicular hyperkeratosis, especially on the back of the arms, legs, and on the shoulder and lower abdomen, giving the appearance of the skin of a toad.
2. Anorexia and growth retardation.
3. Even the mild vitamin A deficiency causes an increase in morbidity and mortality due to respiratory and intestinal infection.

Absorption and Storage of Vitamin A

Vitamin A is absorbed in the small intestine and pass along with fate through the lymphatic system into the bloodstream; from bloodstream, liver can store large amount of vitamin A, when fed on diet rich in vitamin A.

The liver has an enormous capacity for storing vitamin A, mostly in the form of retinol palmitate. A well-fed person has sufficient vitamin A reserves to meet his/her needs for 6–9 months or more. In severe protein deficiency, decreased production of retinol-binding protein prevents mobilization of liver retinol reserves.

Vitamin D

The nutritionally important forms of vitamin D in man are calciferol (vitamin D_2) and cholecalciferol (vitamin D_3). Calciferol may be derived by irradiation of the plant sterol, ergosterol. Cholecalciferol is the naturally occurring vitamin D, which is found in animal fats and fish liver oils. It is also derived from exposure to ultraviolet rays of the sunlight, which converts the cholesterol in the skin to vitamin D. Vitamin D is stored largely in the fat depots.

Functions of Vitamin D

The functions of vitamin D and its metabolites are as follows:

1. **Intestine:** Promotes intestinal absorption of calcium and phosphorus.
2. **Bone:** Stimulates normal mineralization. Enhances bone reabsorption and affects collagen maturation.
3. **Kidney:** Increase tubular reabsorption of phosphate, variable effect on reabsorption of calcium.
4. **Other:** Permits normal growth.

Sources of Vitamin (Table 18.4)

Vitamin D is derived both from sunlight and foods.

Sunlight: Vitamin D is synthesized in the body by the action of ultraviolet rays of sunlight on 7-dehydrocholesterol, which is stored

Table 18.4: Vitamin D content in certain foods

Sources	IU/100 g
Fish liver oil	20,000–400,000
Halibut liver oil	–
Cod liver oil	8,000–30,000
Cod liver oil (BP)	8,000
Shark liver oil	1,200–4,000
Fat fish (sardine, salmon, herring)	200–1,200
Egg (hen—whole)	50–60
Butter	20–60
Ghee (sardine, butter fat)	20–60
Milk powder (full fat)	15–25
Milk (fresh—whole)	2–4

in large abundance in the skin. Dark skin filters off up to 95% of ultraviolet rays.

Foods: Vitamin D occurs only in foods of animal origin, e.g. liver, egg yolk, butter and cheese, fish liver oils; these are the richest source of vitamin D.

Other sources: Other sources of vitamin D are foods that are artificially fortified with vitamin D such as milk, margarine, vanaspati and infant foods.

Deficiency C of Vitamin D

Rickets: Vitamin D deficiency leads to rickets, which is usually observed in young children between the age of 6 months and 2 years. The disease is characterized by growth failure, bone deformity, muscular hypotonia, tetany and convulsions due to hypocalcemia.

The bony deformities include curved legs below the knee, deformed pelvis, pigeon chest, Harrison's sulcus, rickety rosary, kyphoscoliosis, etc. The milestones of development such as walking and teething are delayed.

In adults: Vitamin D deficiency may result in osteomalacia, which occurs mainly in women, especially during pregnancy and lactation when requirements of vitamin D are increased (*osteomalacia* means softening of the bones). Bone deformities due to the weight of the body occur in pelvis, legs and ribs. Due to the deformity of the pelvis, normal delivery of the baby becomes difficult.

Prevention Measures

Prevention measures include the following:

1. Educating parents to expose their children regularly to sunshine.
2. Periodic dosing of young children with vitamin D and vitamin D fortification of foods, especially milk. Periodic dosing and education appear to be the most practical approaches in developing countries.

Signs of vitamin D toxicity: Are related to hypercalcemia such as thirst, anorexia, polyuria and the risk of metastatic calcification.

Daily Requirements

The daily requirements of vitamin D for:

- **Adults:** 100 IU

- **Infants and children:** 200 IU
- **Pregnancy and lactation:** 400 IU.

The daily requirements of vitamin D for infants, children, pregnant and nursing women have been estimated to be 400 IU (10 mg), and for older children and adults about 200 IU (5 mg). In tropical climates, half the above requirements will be adequate, if the subjects are exposed to direct sunlight for some hours daily.

Absorption and Storage of Vitamin D

Vitamin D is stored in the body in fatty tissues and in the liver.

Toxic Effects

Vitamin D, in excess, produces toxic symptoms. These include loss of appetite, nausea, vomiting and calcification of soft tissues such as arteries, kidneys and lungs.

Treatment for Vitamin D Deficiency

For the treatment of rickets and osteomalacia, about 1,000–5,000 IU of vitamin D should be administered orally for about 1 month, followed by 800 IU daily for 6 months. These diseases can be prevented by supplementing the diet with 400 IU of vitamin D.

Vitamin E

Vitamin E is the generic name for a group of closely related and naturally occurring fat-soluble compounds—the tocopherols. Of these, α-tocopherol is biologically the most potent.

Sources of Vitamin E

Vitamin E is widely distributed in various foods. The richest sources of vitamin E are vegetable oils, cotton seeds, sunflower seeds, egg yolk, butter and sprouted grams. Food rich in polyunsaturated fatty acids are also rich in vitamin E.

Deficiency of Vitamin E

There is no clear indication of dietary deficiency.

Daily Requirement of Vitamin E

The current estimate of vitamin E requirement is about 10 mg/day per adult.

Toxic Effects

The cytotoxic effect of vitamin E on human lymphocytes is in vitro high concentrations has been reported.

Absorption and Storage of Vitamin E

Vitamin E, similar to other fat-soluble vitamins, is absorbed along with fat in the intestine. It is stored in the liver, muscles and body fat.

Functions of Vitamin E

The important functions are as follows:

1. Vitamin E prevents peroxidation of polyunsaturated fatty acids in tissues and cell membranes.
2. It protects red blood cells from hemolysis by oxidizing agents.
3. It offers protection to liver injury caused by carbon tetrachloride poisoning.

Effects of Deficiency

Vitamin E deficiency causes the following disorders in animals:

1. Reproductive failure.
2. Hemolysis of red blood cells.
3. Muscular dystrophy.

Dietary Sources

Cereal germ oils, e.g. wheat germ oil and corn germ oil are the richest natural sources. Vegetable oils and fats are good sources. Cereals and animal foods are fair sources of tocopherol. Vegetables and fruits are poor sources. Vitamin E contents of some oils and fats are detailed below in Table 18.5.

Table 18.5: Vitamin E contents of some oils and fats

Oils and fats	Vitamin E (mg/100 g)	
	Total	Tocopherol
Cotton seed oil	81.0	47.0
Mustard oil	32.0	8.6
Peanut oil	22..0	11.0
Rice bran oil	91.0	58.0
Soybean oil	118.0	15.9
Wheat germ oil	255.5	142.8

Vitamin K

Vitamin K occurs in at least two major forms, i.e. vitamin K_1 and vitamin K_2.

Sources of Vitamin K

1. Vitamin K_1 is found mainly in fresh green vegetables, particularly dark green ones and in some fruits. Cow's milk is a richest source (60 µg/L) of vitamin K than human milk (15 µg/L).
2. Vitamin K_2 is synthesized by the intestinal bacteria, which usually provide an adequate supply for humans.
3. Long-term administration of antibiotic doses for more than a week may temporarily suppress the normal intestinal flora (a source of vitamin K_2) and may cause a deficiency of vitamin K.
4. Vitamin K is stored in liver.

Functions of Vitamin K

The role of vitamin K is to stimulate the production and/or the release of certain coagulation factors.

Deficiency of Vitamin K

In vitamin K deficiency, the prothrombin content in blood is markedly decreased and the blood clotting time is considerably prolonged.

Daily Requirement of Vitamin K

1. The daily requirement appears to be about 0.03 mg/kg for the adult. The average diets provide adequate amounts of vitamin K_1.
2. Newborn infants tend to be deficient in vitamin K due to minimal stress of prothrombin at birth and lack of an established intestinal flora.
3. Soon after birth, those infants with increased risk should receive a single intramuscular dose of a vitamin K preparation, i.e. 0.5 mg of vitamin K, by way of prophylaxis.

Dietary Sources

Vitamin K_1 occurs in plant foods, while vitamin K_2 occurs in microorganisms. The best sources of vitamin K are the green leafy vegetables, e.g. spinach, cabbage, etc. Good sources are cauliflower, soybean, wheat bran, wheat germ, etc. Carrots and potatoes are fair sources. Milk, meat and fish are poor sources.

Absorption and Storage

Vitamin K is absorbed along with fat in the diet. Bile is essential for its absorption. The absorbed vitamin passes through the lymphatic system to the general circulation. Liver stores appreciable amounts of this vitamin.

Vitamin C

Vitamin C (ascorbic acid) is a water-soluble vitamin. It is the most sensitive of all vitamins to heat.

Functions of Vitamin C

1. It is necessary for wound healing, as it helps in the formation of connective tissues.
2. It is necessary for the absorption of iron.
3. It is needed for the formation of collagen, which accounts for 25% of total body protein. Collagen provides a supporting matrix for the blood vessels and connective tissue, also for bones and cartilage.

This explains why vitamin C deficiency results in local hemorrhages. Vitamin C, by reducing ferric iron to ferrous iron, facilitates the absorption of iron from vegetable foods.

Sources of Vitamin C

- Amla or Indian gooseberry
- Lemon
- Tomato
- Guavas
- Orange
- Green leafy vegetables.

Amla and guavas are the rich sources of vitamin C; germinating pulses contain good amounts of vitamin C (Table 18.6).

Deficiency of Vitamin C

Deficiency of vitamin C results in scurvy.

Signs and symptoms of infantile scurvy

1. Loss of appetite.
2. Listlessness.
3. The infant cries when its legs and arms are moved.
4. Swelling is observed at the ends of long bones.
5. Hemorrhages occur under the skin.
6. Gums are swollen and spongy.
7. Convulsions may occur, resulting in death of the infant.

Table 18.6: Ascorbic acid contents of foods

Sources	Ascorbic acid (mg/100 g)
Fruits	
Rich sources	
Amla	700
Guava	300
Good sources	
Lime juice	63
Orange	68
Pineapple	63
Mango (ripe)	24
Papaya (ripe)	46
Cashew fruit	60
Fair sources	
Apple	2–8
Banana (plantain ripe)	2–6
Jack fruit	10
Green leafy vegetables	
Amaranth leaves	173
Cabbage	124
Drumstick leaves	220

Vitamin C Requirements (Table 18.7)

Table 18.7: Vitamin C requirements

Age	Requirements
Newborn	
0–0.5 month	20 mg
0.5–1.0 month	40 mg
Children	
1–3 year	40 mg
4–6 year	40 mg
7–9 year	40 mg
Adolescents	
10–18 year	40 mg
Adults	40 mg

Signs and symptoms of scurvy in adults

1. General weakness.
2. Spongy and bleeding gums.
3. Loose teeth.
4. Swollen tender joint.
5. Hemorrhages (bleeding in various tissues under skin).

Thiamine

Thiamine (vitamin B_1) is a water-soluble vitamin.

Functions of Thiamine (Vitamin B1)

1. It is essential for utilization of carbohydrates. Thiamine pyrophosphate plays an important part in carbohydrate metabolism. It is essential for oxidation of pyruvic acid, which is an intermediate product in carbohydrate metabolism.
2. It is essential to maintain the nerve in healthy condition.
3. It helps in maintenance of good appetite and normal digestion.

Sources of Thiamine

1. Important sources are whole grain cereals, wheat germ, yeast, pulses, oilseeds and nuts, especially groundnut.
2. Milk is an important source of thiamine for infants, provided, the thiamine status of their mothers is satisfactory.
3. Rich sources are dried yeast, rice polished and wheat germ.
4. The main source of thiamine in the diet of Indian people is cereals (rice and wheat), which contribute around 60–85% of the total supply.

Thiamine Losses

Thiamine is readily lost from rice during the process of milling, washing and cooking. Thiamine is also destroyed in toast and in cereals cooked with baking soda.

Effects of Thiamine Deficiency

The two principal deficiency diseases are beriberi and Wernicke's encephalopathy. There are two forms of beriberi namely:

1. Wet beriberi.
2. Dry beriberi (occurs in adults).

Another form of beriberi, which affects infants, is called infantile beriberi.

Dry beriberi: The signs and symptoms of this disease include the following:

1. Loss of appetite.
2. Tingling and numbness of the legs and hands.
3. Wasting of muscle and difficulty in walking.

Wet beriberi: In addition to the above signs and symptoms, the other features present include:

1. Edema in the legs.
2. Enlargement of the heart.
3. Palpitation and breathlessness.

Infantile beriberi: The early symptoms are restlessness, sleeplessness and loss of appetite. Palpitation and breathlessness, and loss of appetite develop, as the disease advances, due to the enlargement of the heart. Death may occur suddenly if treatment is delayed.

Wernicke's encephalopathy (seen often in alcoholics): It is characterized by ophthalmoplegia, polyneuritis, ataxia and mental deterioration. It occurs occasionally in people who fast. Manifestations of minor degrees of thiamine deficiency include loss of appetite, absence of ankle and knee jerks, and presence of calf tenderness. Frank beriberi used to be frequently seen in people who eat highly polished rice. In thiamine deficiency, there is accumulation of pyruvic and lactic acids in the tissues and body fluids.

Prevention of Thiamine Deficiency

1. Beriberi can be eliminated by educating people to eat well balanced, mixed diets containing thiamine-rich foods, e.g. parboiled and undermilled rice, and to stop taking alcohol.
2. Direct supplementation of high-risk groups, e.g. lactating mothers is another approach.
3. Beriberi tends to disappear, as the economic conditions improve and diets become more varied.

Recommended Allowances

1. Daily requirement of thiamine is 0.5 mg/1,000 kcals of energy intake.
2. The body content of thiamine is 30 mg and if more than this is given, it is merely lost in the urine.

3. Patients on regular hemodialysis should routinely be given supplements of thiamine.
4. Thiamine should also be given prophylactically to people with persistent vomiting or prolonged gastric aspiration and those who go on long fast.

Riboflavin (Vitamin B2)

Riboflavin (vitamin B_2) is a member of the B-group vitamins.

Functions of Riboflavin

Riboflavin has a fundamental role in cellular oxidation. It is a cofactor in a number of enzymes involved with energy metabolism. Riboflavin plays an important role in many enzyme systems involved in the metabolism of carbohydrates, fats and proteins.

Sources of Riboflavin Deficiency

The most common lesion associated with riboflavin deficiency is angular stomatitis. Other clinical signs include cheilosis, glossitis, nasolabial seborrhea (cheilosis—cracking of the lips, glossitis—soreness of the tongue). Riboflavin deficiency almost always occurs in association with deficiencies of other B-complex vitamins such as pyridoxine. It is usually a part of multiple deficiency syndrome.

Requirement of Riboflavin

Daily requirement is 0.6 mg/1,000 kcal of energy intake. There are no real body stores of riboflavin.

Niacin (Nicotinic Acid)

Functions of Niacin

Niacin or nicotinic acid is essential for the metabolism of carbohydrate, fat and protein. It is essential for the normal functioning of the skin, intestinal and nervous systems. This vitamin differs from other vitamins of the B-complex groups; in that an essential amino acid, tryptophan serves as its precursor.

Sources of Niacin (Box 18.1)

Foods rich in niacin and/or tryptophan are liver, kidney, meat, poultry, fish, legumes and groundnut.

Box 18.1: Sources of niacin

Rich sources:	Good sources:	Fair sources:
• Dried yeast • Liver • Rice polished • Peanut (groundnut) • Peanut flour	• Whole cereals • Legumes • Meat • Fish	• Milled cereals • Maize • Roots and tubers • Other vegetables • Milk • Egg

Functions of Nicotinic Acid

1. Nicotinic acid is essential for the normal functioning of the skin, intestinal tract and nervous system.
2. Nicotinamide is a component of two coenzymes, which are essential for the metabolism of carbohydrates, fats and proteins.

Effects of Niacin Deficiency

Niacin deficiency results in pellagra. The disease is characterized by three D's:

- Diarrhea
- Dermatitis
- Dementia.

In addition, glossitis and stomatitis usually occur. The dermatitis is bilaterally symmetrical and is found only on those surfaces of the body exposed to sunlight, such as back of the hands, lower legs, face and neck, mental changes also occur, which include depression, irritability and delirium. Pellagra is historically a disease of the maize-eating population. Amino acid imbalance caused by an excess of leucine is the cause of pellagra in both jowar and maize eaters. Excess of leucine appears to interfere in the conversion of tryptophan to niacin.

Prevention

Pellagra is a preventable disease. A good mixed diet containing milk and/or meat is universally regarded as an essential part of prevention and treatment, which aides in agricultural and social development; there is every reason to hope that this disease could be eliminated.

Requirement

The recommended daily allowance is 6.6 mg/1,000 kcal of energy intake.

Pyridoxine (Vitamin B_6)

Pyridoxine (vitamin B_6) exists in three forms:

- Pyridoxine
- Pyridoxal
- Pyridoxamine.

Functions of Pyridoxine

Pyridoxine plays an important role in the metabolism of amino acids, fats and carbohydrates. Pyridoxal phosphate acts as a coenzyme in the metabolism of amino acids. Pyridoxine is essential for maintaining the nerves in normal condition.

Sources of Pyridoxine

Pyridoxine is widely distributed in foods, e.g. milk, liver, meat, egg yolk, fish, whole grain, cereals, legumes and vegetables. Rich sources of pyridoxine are dried yeast, rice polishings, wheat germ and liver.

Effects of Pyridoxine Deficiency

Pyridoxine deficiency is associated with peripheral neuritis. Riboflavin deficiency impairs the optimal utilization of pyridoxine.

Requirement

Adults may need 2 mg of pyridoxine. During pregnancy and lactation, the requirement is 2.5 mg/day. The requirement of adults vary directly with protein intake. Balanced diets usually contain pyridoxines, therefore deficiency is rare.

Folate (Vitamin B_9)

The recommended name is folate. Alternative name is folacin and the usual pharmaceutical preparation is folic acid. Folic acid occurs in food in two forms, i.e. free folates and bound folates. It was found effective in curing tropical macrocytic anemia in human beings.

Functions of the Folate

Folic acid plays a role in the synthesis of the nucleic acids (which constitute the chromosomes). It is also needed for the normal development of blood cells in the marrow. It is also essential for the maturation of red blood cells.

Sources of Folate

The name comes from Latin word folia, means leaf. All leafy vegetables are good dietary sources of folate. Foods such as liver, meat, dairy products, eggs, milk, fruits and cereals are as good dietary sources as leafy vegetables. Overcooking destroys much of folic acid and this contributes to folate deficiency in man.

Absorption of Folate

Free folate is rapidly absorbed from the proximal part of the small intestine.

Effects of Folate Deficiency

Folate deficiency is commonly found in pregnancy and lactation, where requirements are increased. It results in megaloblastic anemia, glossitis, cheilosis and gastrointestinal disturbances such as diarrhea, distension and flatulence. In early pregnancy, folate deficiency may produce abortions or congenital malformations.

Severe folate deficiency may cause infertility or even sterility. There is also evidence about the administration of folic acid antagonists, e.g. alcohol, pyrimethamine and cotrimoxazole. Folic acid supplementation during pregnancy has been found to increase the birth weight of infants and decrease the incidence of low-birth-weight babies. Folic acid requirements are greatest in conditions where there is rapid cell multiplication such as during growth in young children and during pregnancy (Table 18.8).

Table 18.8: Folate requirement

Stages	Requirement/day (mg)
Healthy adults	100
Pregnancy	300
Lactation	150
Children	100

Megaloblastic anemia of pregnancy

Megaloblastic anemia is the severe form of anemia, which results due to insufficiency of folic acid, from the demands of the fetus or some factors interfering with the absorption of metabolism of folic acid. It tends to occur when the hemoglobin is below 7 g (50%). Therefore, the administration of iron prophylactically should reduce the incidence of megaloblastic anemia significantly.

Signs and Symptoms

Pallor is marked, the woman complains of extreme form of weakness, vomiting, dyspnea, and sometimes diarrhea and persistent swelling of the ankles.

Treatment

A striking improvement is the evidence following the administration of folic acid 5 mg three times daily with iron, throughout pregnancy and continued 6 weeks postpartum rest in bed; and a light diet high in proteins, iron and other minerals are essential.

A blood transfusion will be necessary, if anemia is severe or in untreated cases, if delivery is imminent; extreme case is exercised with this product. Patients with anemia fails to respond to iron therapy in 4 weeks and cases in which hemoglobin is less than 10 mg (70%), should have blood investigation made to determine if megaloblastic anemia is present.

Megaloblastic anemia in infants and children

Megaloblastic anemia has been reported to occur among malnourished children in the developing countries.

Signs

The hemoglobin content is usually low, i.e. 5–8 g/100 mL blood and red blood corpuscle (RBC) count of 2.5–3 million per mm.

Dietary sources

Dried yeast, hen's egg and liver are rich sources. Whole cereals, legumes and green leafy vegetables are good sources.

Vitamin B_{12} (Cyanocobalamin)

Vitamin B_{12} is a complex organometallic compound with a cobalt atom. The preparation, which is therapeutically used is cyanocobalamin, which is relatively cheap.

Functions of Vitamin B_{12}

1. Vitamin B_{12} stimulates the formation of RBC and promotes the maturation of RBC.
2. It cooperates with folate in the synthesis of DNA; so deficiency of either leads to megaloblastosis.
3. It has a separate biochemical role in the synthesis of fatty acids in myelin.

Sources of Vitamin B_{12}

Good sources are liver, kidney, meat, fish, eggs, milk and cheese. Liver is the main storage site of vitamin B_{12}; about 2 mg is stored in liver and another 2 mg elsewhere in the body. Unlike folic acid, vitamin B_{12} is relatively heat stable.

Effects of Vitamin B_{12} Deficiency

Vitamin B_{12} deficiency is associated with megaloblastic anemia (pernicious anemia) demyelinating neurological lesions in the spinal cord. Vitamin B_{12}, formerly known as the extrinsic factor of castle, requires an enzyme-like substance, the intrinsic factor present in gastric juice for its absorption. There is no evidence of chemical combination between the extrinsic factor and intrinsic factor.

Vitamin B_{12} is not effective, if taken by mouth in most cases of pernicious anemia, which show lack of intrinsic factor in the gastric juice, but functions if given by infection. In 1948, the antipernicious anemia factor, now known as vitamin B_{12} was isolated and found effective for the blood condition, gastrointestinal symptoms and nervous symptoms of pernicious anemia. Pernicious anemia—severe anemia due to lack of substance in gastric juice results in failure to absorb vitamin B_{12}.

Absorption

Vitamin B_{12} (the antianemic factor) is necessary for the development of the red blood cells. It is present in foods mainly of animal origin and requires a substance present in the normal gastric juice, the intrinsic factor (being inside the body) for its absorption. The complex is absorbed only at a special site in the terminal ileum.

Effects of Deficiency

Vitamin B_{12} deficiency causes the disease 'pernicious anemia.' Vitamin B_{12} is not absorbed in this disease due to the absence of intrinsic factor (IF) in the stomach. The principal signs and symptoms of the disease are as follows:

1. The RBC count is low (1.5–2.5) million per mm and the hemoglobin is also low (8–9%).
2. Maturation of the RBC is affected.
3. Soreness and inflammation of the tongue are commonly observed.
4. Numbness and tingling of fingers and toes, and signs of degeneration of the special spinal cord are observed.

Dietary Sources

Vitamin B_{12} is present only in foods of animal origin. It is not present in foods of vegetable origin. Important dietary sources of vitamin B_{12} are as follows:

1. **Rich sources:** Liver—120 mg/100 g.
2. **Good sources:** Meat and sheep—30 mg/100 g.
3. **Fair sources:** Skimmed milk powder—3.2 mg/100 g.

Biotin

The factor was called anti-egg white injury factor. Later Gyorgy (1931) gave the name 'vitamin H' to this factor.

Physiological Functions

1. It helps to maintain the skin and the nervous system in sound condition.
2. It is essential for the synthesis of malonyl-CoA from acetyl-CoA and oxaloacetic acid from pyruvic acid.

Effects of Deficiency

Biotin deficiency has been reported in an adult who consumed daily 4–12 raw eggs and 1–4 quarts of wine.

Egg white injury factor (avidin)

The active principle present in egg white is responsible for producing 'egg white injury'. It is a protein called 'avidin', which binds biotin. Avidin present in egg white or in purified form is denatured and inactivated by prolonged heating (steaming at 100°C for 60 minutes).

Dietary Sources (Table 18.9)

Biotin occurs widely both in foods of vegetables and animal origin.

Table 18.9: Dietary sources of biotin

Dietary sources	Biotin content of foods	Biotin (µg/100 g)
Rich sources	Dried yeast Liver Soybean Peanut	100–200 100–122 45–55 35–40
Good sources	Whole cereals Legumes Mutton Eggs	6–15 12–18 5–8 20–22
Fair sources	Vegetables	3–5

Requirements

The daily biotin requirement of adults may range from 50 to 60 μg; for children, 20 to 40 μg and for infants, 10 to 15 μg. The biotin content or poor diets consumed in the developing countries is about 50-60 μg, while that of diets consumed in the developed countries vary from 150 to 300 μg. Cow's milk contain approximately 50 μg biotin per liter, while human milk contains only 4 μg/L. Cases of biotin deficiency occurring in infants fed on breast milk and suffering from diarrhea have been reported.

Choline

Choline is an integral part of phospholipids, which is present in nervous tissues and is essential for the life processes. In view of its importance in nutrition, it is usually considered as a member of the vitamin B complex.

Physiological Functions

Choline prevents accumulation of fat in the liver. It is a constituent of phospholipids, which is essential constituents of cells in the body. Acetylcholine plays an important part in the humoral transfer of nerve impulses.

Dietary Sources (Table 18.10)

Table 18.10: Important dietary sources of choline

Dietary sources	Food	Choline (μg/100 g)
Rich sources	Liver	550–660
	Wheat germ	406–450
	Egg yolk	1,490
	Legumes	210–340
Good sources	Rice polishings	150–180
	Whole cereals	110–146
Fair sources	Milled cereals	50–60
	Vegetables	20–80
	Fruits	12–24
	Milk	15–18

Effects of Deficiency

Choline deficiency in rats produces fatty liver and hemorrhage degeneration of the kidney.

Requirement

Choline requirement of human beings is not known.

Bioflavonoids (Vitamin P)

Many investigators have confirmed the value of vitamin P (bioflavonoids) along with ascorbic acid in preventing capillary fragility. The term 'bioflavonoids' was proposed for these group of compounds having vitamin 'P' activity.

Physiological Functions

1. Studies with experimental animals have shown that bioflavonoids control capillary permeability in experimental animals.
2. Citrine also cures intestinal hemorrhages when administered with ascorbic acid.

Effects of Deficiency

The signs of bioflavonoid deficiency are:

1. Decreased capillary resistance leading to petechial bleeding, accompanied by pain across the shoulder and in legs.
2. Lassitude.
3. Fatigue administration of bioflavonoids is effective in curing the above symptoms.

Treatment

Bioflavonoids are generally given orally in doses of about 200 mg four times a day. They have been found effective in curing decreased capillary resistance in allergic subjects.

Dietary Sources

Bioflavonoids occur mainly in fresh fruits and vegetables. Bioflavonoid activity (vitamin P) of some fruits and vegetables (1 U activity per mg citrin frome lemon peel) is given in Table 18.11.

Requirements

The bioflavonoid requirement for human beings is not known.

Table 18.11: Dietary sources of bioflavonoids

Food	Vitamin P content (U)
Lemon peel	500
Lemon juice	450
Orange (juice and peel)	490
Rosehip syrup	240–350
Walnut	100
Spinach	130
Tomato	60–70
Cabbage	60
Apple	60

Pantothenic Acid

Pantothenic acid is one of the vitamins of the vitamin B_2 complex, which can prevent or cure a specific type of dermatitis called chick pellagra. There is a long-standing evidence for relation between pantothenic acid and adrenal cortical function. Pantothenic acid is used in the biosynthesis of corticosteroids. Human blood normally contains 18–35 mg of pantothenic acid per 100 mL, mostly present in the cells as coenzyme. Dried yeast, liver, legumes, etc. are the sources of pantothenic acid (Table 18.12).

Table 18.12: Pantothenic acid content of foods

Sources	Food	Pantothenic acid (μg/100 g)
Rich sources	Dried yeast	10–11
	Liver	7–8
Good sources	Whole cereals	0.6–1.5
	Legumes	0.6–2.2
	Nuts and oilseeds	0.6–2
Fair sources	Vegetables	0.2–1.0

Physiological Functions

Pantothenic acid acts in the form of coenzyme that takes part in the metabolism of carbohydrates and fats. It is essential for the oxidation of pyruvic acid.

Effects of Deficiency

In human beings, the visible signs of deficiency include nausea, vomiting, tremor of the outstretched hand and irritability.

Requirements

The daily allowances of pantothenic acid for humans recommended by National Research Council (NRC) USA is given in Table 18.13.

Table 18.13: Requirement of daily allowances

Humans	Pantothenic acid (mg/day)
Infant	1.5–2.5
Children	5–8
Adolescents	5–9
Adults	10
Pregnant and lactating women	5–10

Chapter 19

Minerals

CHEMICAL ELEMENTS

More than 50 chemical elements are found in the human body, which are required for growth, repair and regulation of vital body functions. These can be divided into three major groups:

1. **Major minerals:** These include calcium, phosphorus, sodium and sodium chloride, potassium and magnesium.
2. **Trace elements:** These are elements required by the body in quantities of less than a few milligrams per day, e.g. iron, iodine, fluorine, zinc, copper, cobalt, chromium, manganese, molybdenum, selenium, nickel, tin, silicon and vanadium (Table 19.1).
3. **Trace contaminants with no known function:** These include lead, mercury, barium, boron and aluminum.

Trace elements are those minerals required by the body in microquantities. The World Health Organization (WHO) Expert Committee on Trace Elements in Human Nutrition (1973) recognized iron, iodine, fluorine, zinc, copper, cobalt, chromium, manganese, molybdenum, selenium, nickel, tin, silicon and vanadium.

The functions of many of these trace elements in our body are not completely understood. Man is not likely to suffer from trace element deficiencies as long as he is omnivorous. Trace elements should not be used as dietary supplements, since excessive amounts can have injurious effects.

Calcium

Calcium is a major mineral element of the body. Calcium occurs in the highest amounts in the body. It constitutes 1.5–2% of the body weight of an adult human. An average adult body contains about 1,000–1,200 g of calcium of which over 99% is found in the bones and

Table 19.1: Summary of minerals

Trace elements	Functions	Recommended daily allowance (RDA)	Deficiency	Toxicity
Calcium	Bone and tooth formation, blood clotting, muscle and nerve action	Average adult body contains 1,000–2,000 g	Osteoporosis, osteomalacia in adults, rickets in children	Tingling of fingers, muscle cramps, fractures
Phosphorus	Formation of bones and teeth, activation of B vitamins, transfer of energy in cells	The adult human body contains about 400–700 mg	In rickets, serum phosphate level is decreased, acidosis	Erosion of jaw and calcium loss
Sodium	Regulation of acid-base equilibrium	The adult human body contains about 100 g of sodium ion	Edema, hyponatremia	Weakness, cramps, dyspnea
Potassium	Regulation of acid-base balance in the cell, growth and building of tissues	An adult human body contains about 250 g K^+	Hypokalemia, hyperkalemia	Weakness, muscular paralysis, vomiting, diarrhea
Magnesium	Helps in utilization of Ca, K, protein and maintenance of electrical activity in nerves and muscles	The adults human body contains about 25 g of magnesium	Kwashiorkor in children, diarrhea	Depression, muscular weakness and neuromuscular irritability
Iron	Component of hemoglobin, metalloprotein, oxygen transport	Premenopausal—18 mg/day; postmenopausal female and male—8 mg/day	Iron deficiency anemia	Hemosiderosis, hemochromatosis

Contd...

Contd...

Trace elements	Functions	Recommended daily allowance (RDA)	Deficiency	Toxicity
Zinc	Protein synthesis, zinc finger protein, component of enzymes	Female: 10 mg/day Male: 12 mg/day	Ageusia, growth retardation, dermatitis hypogonadism, acrodermatitis enteropathica	Copper deficiency, nausea and vomiting
Copper	Cellular respiration, collagen synthesis, component of enzymes, antioxidant	Adults: 2 mg/day	Menkes kinky hair syndrome; hypochromic anemia, skeletal defects	Wilson's disease
Chromium	Glucose tolerance factor	Female: 25 µg/day Male: 35 µg/day	Hyperglycemia, neuropathy, encephalopathy	Dermatitis, eczema, bronchogenic carcinoma
Fluorine	Prevents tooth decay	1.5–4 mg/day	Dental caries	Fluorosis, mottled enamel
Manganese	Component of metalloenzymes, manganese superoxide dismutase	Female: 1.8 mg/day Male: 2.3 mg/day	Hypocholesterolemia, hair and nail changes, impaired clotting factors	Parkinsonism-like features
Molybdenum	Cofactor for xanthine and sulfite oxidase	45 µg/day	Hypercupremia, low-sulfate excretion and hypouricemia	Risk of gout, anemia, thyrotoxicosis

Contd...

Contd...

Trace elements	Functions	Recommended daily allowance (RDA)	Deficiency	Toxicity
Selenium	Component of glutathione peroxidase, superoxide dismutase	55 µg/day	Keshan disease Kashin-Beck disease Myxedematous endemic cretinism	Hair and nail loss, neuropathy, liver failure
Iodine	Component of thyroid hormone	150 µg/day	Hypothyroidism	Thyrotoxicosis
Cobalt	Component of vitamin B_{12}	–	Vitamin B_{12} deficiency anemia	Cardiomyopathy, heart failure, goiter, hypothyroidism vomiting and diarrhea
Boron	Calcium, magnesium, vitamin D metabolism	–	Osteoporosis, low estrogen, testosterone levels	Reduce fertility in men
Germanium	Immunostimulant	–	Hypertension and heart disease	–
Vanadium	Insulin signal enhancer, lipid metabolism	Infants: 10–50 µg/day Adults: 50–100 µg/day	–	Greenish tongue, nephrotoxic
Silicon	Bone and connective tissue formation	–	Risk of osteoporosis	Silicosis of lungs

remaining 1% in soft tissues. The amount of calcium in the blood is usually about 10 mg/dL. The developing fetus requires about 30 g of calcium. The body of the infant at birth contains about 27.5 g of calcium. There is a dynamic equilibrium between the calcium in the blood and that in the skeleton; this equilibrium is maintained by the interaction of vitamin D, parathyroid hormone and probably calcitonin (Table 19.2).

Table 19.2: Recommended intake of calcium by Indian Council of Medical Research (ICMR)

Years	Calcium (g)
0.0–1.0	0.6
1–9 year	0.5
Adolescents	
10–12	0.5
13–15	0.7
16–18	0.6
Adults	
Males and females	0.5
Pregnancy	1.0
Lactation	1.0

Functions of Calcium

The important physiological functions of calcium are:

1. It is essential for the:
   a. Formation of bones and teeth.
   b. Coagulation of blood.
   c. Contraction of muscles and the heart.
   d. For cardiac action.
   e. Keeping the membranes of cells intact.
   f. In the metabolism of enzymes and hormones.
2. It regulates the permeability of capillary walls.
3. It regulates the excitability of nerve fibers and nerve centers.
4. It also plays a crucial role in the transformation of light to electrical impulses in the retina.

In short, the calcium, iron controls many life processes ranging from muscles contraction to cell division.

Sources of Calcium

The best natural sources are milk and milk products, e.g. cheese, curd, skimmed milk and butter milk. A liter of cow's milk provides about 1,200 mg of calcium and human milk about 300 mg. Calcium occurs in milk as calcium caseinate, which is readily assimilated by the body. Mutton has the highest calcium content of the flesh foods with the exception of crab muscle.

The cheapest dietary sources of calcium are green leafy vegetables, cereals and millets. Ragi is particularly rich in calcium. Drinking water provides up to 200 mg/day. Sitaphal (custard apple) fruit contain good amount of calcium. Ladies finger, carrot, beetroot, onion are also the good vegetable sources of calcium.

Effects of Calcium Deficiency

Absorption of calcium is enhanced by vitamin D. It has been established that if the intake of vitamin D is adequate, the problems of rickets and osteomalacia do not arise even with low-calcium intake.

Young animals and children

The effect of deficiency in young animals and children are:

1. Decreased rate of growth.
2. Negative calcium balance.
3. Loss of calcium from bone leading to the development of osteoporosis.
4. Hyperplasia (a diffuse overgrowth) of parathyroid glands.
5. Hyperirritability and tetany to death.

Adults

Osteoporosis in adults, is a condition in which parafunction (decalcification) of the bone occurs due to calcium in the diet. Fractures of the brittle bones occur ever after minor accidents. The treatment consists of giving a well-balanced diet containing about 1–1.5 g calcium with vitamin D (400–800 IU).

Calcium Requirements

A daily intake of 400–500 mg of calcium has been suggested for adults. The physiological requirements are higher in children, expectant and nursing mothers.

Absorption of Calcium

About 20–30% of dietary calcium is normally absorbed. Absorption of calcium is enhanced by vitamin D and decreased by the presence of phytates, oxalates and fatty acids in the diet. Factors that may hinder the absorption of calcium or factors limiting the use of calcium are:

1. Too much phosphorous in the form of phosphate in food.
2. Anything which causes food to pass quickly through the intestine, e.g. infection causing diarrhea, too much roughage in food.
3. Any substance, which forms an insoluble salt with calcium, e.g. excess fatty acids.
4. Deficiency of vitamin D may hinder absorption of calcium.
5. Purgatives, oxalates, excess phosphorus or fatty acids, ptyalin, and deficiencies of vitamin D hinders the absorption of calcium and this affects the use of calcium.

Calcium Content of Blood

The calcium content of blood serum is fairly constant ranging from 9 to 11 mg/100 mL. This level is maintained constant in healthy subjects by the following factors:

1. Calcium absorbed from food through the intestines.
2. The rate of secretion of parathyroid hormone, which controls the level of calcium in blood.

Phosphorus

Adult human body contains about 400–700 g of phosphorus as phosphates. A greater part of this is present in the bone and teeth, and the rest in tissues; phosphorus is present in the body as inorganic salts of phosphoric acid or in combination with organic compounds. Inorganic phosphorus is present as calcium phosphate in bones and teeth; as phosphates of sodium and potassium in soft tissues and body fluids.

Organic Phosphorus

The important organic compounds containing phosphorus are the following:

1. Phospholipids, e.g. lecithin, cephalin.
2. Nucleoproteins and nucleic acid.
3. Creatine phosphate.
4. Hexose phosphates, triose phosphates and glycerophosphates.

Food Sources

The important food sources are milk, eggs, meat and fish. Vegetables are fair sources. A greater part of the phosphorus present in cereals, pulses, nuts and oilseeds exist in the form of phytic acid or phytin. Phytic acid is a compound of inositol and phosphoric acid, and phytin is a salt of phytic acid.

Functions of Phorphorus

The important functions are as follows:

1. Phosphorus is necessary for the formation of bone and teeth.
2. It is necessary for the formation of phospholipids—lecithin and cephalin, which are the integral parts of cell structure and also intermediates transport and metabolism.
3. It is a constituent of certain coenzymes, e.g. coenzyme I, and cocarboxylase, which take part in the enzyme systems concerned in the oxidation of carbohydrates, fats and proteins.
4. It is an essential constituent of nucleic acid and nucleoproteins, which are integral parts of the cells.

Phosphorus Metabolism

Phosphorus is absorbed in the small intestine as inorganic phosphates. Phosphorus present in organic combination, e.g. phytic acid should be hydrolyzed to inorganic phosphate before absorption, since the enzyme phytase is not present in human digestive juices. Phytin phosphorus is absorbed only to a very slight extent in human beings. Phosphorus present in animal foods such as milk, meat and eggs is absorbed to a greater extent than that present in cereals and legumes, as the latter exists mostly in the form of phytic acid. The kidney is the major pathway of excretion of the phosphorus absorbed. The retention of phosphorus in children on different diets has been reported to vary from 10 to 40%. The retention of phosphorus will depend on the following factors:

1. Quantity of phosphorus ingested.
2. Calcium content of the diet.
3. Form in which phosphorus exists in the diet.
4. Vitamin D intake.

Phosphorus Content of Blood Serum

The inorganic phosphorus content of blood serum in normal human adults ranges from 2.5 to 4.0 mg/100 mL and in children from 4.0 to

5.0/100 mL. In rickets, the level of phosphorus is reduced to less than 3 mg/100 mL.

Phosphorus Requirements

Phosphorus requirements depend on the availability of phosphorus present in diets. Phosphorus present in cereals and legumes are available to a lesser extent (as it is present in the form of phytic acid) than that present in milk, meat, eggs and fish. In view of this, phosphorous requirements of persons consuming predominantly cereal-based diets, will be greater than those consuming large quantities of milk, meat, eggs and fish. The optimal calcium:phosphorus ratio for infants and children is 1:1 and for adults 1:2.

Sodium

The adult human body contains about 100 g of sodium iron. It is distributed entirely in the extracellular fluid (plasma, tissue fluid and lymph) of the body. On an average, 5–10 g sodium chloride is ingested per day in an average diet.

Function of Sodium Ion

Sodium (Na) ion exists in the body in association with the following anions, i.e. chloride bicarbonate, phosphate, lactate and proteinate. The functions of sodium ion are:

1. Regulation of acid-base balance of the body.
2. Regulation of the osmotic pressure of the plasma or tissue fluids.
3. Sodium ions play a special role in originating and maintaining the heartbeat.

Excretion

On an average diet, about 3–5 g of sodium (corresponding to 8–12 g NaCl) is excreted in urine. On a low-salt diet and in starvation, urinary excretion may fall to very low levels.

Low-sodium Diets

Low-sodium diets are prescribed for patients suffering from high blood pressure. Depletion of sodium causes muscle cramps.

Sodium Chloride

All minerals except sodium chloride (NaCl) are usually present in sufficient amounts in a well-balanced diet. Sodium chloride is the only mineral, which is taken in more or less pure form in addition to the amount present in natural foods.

Sodium Chloride Intake and Excretion

A healthy adult excretes daily about 10–15 g sodium chloride in urine. All this is derived from the salt taken in food. Sodium chloride is also excreted in sweat. During excessive sweating in hot climates, while doing hard work, the loss of sodium chloride in sweat may vary from 10 to 20 g daily. During fasting or on salt-free diets, the excretion of chlorides in urine may be decreased and only a trace of sodium chloride may be found. Absence of sodium chloride in urine is an indication for adding more sodium chloride to the diet. Sodium chloride is stored in the subcutaneous tissue. During sodium chloride deprivation, the stored form is used up (Table 19.3).

Table 19.3: Sodium chloride (NaCl) requirements (g/day) for tropical countries

Age groups	NaCl (g)
Adults	
Light work	10–15
Hard work	15–20
Very hard work	25–30
Children	
Adolescent boys and girls	10–25
Women	
Pregnancy First half Second half	 10 5
Lactation	15

Heat Cramps due to Sodium Chloride Deficiency

Men doing hard work in not humid climates, e.g. as in mines, suffer from heat cramps, i.e. intense and painful contractions of skeletal muscle. This is due to sodium chloride deficiency caused by loss of sodium chloride from the body by excessive sweating. The loss may be about 2–5 g of sodium chloride per hour of very hard work or 10–20 g sodium chloride per day. Heat cramps may be prevented by taking 10–20 g/day by adding NaCl (0.3–0.5%) to drinking water. Drinking pure water without replacing the salt loss, aggravates the deficiency.

Excessive Intake of Sodium Chloride

Consumption of excessive amounts of sodium chloride causes edema in protein deficiency and increases blood pressure in hypertension patients.

Sodium Chloride Equirements

Sodium chloride requirements depend on the climate and occupation. Foods of animal origin contain more sodium chloride than those of vegetable origin.

Potassium

The adult human body contains about 250 g of potassium, which is present almost entirely in the cells of different tissues, muscle, etc. Only small quantities are present in extracellular fluid. While plasma contains only traces of potassium, the red blood cells (RBCs) contain large amounts of potassium ion (Table 19.4). Potassium is the major

Table 19.4: Potassium content of foods

Foods	Potassium (per 100 g/mg)
Rice sources	
Pulses	
Peas	980
Black gram dal	643
Green gram dal	643
Green gram (with huge)	583
Black gram	523
Red gram dal	482
Cereals	
Bajra	402
Cholam or kaffir corn	321
Maize or corn	290
Wheat	349
Leafy vegetables	
Spinach	570
Coriander leaves	453
Lettuce	329
Roots tubers	
Carrot	482
Colocasia	464
Beetroot	300

basic ion of the body cells and separately serves in cells the same functions as sodium in the extracellular fluids. Potassium occurs in abundance in foods and so potassium deficiency seldom occurs in normal human beings.

Functions of Potassium

The important functions of potassium are:

1. Regulation of pH of cell contents.
2. Regulation of the osmotic pressure of cell contents.
3. Potassium ion increases the relaxation of heart muscle, which is antagonized by calcium (Ca) ion.

Potassium Deficiency and Excess

Potassium deficiency causes weakness and muscular paralysis. In animals, hypertrophy of the heart has been observed. Consumption of excessive amounts of potassium causes muscular weakness and apathy—symptoms similar to those of potassium deficiency.

Magnesium

The adult human body contains about 25 g of magnesium. About half of this quantity is present in the bones in combination with phosphate and carbonate, and about one fifth of the total magnesium in the body is present in the soft tissues.

Functions of Magnesium

1. Magnesium is found in certain enzymes, e.g. cocarboxylase, which decarboxylates pyruvic acid.
2. It acts as an activator of several enzymes, e.g. alkaline phosphatase, all phosphorylating enzymes.
3. It is required as a cofactor for oxidative phosphorylation.

Magnesium Metabolism

The average intake from the diet by adults is about 300–400 mg. A greater part of this (40–50%) is not absorbed and hence excreted in the stools. About one third of the amount ingested is excreted in urine. The magnesium content of normal human serum is about 2–3 mg/100 mL and of whole blood is 1.56 mg/100 mL.

Effects of Magnesium Deficiency

The principal clinical features are depression, muscular weakness, vertigo and liability to convulsions. All these clinical symptoms were occurred when the magnesium level was below 1 mg/100 mL. All the clinical symptoms were cured by the parenteral and administration of magnesium salts (100 mg magnesium chloride) within 4 hours.

Magnesium deficiency has also been observed in chronic alcoholics as indicated by low-serum magnesium and muscular weakness. In children, it is possible that magnesium deficiency exists in cases of kwashiorkor, as the serum magnesium (Mg) level has been reported to be low. Magnesium deficiency may contribute to some extent to apathy and weakness in kwashiorkor.

Magnesium Requirements

Magnesium requirements for different age groups are given below:

- **Adults:** 200–300 mg/day
- **Older children:** 150–200 mg/day
- **Infants and preschool children:** 100–150 mg/day.

TRACE ELEMENTS

- Iron
- Iodine
- Zinc
- Copper
- Cobalt
- Chromium
- Manganese
- Molybdenum
- Selenium
- Nickel
- Tin
- Fluorine
- Silicon
- Vanadium.

Iron

Iron is of great importance in human nutrition. The adult human body contains about 4–5 g of iron of which about 60–70% is present in the blood [hemoglobin (Hb) iron] as circulating iron and the rest (1–15 g) as storage iron. Each gram of hemoglobin contains about 3.34 mg of iron.

Functions of Iron

Iron is necessary for the:

- Formation of hemoglobin
- Brain development and function
- Regulation of body temperature
- Muscle activity and catecholamine metabolism
- A lack of iron directly affects the immune system; it diminishes the number of T cells and the production of antibodies
- Iron is a component of myoglobin, cytochromes, catalase and certain enzyme systems
- Iron is essential for binding oxygen to the blood cells. The central function of iron is 'oxygen transport' and cell respiration.

Sources of Iron

There are two forms of iron:

- Heme iron
- Non-heme iron.

Heme iron is better absorbed than non-heme iron. They are not only important sources of readily available iron but they also promote the absorption of kidney, non-heme iron in plant foods eaten at the same time.

Foods rich in heme iron are liver, meat, egg yolk and poultry. Iron content milk is low. Foods containing non-heme iron are those of vegetable origin, e.g. cereals, i.e. ragi, green leafy vegetables, oilseeds, e.g. gingelly seed, jaggery and dried fruits. They are important sources of iron in the diets of a large majority of Indian people.

The bioavailability of non-heme iron is poor owing to the presence of phytates, oxalates, carbonates, phosphates and dietary fiber, which interfere with iron absorption. Other foods, which inhibit iron absorption are milk, eggs and tea. The Indian diet, which is predominantly vegetarian, contains large amounts of these inhibitors, e.g. phytates in brain, phosphates in egg yolk, tannin in tea and oxalates in vegetables.

Effects of Iron Deficiency

The end result of iron deficiency is nutritional anemia, which is not a disease entity. It is rather a syndrome caused by malnutrition. Besides anemia, there may be other functional disturbances such as impaired cell-mediated immunity, reduced resistance to infection, increased morbidity and mortality and diminished work performance.

Diagnosis of Anemia

A WHO Expert Group proposed that 'anemia or deficiency should be considered to exist' when hemoglobin is below the following levels as detailed in Table 19.5.

Table 19.5: Cutoff points for the diagnosis of anemia

Age groups	Venous blood (g/dL)	MCHC* (%)
Adult males	13	34
Adult females (nonpregnant)	12	34
Adult females (pregnant)	11	34
Children (6 month to 6 year)	11	34
Children (6–14 year)	12	34

*MCHC, mean corpuscular hemoglobin concentration

At all ages, the normal mean corpuscular hemoglobin concentration (MCHC) should be 34; values below that indicate that red cells are hypochromic, which occurs in iron deficiency anemia. A hemoglobin level of 10–11 g/dL has been defined as early anemia, a level below 10 g/dL as marked anemia.

Classification of Iron Deficiency

Three stages of iron deficiency have been described:

1. **First stage:** Characterized by decreased storage of iron without any other detectable abnormalities.
2. **An intermediate stage or latent iron deficiency:** Here, iron storages are exhausted, but anemia has not occurred as yet.
3. **Third stage or overt iron deficiency:** When there is a decrease in the concentration of circulating hemoglobin due to impaired hemoglobin synthesis.

Absorption of Iron

Iron is mostly absorbed from duodenum and upper small intestine in the ferrous state, according to body needs. The rate of iron absorption is influenced by so many factors such as iron reserves of the subjects, the presence of inhibitors, for exampe, phosphates and promoters, e.g. ascorbic acid-rich food of iron absorption, and disorders of duodenum and jejunum, e.g. celiac disease, tropical sprue. Iron absorption is greater when there is an increased demand for iron. Iron absorption from habitual Indian diet is less than 5%, the bioavailability being poor.

Storage of Iron

The absorbed iron is transported as plasma ferritin and stored in liver, spleen, bone marrow and kidney. The characteristic feature of iron metabolism is conservation. When red cells are broken down, the liberated iron is reutilized in the formation of new red cells.

Iron Requirement

Because of recycling of iron, only a small amount of iron is needed by the body. In general, iron requirements are greater when there is rapid expansion of tissue and red cell masses, e.g. during pregnancy, childhood and adolescence (Table 19.6).

Table 19.6: Recommended daily intake of iron

Age group	Iron (mg)
Infants and children (year)	
0.0–1.0	1.0/kg
1–7	20–25
Adolescents (year)	
10–15	20–25
16–18	35
Adults	
Male	24
Female	32
Pregnancy	40
Lactation	32

Metabolism of Iron (Fig. 19.1)

The metabolism of iron is closely linked with the life cycle of RBCs in the body and with the condition of anemia. Anemia may be caused in various ways, but in nutrition, it is the dietary causes, which are of particular importance. The following should be noted:

1. Iron is a necessary constituent of hemoglobin. Deficiency of iron in the diet or failure of absorption in the small intestine may lead to anemia.
2. Protein is combined with iron to form hemoglobin and is also necessary for the formation of the actual RBCs, which are to contain the hemoglobin.

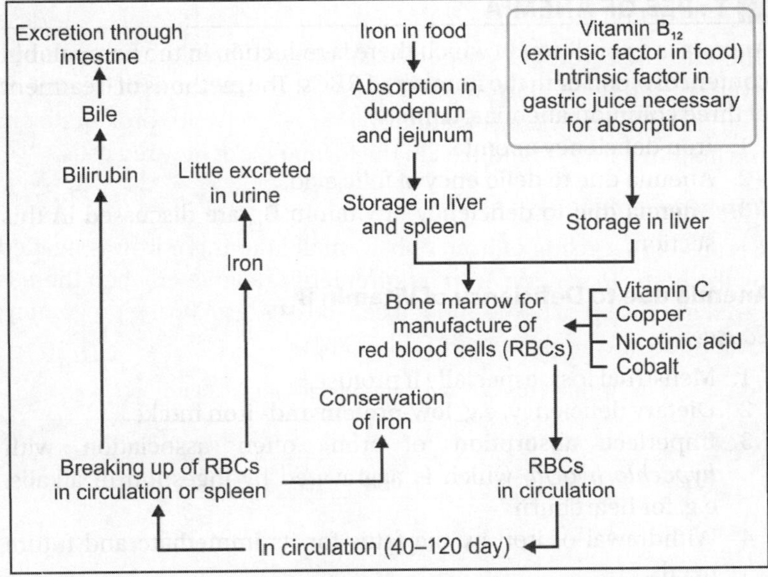

Figure 19.1: Diagram illustrating the metabolism of iron

3. 'Vitamin B_{12}' (the antianemic factor) is necessary for the development of the RBCs. It is present in foods mainly of animal origin and requires a substance present in the normal gastric juice, the intrinsic factor, for its absorption. 'Folic acid' has an action similar to vitamin B_{12}.
4. It has been claimed that other vitamins of B group and ascorbic acid also have an effect on development of the RBCs. Copper is believed to be a catalyst in the formation of hemoglobin. There is only a very small amount of copper in the human body and in a diet, which is adequate in all other nutrients there is not likely to be a deficiency of copper.

The life of the RBCs has been estimated to be between 40 and 120 days. The cells are then broken down and the hemoglobin is split into bilirubin and iron compounded. The bilirubin is carried to the liver and excreted in the bile, while the iron compounds are stored in the liver or spleens for future use. This is known as conservation of iron in the body.

TYPES OF ANEMIA

Anemia is a condition in which there is reduction in the hemoglobin content of blood or in the number of RBCs. The methods of treatment of three common anemias, namely:

1. Iron deficiency anemia.
2. Anemia due to deficiency of folic acid.
3. Anemia due to deficiency of vitamin B_{12} are discussed in this section.

Anemia due to Deficiency of Vitamin B_{12}

Causes

1. Menstrual loss, especially if profuse.
2. Dietary deficiency, e.g. low-protein and- iron intake.
3. Imperfect absorption of iron, often association with *hypochlorhydria,* which is aggravated by ingestion of alkalis, e.g. for heart burn.
4. Withdrawal of iron by the fetus for its immediate and future needs.
5. Loss of blood during third stage of labor.
6. Intestinal worm infestation.

Signs and Symptoms of Anemia

1. Pallor of mucous membranes.
2. Lassitude (always tired).
3. Breathlessness.
4. Palpitation and rapid pulse in some cases.
5. Poor appetite, gastrointestinal upsets.

Treatment

Mild cases of anemia respond well to the oral administration of medicinal iron, but digestive disturbances and constipation may occur. All iron tablets should be taken after meals with a little water. A diet rich in first class proteins, vitamins C and B_{12}, iron and other minerals should also be taken apart. The need for fresh air and sunshine ought to be stressed.

Iron Deficiency or Microcytic Anemia

Iron is essential for the formation of hemoglobin. Hence in iron deficiency anemia, there is a marked reduction in the hemoglobin content (6–8%) depending on the severity of anemia. It occurs very frequently among the pregnant women, the incidence being as high as 60%.

Causes

The important causes of iron deficiency anemia are:

1. Inadequate iron intake.
2. Poor absorption of dietary iron due to presence of excess of phytates, phosphates and oxalates.
3. Decreased absorption due to hypoacidity in the stomach.
4. Increased requirements, e.g. pregnancy, childhood and adolescence.
5. Increased blood loss due to physiological or pathological causes, excess blood loss in menstruation, hookworm infestation, etc.
6. Poor absorption due to defect in intestinal mucosa, e.g. malabsorption syndrome.

Signs and Symptoms

Woman

The clinical features of anemia include diminished oxygen supplies to tissues as a result of low-hemoglobin content of blood. The clinical features commonly observed are general fatigue, breathlessness on exertion, giddiness and pallor of the skin. In severe cases, edema of ankles may be present.

Weaned infant and young children

Iron deficiency anemia occurs commonly among weaned infants and young children. The hemoglobin levels are low (5–8%). The children are weak, inactive and show pallor of the skin.

Treatment

The diet should be well balanced and provide adequate amounts of all dietary essentials including iron. The composition of balanced diets suitable for different age groups is given in chapter on 'Diet in Anemia'.In the case of adults and adolescents, ferrous sulfate tablets (0.2 g providing 60 mg iron) should be given four times a day. In the case of older children, ferrous sulfate tablets should be given twice daily. In the case of weaned infants, a sweetened syrup containing 0.2 g ferrous ammonium citrate (providing 20 mg iron) should be given thrice daily. The treatment should be continued for a month or longer till the anemia is cured.

Megaloblastic Anemia due to Folic Acid Deficiency

Megaloblastic anemia due to folic acid deficiency occurs commonly among pregnant woman and to a lesser extent in preschool children.

Blood Picture

The RBC count is low; 2–3 millions/mm and hemoglobin is 6–9%. The diameter of the RBC is greater than normal hence the anemia is greater than normal and hence the anemia is called macrocytic anemia. Examination of the bone marrow aspirates reveals the presence of characteristic megaloblasts, indicating that maturation of the RBC is affected in folic acid deficiency.

Clinical Signs

The clinical signs are similar to those observed in iron deficiency anemia.

Treatment

The subjects should receive a well-balanced diet providing all dietary essentials. Diets for different age groups are given in chapter on 'Diet in Anemia'. In addition, the subjects should be given folic acid.

Preschool children

Folic acid (1–2 mg) orally daily, ferrous ammonium sulfate mixture to provide 6 mg iron per kg body weight daily should be given for a period of 1 month or longer till the anemia is cured.

Adults

Folic acid 5 mg once daily and ferrous sulfate tablets (0.2 g) thrice daily for 10 days; and folic acid 2 mg once daily and ferrous sulfate (0.2 g) twice daily from 11th to 40th day should be administered.

Pernicious Anemia due to Vitamin B_{12} Deficiency

Pernicious anemia is caused by the lack of intrinsic factor in the stomach with consequent failure in the absorption of vitamin B_{12} in the intestines.

Blood Picture

The RBC count is low (1.5–2.5 million/mm) compared with normal count of 4.5–5.5 millions. The average diameter of the RBC is greater than normal. The anemia is macrocytic. There is evidence that the abnormal circulating RBC are undergoing excessive destruction with consequent increase in serum bilirubin content. The hemoglobin content is also low (7–9%).

Effects of Deficiency on Body Parts/Organs

Bone marrow

The megaloblasts in bone marrow aspirate are high. If the successive stage of the maturation of RBC are called stages I, II and IV, then in pernicious anemia I and IV, it is 30%; while in normal persons, it is reverse.

Stomach

The cells, which secret acid and enzymes are atrophied; the gastric secretions are devoid of acid, pepsin and intrinsic factor (IF).

Mouth

Soreness and inflammation of the tongue are commonly observed.

Nervous system

In about 80% of the cases, paresthesia (numbness and tingling) occurs in fingers and toes. There is also evidence of the involvement of spinal cord. In advanced cases, demyelination of the white fibers of the spinal cord occurs, affecting the dorsal column and later, the lateral column (subacute combined degeneration of the cord).

Treatment

The subject should receive a well-balanced diet providing all dietary essentials. Diets for different age groups are given in Chapter 30 on 'Calculation of Balanced Diets for Different Categories'. In addition, the subjects should be given vitamin B_{12}. This vitamin (1,000 μg) should be administered by injection twice a week for 2 weeks and then once a week till the anemia is cured. Ferrous sulfate (0.2 g) three times daily and folic acid (5 mg) once a week orally should be administered till the anemia is cured. After the anemia is cured, the subject should receive 1,000 μg of vitamin B_{12} by injection once in 2 months to prevent recurrence of the disease.

Anemia Prevention and Control

The following plan will provide the essential nutrients necessary for blood building:

1. Include daily one serving of dried fruits such as raisins, dates, pistachio, etc.
2. Use cereals, which are whole grain and not finely milled.
3. Include weekly 1–2 servings liver, kidney and two or more servings of pulses such as dal.
4. Use plenty of jaggery and green leafy vegetables daily.
5. Provide high-protein diet, including milk, eggs, meat and fish.

Iodine

Iodine is a constituent of thyroxine, the active principle of the thyroid gland. The thyroid gland, weighing about 25 g in a normal adult, contains only about 10 mg of iodine. The adult body as a whole contains about 50 mg of iodine. The thyroid gland plays an important part in energy metabolism and in the growth of the body.

Food Sources of Iodine

The best sources of iodine are sea foods, e.g. sea fish, sea salt and cod liver oil. The iodine content of fresh water is small and vary/variable about 1–50 μg/L. Small amounts occurs in other foods such as milk, meat, vegetables, cereals, etc. About 90% of iodine comes from foods eaten; the remaining from drinking water. The iodine content of the soil is determined by its presence in both water and locally grown foods. The deficiency is geochemical in nature.

Goitrogens

Goitrogens are chemical substances leading to the development of goiter. They interfere with iodine utilization by the thyroid gland. They may occur in food and water. The brassic a group of vegetables, e.g. cabbage, cauliflower and radish contain substances known as goitrogens. Consumption of large quantities of these foods leads to the development of goiter by making the iodine present in the food not available to the body.

Iodine Deficiency in Human Beings (Table 19.7)

If sufficient iodine is not taken in the diet, enlargement of the thyroid takes place, resulting in the disease called *goiter*. The thyroid gland of the adult, which normally weighs about 25 mg, may weigh as much as 200–500 g or even more in goiter.

Histological examination shows diffuse overgrowth of the glandular tissue known as general hyperplasia of the glands. The vehicles contain little or no colloid. If treatment with iodine is started very early, the thyroid may become normal. But if treatment is delayed, the enlargement of the gland persists. In children, severe iodine deficiency may result in serious retardation of growth. This condition is known as *cretinism*. Other severe forms of iodine deficiency include:

1. Hypothyroidism.
2. Retarded physical development and impaired mental function.

Table 19.7: Spectrum of iodine deficiency disorders in approximate order of increasing severity

Disorders	Levels of severity
Goiter	Grade I Grade II Grade III Multinodular
Hypothyroidism	
Subnormal intelligence, delayed motor milestones Mental deficiency Hearing defects Speech defects	Variable severity
Strabismus (squint)	
Nystagmus	Unilateral
Spasticity (extrapyramidal)	Bilateral
Neuromuscular weakness	
Muscle weakness in legs, arms, trunk Spastic diplegia Spastic quadriplegia	
Endemic cretinism	
Hypothyroid cretinism Neurological cretinism	
Intrauterine death	
Spontaneous abortion Miscarriage	

3. Increased rate of spontaneous abortion and stillbirth.
4. *Neurological cretinism* including deaf and mutism.
5. Myxedematous cretinism, including dwarfism and severe mental retardation.

To refer to all effects of iodine deficiency on human growth and development, the term iodine deficiency disorders (IDD) is now replaced. The IDD can be prevented by correction of iodine deficiency.

Iodine Requirement (Table 19.8)

The daily requirement of iodine for adults is placed at 150 μg or 0.15–0.2 mg, and for infant and children 0.05–0.10 mg/day.

Table 19.8: Recommended daily dietary intake of iodine

Stage	Iodine (μg)
Infants and children (year)	
0.0–1.0	40–50
1–3	70
4–6	90
7–9	120
Adolescents	
10–18 year	140
Adults	150
Males/Females	150
Pregnancy	150 + 25
Lactation	150 + 25

The amount is normally supplied by well-balanced diets and drinking water, except in regions where food and water are deficient in iodine.

Fluorine

Fluorine is the lightest member and one of the most active elements of the halogen group. It is never found free in the nature. About 96% of the fluoride in the body is found in the bones and teeth. Fluorine is essential for the normal mineralization of bones and formation of dental enamel.

Sources

1. **Drinking water:** The main source of fluoride to man is drinking water. The fluoride content of drinking water in this country is about 0.5 mg/L, but in fluorosis-endemic areas, the natural waters have been found to contain as much as 3-12 mg of fluorides per liter.
2. **Foods:** Fluorides occur in traces in many foods, but some foods such as sea fish, cheese and tea are rich in fluorine. The average adult man ingest about 1 mg of fluoride daily from drinking water. In addition to this, the daily diet may provide 0.25–0.35 mg of fluorine.

Requirements

Since drinking water is the main source of fluorine to man, a concentration of 0.5–0.8 mg/L in water is considered a safe limit in this country. In temperate climates where the intake of water is low, the optimum level of fluorine in drinking water is accepted as 1 mg/L.

Fluorine in Human Health

Fluorine is often called two-edged sword. Ingestion of large amounts is associated with dental and skeletal fluorosis, and inadequate amounts with dental caries.

Dental Fluorosis

In young children, the disease affects only the teeth. This is known as 'dental fluorosis.' The teeth lose their shiny appearance and chalky white patches develop on them. This is known as 'mottled enamel' and is an early sign of dental fluorosis. The white patches later become yellow and sometimes brown or black. In severe cases, loss of enamel is accompanied by 'pitting,' which gives the tooth a corroded appearance. Mottling is best seen on the incisors of the upper jaw. It is almost entirely confirmed to the permanent teeth and develops only during their period of formation.

Skeletal Fluorosis

In older people, the disease affects the bones, tendons and ligaments. This is known as 'skeletal fluorosis.' This is followed by pain and stiffness of the back, and later of joints of both limbs and limitation of neck movements. Early detection of the disease many escape till radiological help is sought. Radiological changes are quite characteristic—there is formation of new bone (exostosis), and calcification of tendons and ligaments as well as interosseous membranes. Skeletal fluorosis has been reported to be a public health problem of considerable magnitude in several districts of Andhra Pradesh, Haryana, Karnataka, Kerala, Punjab, Rajasthan and Tamil Nadu.

Dental Caries

Fluoride levels below 0.5 mg/L are usually associated with a high prevalence of dental caries.

Prevention and Control

It is of utmost importance to prevent the development of fluorosis as there is no specific treatment. The normal content of fluoride in water should be below 1 mg/L. Drinking water with safe levels of fluoride should be supplied to the community. The National Environmental Engineering Research Institute, Nagpur has developed a simple technique known as 'Nalgonda Technique' for defluoridation of water. It involves addition of two readily available chemicals, viz. lime and alum in sequence followed by flocculation.

Sedimentation and filtration

Lime powder is added first (30 mg/L) and mixed well with water. Generally the lime dose is 1/20th the alum dose. Alum (500 mg/L) is then added and the water is stirred for 10 minutes. The contents are allowed to settle for 1 hour. The settled water will contain fluorides within permissible limits. This technique is suitable both for domestic and community water treatment. Dental caries may be prevented by fluoridation of community water supplies where the fluorine intake from water and other sources for the given population is below optimum levels.

Zinc

Zinc is present in small amounts in all tissues, and is a constituent of insulin and of many enzymes in the body. Zinc-plasma level is about 96 μg/100 mL for healthy adults, and 89 μg/100 mL for healthy children. The average adult body contains 1.4–2.3 g of zinc.

Functions of Zinc

Zinc is required for the synthesis of insulin by the pancreas and for the immunity function. It is active in the metabolism of glucosides and proteins.

Effects of Zinc Deficiency

Zinc deficiency leads to retarded growth, sexual infantilism, multiple infections, disorders in taste and skin disorders:

- Skin disorders—scaling and cracking of the paws
- Alopecia (loss of hair)—accompanied by gross epithelial, especially cutaneous lesions
- Retardation or growth failure
- Degenerative changes in the female and male reproductive organs
- Anemia.

Sources

Zinc is widely distributed in foodstuffs, both vegetable and animal origin. But the bioavailability of zinc vegetable foods is low. Animal foods such as meat, milk and fish are dependable sources.

Requirements

Suggested daily intake are as follows:

- **Infants:** 3.5 mg
- **Children:**10–15 mg
- **Adult:** 15 mg
- **Pregnancy and lactation:** 20–25 mg.

Most human diets provide these amounts.

Copper

Copper is essential, as it is incorporated in several enzymes. The amount of copper in an adult body is estimated to be between 100 and 150 mg.

Sources

Copper is widely distributed in nature; even poor diets provide enough copper.

Human needs: Red gram dal contains 1.25 mg/100 g, about 1.13 mg, horse gram 1.03 mg. Either deficiency or excess of these elements is very rare.

Hypercupremia may reflect excessive intake, which may result from eating food prepared in copper cooking vessels. Or it may to associated with several acute and chronic infections (leukemia, Hodgkin's disease, severe anemia hemochromatosis, myocardial infarction and hyperthyroidism). Hypercupremia occurs in patients with nephrosis, Wilson's disease and protein-energy malnutrition (PEM), and in infants fed for long period exclusively on cow's milk. Neutropenia is the best-documented abnormality of copper deficiency.

Requirements

The copper requirements are given below:

- **Adults:** 2 mg/day/caput
- **Pregnancy:** 3 mg/day/caput
- **Lactation:** 3 mg/day/caput
- **Infants (1–12 month):** 0.5–1.0 mg/day/caput

- **Children:** 2 mg/day/caput
- **Adolescents:** 3 mg/day/caput.

Manganese

The body of a normal man weighing 70 kg contains about 12–20 mg manganese. It is distributed throughout the body tissues and fluids. The following tissues, viz. bone, kidney, liver, pancreas and pituitary contain more manganese than other tissues. The manganese content of human blood is very low (2–3 μg/100 mL).

Manganese Metabolism

Only 3–4% of the manganese present in the diet is absorbed, the remaining being excreted in the feces. The urine contains only traces of manganese.

Deficiency of Manganese

Manganese deficiency in animals: The most important deficiency effects observed are impaired growth, skeletal abnormalities, depressed reproductive function and ataxia of the newborn.

Manganese toxicity in human beings: Toxic symptoms have been reported to occur in mine workers due to inhalation of dust from manganese ores. The signs and symptoms are:

- Blurred speech
- Tremors of the hands
- Spastic gait.

Cobalt

Cobalt occurs in small amounts in all tissues, highest concentration occurring in liver and kidneys. Most of the cobalt is present in vitamin B_{12}.

Cobalt Metabolism

Cobalt present in the diet is absorbed to the extent of 70–80% and about half the absorbed cobalt is excreted in the urine. The excretion in the feces is 20–30% of the intake.

Cobalt Functions

Cobalt may be necessary for the first stage of hormone production and capture of iodine by the gland.

Effects of Cobalt Deficiency

Cobalt deficiency and cobalt iodine ratio in the soil have shown to produce goiter in humans. Cobalt may interact with iodine and affect its utilization. Human beings require a dietary source of vitamin B_{12} and cannot synthesize it in the body.

Cobalt Requirements

Cobalt requirements appear to be met by traces of cobalt found in foods.

Cobalt Toxicity

Cobalt administered in excess causes a condition known as polycythemia, i.e. increased number of RBCs in blood.

Chromium

Chromium occurs in traces in human and animal tissues. Total body content of chromium is small, i.e. 6 mg.

Functions

Current interest in chromium is based on the occurrence of unusual glucose tolerance curves that are responsive to chromium. Thus there is suggestive evidence that chromium plays a role in relation to carbohydrate and insulin function.

Effects of Deficiency of Chromium

Chromium deficiency is characterized by impaired growth and disturbances in glucose, lipid and protein metabolism.

Requirements

The exact requirements are not known; average diets appear to meet the chromium requirements.

Selenium

Until recently, little attention had been given to Selenium in human nutrition. The first report that Selenium deficiency may occur in man appeared in 1961 and a similar report in 1967. Selenium administration to children with kwashiorkor resulted in significant weight increase. Studies indicate that human selenium deficiency may occur in PEM.

Molybdenum

Excess absorption of molybdenum has shown to produce bony deformities. On the other hand, deficiency of molybdenum is associated with mouth and esophageal cancer.

Nutritional Requirements of Special Groups

Pregnancy

1. **Energy intake:** For a reference, Indian woman whose body weight is 45 kg, the total energy cost of pregnancy is estimated to be 62,500 kcal. Since pregnant women do not appear to increase their food intake materially during the first trimester, nutrition experts in India have recommended an additional intake of 300 kcal/day during the second and third trimesters.
2. **Proteins:** About 900 g of proteins are deposited in the fetus and material tissues during pregnancy. The ICMR Expert Committee on Nutrition in 1981 recommended an additional allowance of 14 g/day of dietary protein during the second and third trimesters.
3. **Other nutrients:** There must be a regular and adequate intake of all other nutrients drawn from a wide variety of foods. Special mention must be made of iron and folic acid intake. Balanced diets suitable for women during pregnancy are given in Chapter 30, 'Calculation of Balanced Diet for Different Categories'.

Lactation

1. **Energy intake:** Estimation of additional energy needs during lactation are based on a milk output of 850 mg, and 80% efficiency of conversion of dietary energy into milk energy. On this basis, the additional energy allowance of 550 kcal/day for the first 6 months of lactation has been recommended. Since Indian women continue to lactate beyond 6 months, although with reduced milk output, an extra allowance of 400 kcal/day has been recommended for a period of 6 months to 1 year of lactation.
2. **Proteins:** The ICMR Expert Committee in 1981 recommended an additional allowance of 25 g/day during the period of lactation.
3. **Other nutrients:** A regular and adequate intake of all other nutrients, though balanced diets should be ensured, special

mention must be made of the enhanced requirements of vitamin C (80 mg/day) during lactation.

Infants

Mother's milk is the ideal food for infants. About 850 mg of breast milk would be needed up to 3 moths of age, and 1,200 mL between 3 and 6 months of age. The average breast milk output of Indian women belonging to poor income groups are much lower than these. The protein and calorie requirements of infants are given in Chapter 30.

Weaning

Weaning is not sudden withdrawal of child from the breast. It is a gradual process starting around the age of 5–6 months, when the child is introduced to 'supplementary foods'. These are usually cow's milk, soft cooked rice, mashed potatoes, soft cooked vegetables; because usually after about 6 months of age, mother's milk is no longer sufficient to sustain growth. Supplementation with cereals, pulses, milk and eggs is essential. If this is delayed or not done, children do not grow properly and PEM develops.

At the age of 1 year, the child should receive solid foods consisting of cereals, pulses, vegetables and fruits. The best indicator of infant nutrition is its body weight. An average Indian baby weighs 2.8 kg at birth. The infant nearly doubles its birth weight at the end of 4 months and is three times the birth weight by the end of 1st year.

Preschool Children

Children in the age group of 1–5 years need special attention. They grow rapidly physically and mentally. The energy requirements of a child aged 1 year is about 1,000 kcal daily. After the age of 1 year, the energy needs can be computed by adding 100 kcal for every year of life. Thus a child aged 5 years needs 1,500 kcal daily.

The protein requirements can be calculated either according to body weight or as a percentage of the energy need. If weight is taken into consideration, the expected weight for that age should be used, and not the actual weight, which may or may not be the expected weight. Alternatively, 8–10% of the energy needs may be given as proteins. This is adequate for children of all ages.

Mid-day School Meal

School feeding programs have been in operation in a number of countries for over 100 years. In India, a free school service was introduced in Madras City as early as 1925. School feeding is an integral part of the education system in many countries. For more details on mid-day meal program, refer Chapter 43, 'National Programs Related to Nutrition'.

Chapter 20

Energy

Energy is a prime requisite for body function and growth. When a child's intake of food falls below a standard reference, growth slows and low levels of intake persist, adult stature will be reduced. If adults fail to meet their food requirements, they lose weight. This may lead to reduced ability to work, resist infection and fail to enjoy the normal satisfactory life.

DIETARY SOURCES

The dietary sources of energy are protein, fat and carbohydrate. They supply energy at the following rates:

- **Protein:** 4 kcal/g (17 kJ)
- **Fat:** 9 kcal/g (37 kJ)
- **Carbohydrate:** 4 kcal/g (17 kJ).

Food Sources

- Cereals and millets
- Pulses and legumes:
  - Grams
  - Peas
  - Beans.
- Nuts and oils seeds
- Vegetables:
  - Green leafy vegetables
  - Roots and tubers.
- Other vegetables:
  - Cauliflower
  - Cabbage.
- Fruits
- Fats and oils
- Foods of animal origin (meat, fish and eggs)

- Milk and milk products
- Sugar and jaggery
- Spices and condiment
- Miscellaneous beverages.

ENERGY REQUIREMENTS

The energy requirements of an individual might be defined as that level of energy intake in relation to expenditure, which is least likely to result in obesity or heart disease, or which is most likely to prolong active life. Broadly, the total energy requirement of an individual is made up of three components:

1. Energy required for basal metabolism. This is above 1 kcal/h for every kg of body weight for an adult.
2. Energy required for daily activities such as walking, sitting, standing, dressing and undressing, climbing stairs, etc.
3. Energy expenditure for occupational work. This is further classified as light work (an office clerk), moderate work and heavy work (manual physical labor).

The first component is nearly the same for all individuals. It is the latter two components that vary depending upon the type of activities.

Factors Affecting Energy Requirement

Energy requirements vary from one person to another depending upon interrelated variables acting in a complex way such as age, sex, working condition, body composition, physical activity, physiological state, etc. (Tables 20.1 and 20.2). All these factors lead to difference in food intake.

Table 20.1: Daily intake of energy

Age	Body weight (kg)	Energy in kcal/kg/24 h (approximate)
1 year (average)	–	112
1–3 year	12.0	100
4–6 year	18.8	90
7–9 year	26.3	80
Reference man	55.0	45
Reference woman	45.0	40

Table 20.2: Recommended daily intake for energy

Group	Body weight (kg)	Energy allowance per day	
		kcal/kg/day	MJ
Infancy			
0–6 month	–	118	–
7–12 month	–	108	–
Children			
1–3 year	12.03	1,220	5.1
4–6 year	18.87	1,720	7.2
7–9 year	26.37	2,050	8.6
Adolescents			
10–12 year	34.30	2,420 (males)	10.1
		2,260 (females)	9.5
13–15 year	47.03	2,660 (males)	11.1
		2,300 (females)	9.6
16–18 year	56.50	2,820 (males)	11.7
Adults			
Males (reference)	55.00	2,400 (light work)	10.00
		2,800 (moderate work)	11.70
		3,900 (heavy work)	16.30
Females (reference)	45.00	1,900 (light work)	7.95
		2,200 (moderate work)	9.20
		3,000 (heavy work)	13.10
Pregnancy	–	+ 285 (throughout pregnancy)	+ 1.25
Lactation	–	+ 550 (first 6 month)	+ 2.3
		+ 400 (6–12 month)	+ 1.68

Energy requirements have been laid down by various expert groups of Food and Agricultural Organization (FAO) and World Health Organization (WHO). It has become customary for countries to lay down their own standards. Thus, there are British standards, American standards, Canadian standards, etc. The standards in India are those recommended by the Indian Council of Medical Research. These standards are revised from time to time in the light of newer knowledge.

Vulnerable Groups

Pregnant and Lactating Mothers

The energy requirements of women are increased by pregnancy (+ 285 kcal daily throughout pregnancy) and lactation (+ 550 kcal during first 6 months and + 440 kcal during the next 6 months) over and above their normal requirements. This is to provide for the extra energy needs associated with the deposition of tissues or the secretion of milk at rates consistent with good health.

Children

Because of their rapid growth rate, young children require proportionately more energy for each kilogram of body weight than adults. In order to provide for 'catch-up growth' during childhood, intake should be based on age rather than weight. The Indian Council of Medical Research (ICMR) standards are based on age and not on body weight (except during the 1st year of life).

Children above the age of 13 years need much energy similar to adults. This is because they show a good deal of physical activity, almost equal to hard work by adults. This is also the age when puberty sets in and there is spurt in growth, and an increase in metabolic rate. This fact should be borne in mind when planning dietaries for children.

Adults

The energy requirements decreases with age because of a fall in basal metabolic rate (BMR) and a decrease in physical activity in most persons. In general, there is a 2% decline of resting for each decade for adults. The FAO/WHO committee suggested that after the age of 40 years, requirement should be reduced by 5% each decade, until the age of 60 and 10% for each decade thereafter.

NUTRITIONAL INDIVIDUALITY

The concept of nutritional individuality needs to be stressed and its negligence may result in the overfeeding of some whose needs happen to be less than the 'average standard requirement'.

Standards of Requirements of Calories and Various Nutrients

An expert commission for the League of Nations has drawn-up the following statement about energy requirements:

1. An adult male or female living an ordinary, everyday life in a temperate climate and not engaged in manual work is taken as the basis on which the needs of the other age groups are reckoned. An allowance of 2,400 calories per day is considered adequate to meet the requirements of such an individual.
2. The following supplements for muscular activity should be added to the basic requirements given above:
   - Light work: up to 75 cal/h of work
   - Moderate work: 75–150 cal/h of work
   - Hard work: 150–300 cal/h of work
   - Very hard work: 300 cal/h of work (upwards).

   Example of different types of activities are given below:
   - Light work: Writing, typing and tailoring
   - Moderate work: Shoe making, carpentry, light engineering works and walking
   - Hard work: Cycling, heavy carpentry, light blacksmithing, stone mason's work, ploughing, sawing wood and harvesting
   - Very hard work: Coal mining, heavy blacksmithing, earth work, carrying heavy loads and wood cutting.

UNITS OF ENERGY

1. The energy value of food is expressed in terms of kilocalories (kcal). A kilocalorie is defined as the amount of heat required to raise the temperature of 1 kg of water by 1°C.
2. The kilocalorie is generally expressed as calorie written with a capital 'C' letter.
3. Calorie has been replaced by 'Joule', expressed as 'J', which has been accepted internationally. The international unit of energy is the 'Joule'.
4. However, the use of kcal to measure energy still continues. Scientists and nutritionists are concerned with large amounts of energy, so they use the units:
   - Kilocalorie (kcal)
   - Kilojoule (kJ)
   - Megajoule (MJ) to express energy.

In the metric system, the international unit, which is kilojoules, is used instead of kilocalories; kilojoule is energy expended when 1 kilogram of mass is moved by 1 meter using a force of 1 Newton.

Relationship Between Calorie and Joule

- 1 cal = 4.184 J
- 1 kcal or C = 4.184 kJ
- 1,000 kcal or C = 4.184 MJ
- 1 kJ = 0.239 kcal
- 1 MJ = 239 kcal
- 100 MJ = 23,900 kcal.

Calorie

The standard unit to measure energy is calorie. The energy needs of the body are calculated in terms of calories (sometimes) called kilocalorie or kcal or in Joule:

1. 'Calorie' is defined as the amount of heat required at 1 atmosphere pressure to raise the temperature of 1 kg of water by 1°C.
2. 'Kilocalorie' is defined as amount of heat required to raise the temperature of 1 liter of water by 1°C.
3. In the current day situation, a new unit of energy is being used, which is termed as 'Joules'.
4. Joule (J) is defined as the energy required accelerating with a force of 1 Newton (N) for a distance of 1 meter.
5. The number of calories obtained for a food is its calorific value. Every food varies in its calorific value.

ENERGY VALUES OF FOODS

Carbohydrates are the major source of energy for the body, i.e. 1 g of carbohydrates = 4 kcal (17 kJ).

Relation Between Oxygen Required and Caloric Value

It is important to know the heat produced, when 1 liter of O_2 is used for the oxidation of carbohydrates, fats and proteins. This can be calculated from the data obtained by the oxycalorimeter and bomb calorimeter as explained below:

- 1 g carbohydrate requires about 0.8 L of O_2 for complete oxidation and yields 4.1 kcal of heat
- 1 g fat requires about 1.2 L of O_2 for complete oxidation and yields 5.5 kcal of heat
- 0.8 L of O_2 oxidizes 1 g carbohydrate and produces 4 kcal of heat
- 1 L of O_2 oxidizes 1.25 g carbohydrate and produces 5 kcal of heat
- 2.2 L of O_2 oxidizes 1 g fat and produces 9.5 kcal of heat

- 1 L of O_2 oxidizes 0.49 g fat and produces 4.5 kcal of heat
- 1.2 L of O_2 oxidizes 1 g of protein and produces 5.5 kcal of heat
- 1 L of O_2 oxidizes 0.83 g of protein and produces 4.6 kcal of heat.
- 1 L of oxygen oxidizing carbohydrates, fat and protein to produces nearly the same amount of heat, i.e. 4.5–5 kcal of heat. This is an important conclusion, as this is the basis for indirect determination of energy requirements from oxygen consumed.

Douglas Bag

Energy expenditure during work can be determined by using Douglas bag. The energy metabolism is profoundly influenced by physical work. The general principles underlying this method are as follows:

- Measuring the volume of expired air during work for fixed periods of 5–10 minutes
- Collection of a sample of expired air for the analysis of O_2 and CO_2 contents
- Calculation of O_2 consumption, CO_2 output and respiratory quotient (RQ)
- Calculation of the energy output from the RQ and O_2 consumption.

Douglas bag is made of rubber and usually of 100 L capacity. The subject breaths into the bag for 5–6 minutes. The air in the bag is then measured using a gas meter and a sample is taken for the analysis of O_2 and CO_2. The apparatus is suitable for use in the laboratory, but not in the field.

BASIC METABOLISM

Metabolism is the changes, which take place in nutrients from the time of their absorption until they reach the end products of the various organs through which they pass. The expenditure or using up the energy in the body is known as energy metabolism.

Changes Involved in Metabolism

The changes included in the process of metabolism are of two distinct varieties:

1. **Building-up changes:** This are called 'anabolic changes' or the building up of the muscle from the amino acids obtained from proteins or fat from fatty acid and glycerol.
2. **Breaking-down changes:** This are called 'catabolic changes' or 'catabolism,' e.g. the breaking down of glucose or fat into carbon dioxide and water to release energy for activity.

Factors Affecting Metabolism

The 'principal factors,' which influence the rate of metabolism include body size, age, sex, climate including the degrees of heat, type of clothing and the nature of the work. The rate of metabolism will also depend on the activity of the individual:

1. It will be higher in a manual worker than in an office worker, leading a more sedentary life.
2. The state of nervous tension is a most important factor, as it will affect the rate of breathing and the rate of force of action on heart.
3. Basal metabolism is the metabolism that goes on when the body is at absolute rest.
4. When the body is at complete rest, the energy requirement is at its lowest. This is called the basal metabolic rate, which is the amount of energy required by a person who is awake, but it is as nearly as possible at complete mental and physical rest, and has had no food for 12–14 hours.

BODY MASS INDEX AND BASIC METABOLISM

Obesity is a state in which there is a generalized accumulation of excess adipose tissue in the body leading to more than 20% of the desirable weight. Overweight is a condition, where the body weight is 10–20% greater than the mean standard weight for age, height and sex. The most effective and scientific method is body mass index (BMI). Today, the weight of an individual is assessed on a more scientific basis by a method known as the BMI.

Basal Metabolic Rate

The energy metabolism of a subject at complete physical and mental rest, and having normal body temperature in the post-absorptive state (i.e. 12 hour after the intake of last meal) is known as basal metabolism. The amount of energy required by a person who is awake, but he/she is nearly as much at complete mental and physical rest as possible, and had no food for 12–14 hours is known as basal metabolic rate. It refers to the minimum amount of energy, i.e.:

1. BMR for men = 88.362 + (1.397 × Weight in kg) + (4.779 × Height in cm) – (5.677 × Age in year).
2. BMR for women = 447.593 + (9.247 × Weight in kg) + (3.098 × Height in cm) – (4.330 × Age in year).

The amount of energy required to carry on the involuntary work of the body is also known as basal metabolic rate. It includes the functional activities of various organs such as brain, heart, liver, kidney, lungs and the peristaltic movement of gastrointestinal tract, maintenance of muscle tone and body temperature. The brain and nervous tissue accounts for about one fifth of the energy utilized and the rest by the other parts of body.

Involuntary actions such as expansion and contraction of the heart, respiration and digestion; involuntary actions include energy needed for body maintenance and is known as BMR. This energy must be supplied to the body first, because energy required by the heart for its normal functioning or for the constant supply of blood to the brain are vital functions upon which survival of a living being depends. The BMR is sometimes calculated as an indication of the presence or absence of disease. Since, overactivity of the thyroid gland raises rate and underactivity lowers it.

The basal metabolic rate is calculated by measuring the amount of the heat produced in the body, either directly in a respiratory chamber or indirectly by measuring the amount of CO_2 produced calculating from the quantity of oxygen used. The test is made after resting in bed at night, at least for 12 hours after taking a meal with the individual relaxed and in a tranquil a state of mind; the indirect method is generally used, and in this the expired air is collected in a bag, over a period of time, usually and therefore the amount of heat produced in the body is calculated. The normal BMR is expressed as percentage of the normal rate; thus a BMR of + 10 means that the rate is 10% above the age, weight, height and sex; a BMR of – 10 means that it is 10% below normal. The rate is normally higher in young persons, in males and in persons with a large surface area, and therefore a greater heat loss. Metabolic rate is calculated per meter of the body surface area. The surface area is assessed from a person's height and weight; 1.8/m is an average surface area for an adult male, and 40 calories per meter per hour is an average metabolic rate.

Determination of Basal Metabolic Rate

By Benedict-Roth apparatus

The basal metabolic rate of a person is determined by using Benedict-Roth apparatus. The apparatus is a closed circuit system in which the subject breathes only through mouth (i.e. O_2 from a metal cylinder of about 6 L capacity and CO_2 produced is absorbed by lime present in the tower). The oxygen cylinder floats on water present in an outer tank. The patient wears a nose clip and he/she breathes through the mouth, the oxygen will be present in the cylinder for a period of 6 minutes. The volume of oxygen used is recorded on a graph paper attached to a revolving drum by a pen attached to it. The patient is in the postabsorptive state. The respiratory quotient is assumed to be 0.82 and the calorific value of 1 liter of oxygen consumed is taken as 4.8 kcal:

$$\text{Respiratory quotient (RQ)} = \frac{\text{Volume of } CO_2 \text{ produced}}{\text{Volume of } O_2 \text{ consumed}}$$

By calculations

Basal metabolic rate can be calculated by using the following formulae:

1. **Body weight:**
   - For female = Weight in kg × 0.9 kcal × 24 h
   - For male = Weight in kg × 1 kcal × 24 h.
2. **Harris-Benedict equation:**
   - For female = 65.5 + (9.56 × W) + (1.85 × H) – (4.68 × A)
   - For male = 65.5 + (13.75 × W) + (5.0 × H) – 6.75 × A)
   - Metabolic body size = 70 × Weight in kg × 3/4.
3. **FAO/WHO/UNO equation (Table 20.3):**
   - For female = (30–60 year) – 807 × W + 829
   - For male = (30–60 year) – 11.6 × W + 879.

Note: A is age in years, W is weight in kg and H is height in cm.

Table 20.3: FAO*/WHO†/UNO‡ equations for predicting BMR§ from body weight in kg

Age in year	BMR (kcal/ day)	
	Male	Female
0–3	60.9 × W‖ – 542	61.10 × W – 51
3–10	22.7 × W + 495	22.5 × W + 499
10–18	17.5 × W + 651	12.2 × W + 746
18–30	15.3 × W 6679	14.7 × W + 496
30–60	11.6 × 879	8.7 × W + 829
> 60	13.5 × W + 487	10.5 × W + 596

*FAQ, Food and Agricultural Organization; †WHO, World Health Organization; ‡UNO, United Nations Organization; §BMR, basal metabolic rate; ‖W, weight.

Factors Affecting BMR

Several factors influence the BMR as following:

1. **Surface area of the body:** The larger the surface area of body in relation to bulk, the greater is the heat lost by radiation, e.g. a tall man will have a greater surface area of the body than a short fat man, and will lose more heat by radiation and his BMR will be higher. This may explain at least in part that why a thin man eats more than a fat man of the same weight.
2. **Sex:** Women have lower BMR than men, since a woman's body contains more fat, which is a less active metabolic tissue than muscle or lean body mass, which is found in a larger amount in man. The BMR is 10% higher in males as compared to females. A lean man has a higher BMR than a man who is fatter and has a greater percentage of less active adipose tissue, i.e.:
   - 40 calories per square meter per hour for man
   - 37 calories per square meter per hour for woman.
3. **Diseases:** Some diseases, especially of the thyroid gland, may raise or lower the BMRs. A rase in body temperature of one degree (Fahrenheit) is sound to increase BMR by about 7% . This is important to remember during fever.
4. **Malnutrition:** Under prolonged or chronic undernutrition, the BMR is decreased.
5. **Psychological tension:** This type of tension caused by worry or stress will increase the BMR.
6. **Age:** The BMR is highest during the first 2 years of life. It declines gradually throughout childhood and accelerates slightly in adolescence. Children have higher BMR than adults. As age advances, the BMR falls. Hence, gets older, the food intake must also decrease. During periods of rapid growth, the BMR increases by 15–20%. The BMR is higher in infants and young children than in adults. The BMR increases from birth to 2 years of age and then begins to drop slightly until puberty, then it increases again as the person goes through a growth spurt. After age 20, the BMR decreases by about 2% in every 10 years.

Section VI

Water and Electrolytes

Chapter 21

Water

The body prefers to remain in balance and employs various mechanisms to help maintain homeostasis. Acute rapid changes in fluids and electrolytes are more ominous than slow gradual changes. Water, electrolytes and other substances are present in many different areas of the body, yet serum laboratory values only measure conditions in the intravascular space. So, cellular and other changes often must be inferred. They are vital to life; help to maintain body temperature and cell shape; involved in transporting nutrients, gases and wastes. Principle fluid in body is water. Skin, lungs and kidneys work together to maintain the proper fluid balance.

Water is more important to life than food, since man may live without food for several weeks, but for only a few days without water. It is the largest constituent of the body, about 60–70% of the total body weight consisting of water. The water content of soft tissues ranges from 70 to 80%, while that of bone about 20%.

DEFINITION

Water is a chemical compound consisting of two hydrogen and one oxygen atom. The name water typically refers to the liquid state of the compound. The solid phase is known as ice and gas phase is called steam. Human body contains approximately 70% of water (Fig. 21.1). The cellular and tissue structure divides the organisms into various segments containing water or aqueous solutions.

SOURCES

Water is supplied to the body by exogenous and endogenous sources:

1. **Exogenous:** Water, tender coconut water, buttermilk, fresh fruit juices and clear soups supply water to the body. Water content of solid foods such as vegetables, fruits and water used for

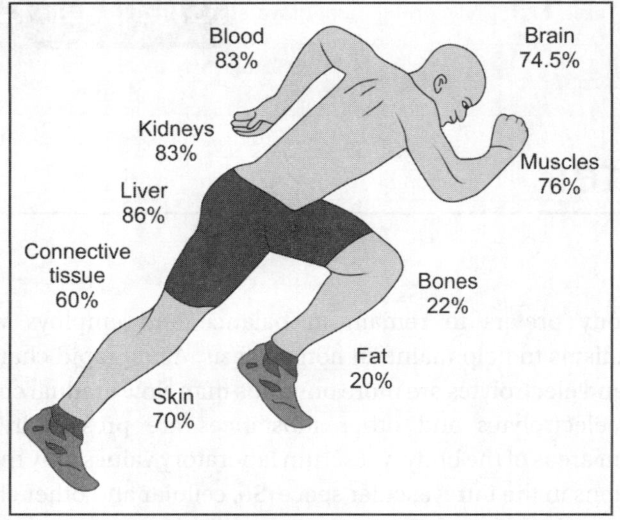

Figure 21.1: Distribution of water (%) in human body

cooking (dal, sambar) are also included. An average man consumes about 1.5–2 L/day.

2. **Endogenous:** Water produced through metabolism of major nutrients such as carbohydrates, fats and proteins amounts to 300 mL/day.

DAILY REQUIREMENT

The body needs a minimum of 1 liter of drinking water (free fluid) per day in order to maintain life and excrete the waste products of metabolism. Additional quantities are required in hot weather and for person doing hard manual labor to make up for extra loss as sweat. Infants require 165 mL of fluid per kg body weight. In infants, the percentage of water in the total body weight is higher than in adults (Table 21.1).

The daily requirement of water is traditionally expressed as milliliter per metabolic kilogram weight. However, in clinical practice, this is a very cumbersome and impractical method, and all calculations are based on the body weight and size.

Estimation of Daily Fluid Requirement

There are three methods that are currently used to estimate the daily fluid requirement.

Table 21.1: Daily requirement of water for various age groups

Age group	Category		Total water adequate intake (food and fluids)
Infants	0–6 month		680 mL/d (through milk)
	6–12 month		800–1,000 mL/d
Children	1–2 year		1,100–1,200 mL/d
	2–3 year		1,300 mL/d
	4–8 year		1,600 mL/d
	9-13 year	Boys	2,100 mL/d
		Girls	1,900 mL/d
	> 14 year		2,200 mL/d
Adults	Men		2,500 mL/d
	Women		2,000 mL/d
	Pregnant		+ 300 mL/d vs adults
	Lactating		+ 600–700 mL/d vs adults
	Elderly		Same as adults

First Method

The first is direct extension of the use of metabolic kilogram weight and utilizes the following formula:

Daily water requirement = 100 mL/kg (for a child weighing less than 10 kg) + 50 mL/kg (for each additional kg up to 20 kg) + 20 mL/kg (for each kg in excess of 20 kg)

Second Method

The second method is based on body surface area and utilizes the following formula:

Daily water requirement = 1,500 mL/m^2 body surface area (BSA)

Third Method

The third method is a refinement of the second and utilizes the following formula:

Daily water requirement = Urine output + Insensible water losses

Based on clinical experience, under normal circumstances, urine output is approximately 1,000 mL/m^2/day and insensible losses amount to 500 mL/m²/day. Thus, for a child weighing 30 kg and 123 cm in height with a BSA of 1.0 m², according to the first method, the daily water requirement is 1,700 mL, while the second method yields 1,500 mL/day. The first method is easier to apply, but it tends to overestimate the water requirement as body weight increases. The third method is the most precise and should be applied in more complicated circumstances such as the patient in the intensive care unit (ICU) with oliguria, secondary to acute kidney injury or the child with increased insensible losses, e.g. diarrhea, increased ambient temperature, tachypnea, burns or cystic fibrosis.

In addition to the daily energy requirement and insensible losses that are represented in the formulas, the amount of water excreted by the kidney on a daily basis is dependent upon the solute load. Because urine has a minimum osmolality, approximately 50 mOsm/kg water, even in the absence of arginine vasopressin (AVP), increased dietary intake of solute will result in a larger obligatory urine volume to accommodate the larger solute load.

The daily sodium and water requirement are generally provided enterally. Intravenous administration of fluids and electrolytes should be resorted to only under clinical circumstance that interfere with normal feeding such as persistent vomiting, gastrointestinal (GI) tract surgery or states of altered consciousness.

Recommendations on Water Requirement

The most recent official recommendation about water requirement has been published by the European Food Safety Authority (EFSA) in 2010. This extensive scientific review has enabled the definition of adequate water intakes, based on European fluid intakes, desirable urine osmolarity and energy intake. The reference values assumed a moderate climate and moderate level of physical activity. These values include water that originates from both consumed fluids and food.

The European Scientific Authority has also stated that the contribution of food to total water intake represents about 20% in adults. On this basis, it means that male adults should drink 2 L/day and female adults 1.6 L/day (Table 21.2). No maximal tolerable intake level has been set by EFSA. This is justified by the great ability of healthy individuals to excrete excess water intakes within a large range of observed intakes. In healthy subjects, the kidneys have the ability to excrete up to 0.7–1 L/h.

Table 21.2: Average daily intake and output in an adult

Intake (mL)	Output (mL)
Oral liquids: 1,300	Urine: 1,500
Water in food: 1,000	Stool: 200
Water produced by metabolism: 300	Water produced in the insensible way: Lungs: 300 Skin: 600
Total: 2,600	Total: 2,600

REGULATION OF WATER

The cells themselves regulate the composition and amount of fluids within and surrounding them. The entire system of cells and fluids remains in delicate, but firmly maintained state of dynamic equilibrium. Imbalances such as dehydration and water intoxication can occur, but the body quickly restores the balance to normal, if it can. The body controls both water intake and water excretion to maintain water equilibrium (Fig. 21.2):

1. The body can survive for only a few days without water. In healthy people, thirst and satiety govern water intake. Thirst is finely adjusted to ensure a water intake that meets the body's needs.
2. When the blood becomes too concentrated (having lost water, but not salt and other dissolved substances), the mouth becomes dry and the brain center known as the hypothalamus initiates drinking behavior.
3. Thirst lags behind the lack of water. A water deficiency that develops slowly can switch on drinking behavior in time to prevent serious dehydration, but a deficiency that develops quickly may not.
4. Also, thirst itself does not remedy a water deficiency, a person must pay attention to the thirst signal and take the time to get a drink. With aging, thirst sensations may diminish. Dehydration can threaten elderly people who do not develop the habit of drinking water regularly.
5. Water intoxication, on the other hand, is rare, but can occur with excessive water consumption and kidney disorders that reduce urine production. The symptoms may include severe headache, confusion, convulsion and even death in extreme cases.

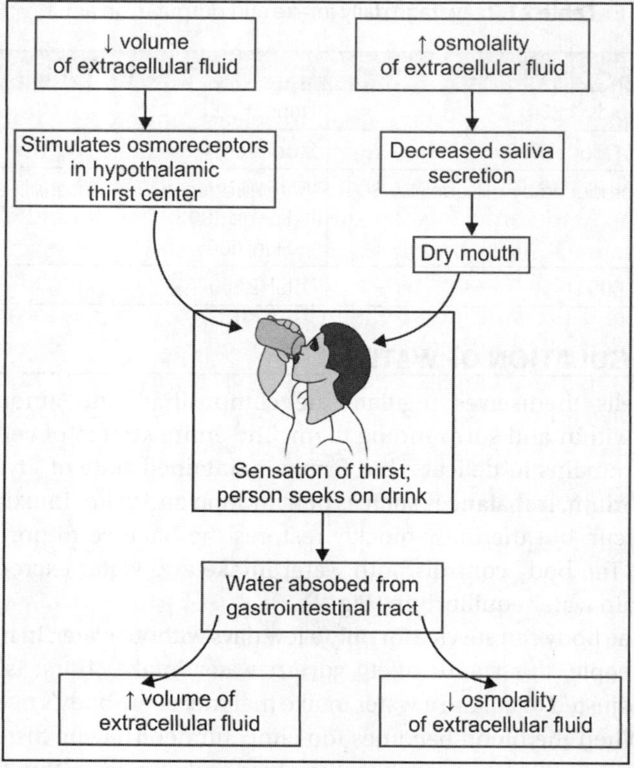

Figure 21.2: Water regulation

Water Intake Regulation

1. The body loses as little as 1% of its water.
2. An increase in osmotic pressure of extracellular fluid due to water loss stimulates osmoreceptors in the thirst center (hypothalamus).
3. Activity in the hypothalamus causes the person to be thirsty and to seek water (H_2O).
4. Drinking and the resulting distension of the stomach by water stimulates nerve impulses that inhibit the thirst center.
5. Water is absorbed through the wall of the stomach, small intestine and large intestine.
6. The osmotic pressure of extracellular fluid returns to normal.

Water Excretion Regulation

1. Water excretion is regulated by the brain and the kidneys. The cells of the brain's hypothalamus, which monitor blood salts, stimulate the pituitary gland to release antidiuretic hormone (ADH) whenever the salts are too concentrated, or the blood volume or blood pressure is too low.
2. The ADH stimulates the kidneys to reabsorb water rather than excrete it. Thus, the more water we need, the less we excrete.
3. If too much water is lost from the body, blood volume and blood pressure fall. Cells in the kidneys respond to the low blood pressure by releasing an enzyme.
4. Through a complex series of events involving the hormone aldosterone, this enzyme also causes the kidneys to retain more water. When more water is needed, less is excreted.

Events in Regulation of Water Output

1. Dehydration.
2. Extracellular fluid becomes osmotically more concentrated.
3. Osmoreceptors in the hypothalamus are stimulated by the increase in the osmotic pressure of body fluids.
4. The hypothalamus signals the posterior pituitary gland to release ADH into the blood.
5. Blood carries ADH to the kidneys.
6. The ADH causes the distal convoluted tubules and collecting ducts to increase water reabsorption.
7. Urine output decreases and further water loss is minimized.

HOMEOSTASIS

Homeostasis is the property of an open system, especially living organisms, to regulate its internal environment to maintain a stable and constant condition by means of multiple dynamic equilibrium adjustments, controlled by interrelated regulation mechanisms. Maintaining homeostasis of fluid in the various compartments of the body involves balancing (Fig. 21.3):

- Fluid intake
- Fluid absorption
- Fluid distribution
- Fluid excretion.

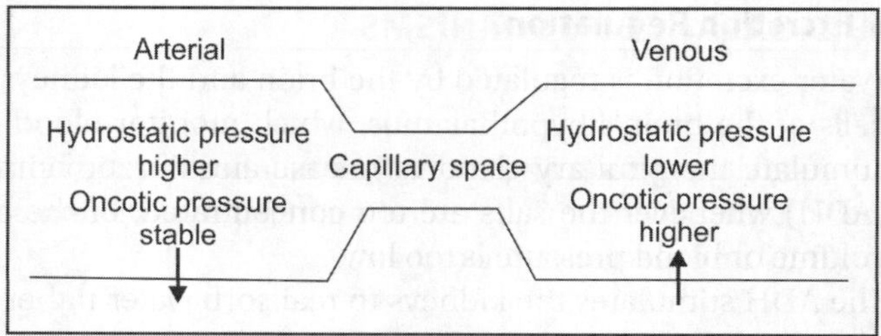

Figure 21.3: Homeostasis of fluid in various compartments of body

A number of body systems contribute to regulation including the kidneys, endocrine system, cardiovascular system, lungs, gastrointestinal system and hormones such as ADH.

Fluid Intake

Normal fluid intake involves drinking fluids orally and ingesting fluids through food. Other methods of fluid intake is tube feeding. IV fluids, water through metabolism or oxidation of nutrients, such as carbohydrates and fat.

Fluid Absorption

An increased osmolality will trigger the thirst center to initiate fluid intake. The fluid intake is then absorbed from the GI tract before reaching the vascular compartment.

Fluid Distribution

Once fluid has been absorbed into the vascular compartment, it is distributed between the vascular and interstitial compartments through filtration. Two forces control movement of fluid from the capillaries into the interstitial area:

- Capillary hydrostatic pressure
- Interstitial fluid osmotic pressure (oncotic).

In addition, two forces—the capillary osmotic pressure and interstitial hydrostatic pressure—move fluid from the interstitial fluid into the capillaries.

Fluid Excretion

The most common areas of the body for fluid excretion are the bowels, skin, lungs and kidneys. The essential urine output of the average individual is approximately 300–500 mL/day, but averages approximately 1,500 mL/day.

FLUID BALANCE MECHANISMS

Kidneys

Primary regulator of fluid and electrolyte balance through changes in urine volume and electrolyte excretion; renal dysfunction causes multiple fluid and electrolyte disturbance.

Thirst

Center in hypothalamus stimulated by hypotension and increased serum osmolality, decreased with hyponatremia; thirst mechanism is less effective in elderly, so more prone to dehydration.

Antidiuretic Hormone

When low blood volume and increased serum osmolality, hypothalamus signals pituitary gland to secrete ADH, which causes the kidneys to retain water, thus increasing blood volume and decreasing serum osmolality. Syndrome of inappropriate ADH (SIADH) results into much water retention, whereas diabetes insipidus (DI) causes diminished ADH secretion and too much water loss.

Renin-angiotensin-aldosterone System

Kidney's juxtaglomerular cells secrete renin when low flow renin converts angiotensinogen to angiotensin I in the liver and angiotensin I is converted into angiotensin II, a potent vasoconstrictor in the lungs; angiotensin II also stimulates the adrenal glands to produce aldosterone, which causes the kidneys to retain sodium and water. High aldosterone is associated with Cushing's disease and hyperadrenocorticism, whereas low aldosterone is associated with Addison's disease and adrenal insufficiency. Angiotensin-converting enzyme (ACE) inhibitors work by blocking this system.

Atrial Natriuretic Peptide

Atrial natriuretic peptide (ANP) is released when atrial pressure increases; ANP decreases serum renin levels, aldosterone whereas ADH release increases glomerular filtration and causes vasodilation. Opposes the renin-angiotensin-aldosterone system by decreasing blood pressure and reducing intravascular blood volume. The amount released rises in response to a number of conditions including chronic renal and heart failure.

Gastrointestinal System and Skin

Gastrointestinal (GI) system is responsible for most of the water intake; diarrhea and vomiting can lead to fluid and electrolyte disturbances, insensible losses are water only whereas sweating causes loss of both fluids and electrolytes.

FUNCTIONS OF WATER

A healthy, sedentary adult living in a temperate climate should drink 1.5 liters of water per day. This threshold of drinking water enables to balance water losses and keep one's body properly hydrated. Water is a major constituent of the body and vital organs:

1. Water is an essential part of body lymph, and all the secretions and excretions of the body.
2. It aids in digestion, absorption and metabolism of food substance in two ways:
    a. By dissolving and transporting substances.
    b. By functioning as a catalyst.

The five vital functions of water in our body are as follows (Fig. 21.4):

1. **Cell life:** Water is a carrier distributing essential nutrients to cells, such as minerals, vitamins and glucose.
2. **Chemical and metabolic reactions:** Water removes waste products including toxins that the organs' cells reject, and removes them through urine and feces.
3. **Transport of nutrients:** Water participates in the biochemical breakdown of what we eat.
4. **Body temperature regulation:** Water has a large heat capacity, which helps to limit changes in body temperature in a warm or a cold environment. Water allows the body to release heat when ambient temperature is higher than body temperature. The body begins to sweat and the evaporation of water from the skin surface cools the body very efficiently. This is carried out in the following ways:
    a. By its specific heat: More heat is required to raise the temperature of 1 g of water through 1°C than almost any other known solid or liquid. Thus, heat produced in chemical changes in the body will cause only very slight rise in temperature.

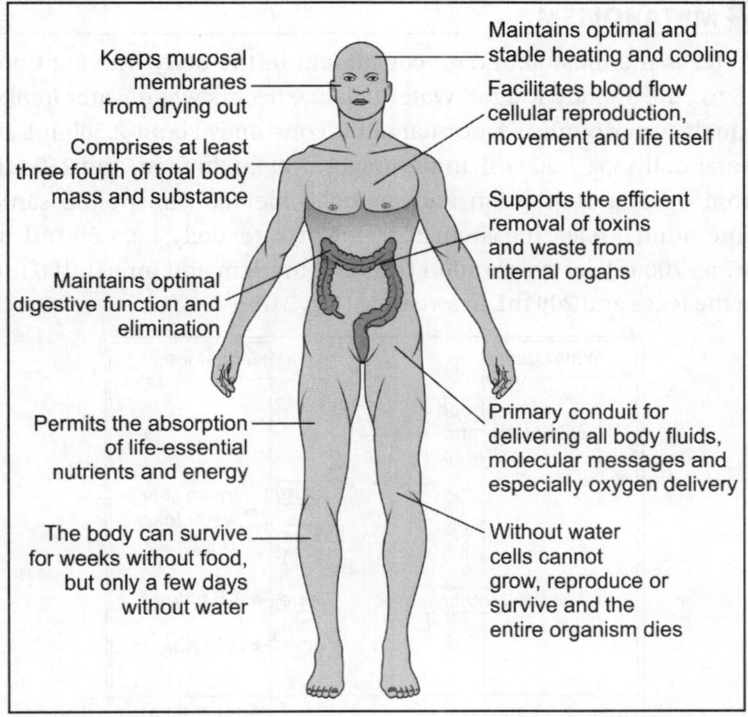

Figure 21.4: Vital functions of water in body

b. By heat conduction: Conduction means passage of heat through matter or substances. Heat conduction of water is greater than that of any known liquid; therefore water is the best possible liquid for conducting heat away from the place where it is produced.

c. By the heat used in the evaporation of water: This heat is removed from the surface of the body by evaporation with a cooling effect. This property of water is made use of in giving a cool sponge bath to a patient with fever.

d. Water acts as a lubricant to joints and mucous membranes, preventing friction.

5. **Elimination of water:** Water is an effective lubricant around joint. It also acts as a shock absorber for eyes, brain, spinal cord and even for the fetus through amniotic fluid. Water is at the center of life. This is why nobody can live more than 3–5 days without any water intake.

METABOLISM

Water is the most abundant constituent in the body, varying from 45 to 75% of body weight. Water balance occurs when water intake equals water output. A normal adult consumes about 2,500 mL of water daily, i.e. 1,500 mL in beverages, 750 mL in food, and 250 mL from cellular respiration and anabolic metabolism. At the same time, adult is releasing about 2,500 mL of water daily, i.e. 1,500 mL in urine, 700 mL by evaporation (through the skin and lungs), 100 mL in the feces and 200 mL in sweating (Fig. 21.5).

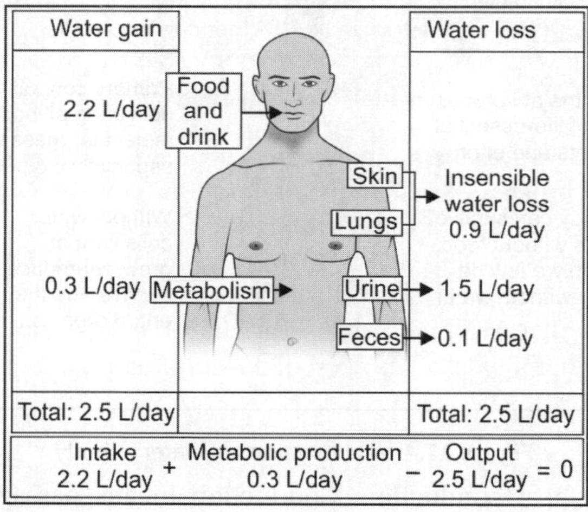

Figure 21.5: Various ways of water gain and water loss

Water Intake and Output (Fig. 21.6)

Water Intake

All the biochemical processes in organism that are necessary for life, take place in aqueous environment. The organism gains water in three ways:

1. **Receiving pure water:** Organism receives 1,200–1,500 mL of pure water daily. This input is easily balanced.
2. **Receiving water by food intake:** The amount of water in food is variable. Organism receives 1,000 mL of water daily in this way. When no food is taken, we have to substitute not only the daily intake of water but the amount of water released from food as well.

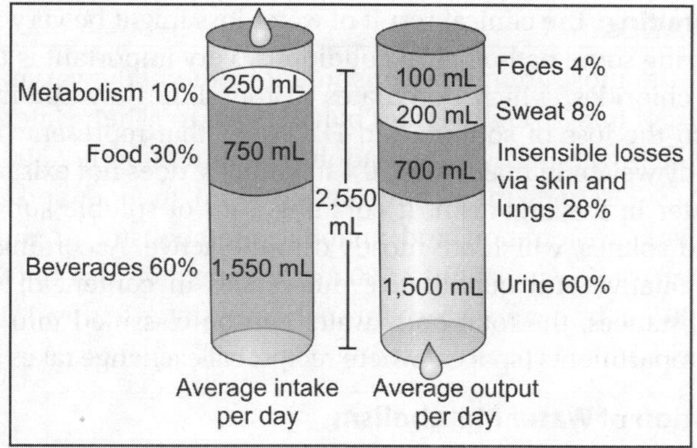

Figure 21.6: Average water intake and output per day

3. **Gaining water from biochemical processes:** Water is released in the process of oxidation. About 35 mL of water is released during oxidation of 100 g of lipids. We can estimate that the daily water intake is 300–500 mL in this way and in case of destructive metabolism, even more. The total water intake is approximately 2,500 mL a day, but it is very variable. The organism adapts to this variability by adaptation of the elimination processes.

Water Output

Water is eliminated by urine, perspiration, respiration, stools and vomiting as detailed below:

1. **Urine:** The kidneys does the most important regulation mechanism for the elimination of water and thus for maintenance of homeostasis. They excrete all superfluous substances to urine and resorb necessary solutes from primary urine. Diuresis ranges between 1,200 and 1,500 mL/day.
2. **Perspiration:** Nearly 600–800 mL of water is lost daily during 'perspiratio insensibilis.' It might be even more in some specific situations. Apart from extreme climatic and working conditions, it is the fever that increases the loss of water during perspiration. Old people with fever may even develop a dehydration.
3. **Respiration:** About 400–500 mL of water is lost daily by respiration. We have to mention that it is the loss of pure water without electrolytes in this case.
4. **Stools:** About 100 mL of water is lost daily by stools. The loss of water and also electrolytes might be extreme during diarrhea.

5. **Vomiting:** The clinical result of water loss might be very serious during some pathological conditions. Very important is the loss of chlorides, which dominates in the clinical symptoms, and also the loss of sodium and H^+. Water that represents 60% of body weight in males and 50% in females, does not exist as pure water in the organism. It contains a lot of soluble substances and solutes, which are mostly osmotic active. According to the qualitative and quantitative differences in content of soluble substances, the total body water can be classified into several compartments (spaces) where reciprocal exchange takes place.

Regulation of Water Metabolism

Water is absorbed rapidly from the small intestine through the portal vein to the general circulation. It rapidly passes to the tissue space as tissue fluid. A greater part of the ingested water is excreted by the kidneys within an hour. The mechanism of exchange of water between blood and tissues is briefly discussed.

Water exchange between plasma and interstitial fluid is controlled by the osmotic pressure of protein in the plasma, which is 25 mm Hg and the arterial capillary pressure (32 mm Hg) at the arterial end. The capillary blood pressure is greater than the protein osmotic pressure of plasma by 7 mm Hg. Hence, fluid passes from capillaries to tissue space. In the venous end, the capillary blood pressure is less than the protein osmotic pressure by 13 mm Hg. Therefore, fluid passes from tissue space into the capillaries; this plasma-interstitial fluid exchange takes place on a large seal, i.e. about 3 L/min.

Effect of Excess Water Intake on Water Balance in the Body

If 2 liters of water is taken, it is distributed rapidly throughout the body. The kidney responds to the increased water intake after about 15–30 minutes. The flow of urine rises from the normal value of 50 mL/h to its peak of 1,500 mL/h. The excess urine output may (in temperate climate) be almost equal to the water ingested. In tropical climate, greater post of the ingested water is lost in the sweat.

Effects of Water Deprivation on Water Balance

Water is being constantly lost from the body in urine, sweat, expired air and feces. If corresponding amounts of water are not ingested, water depletion occurs in the body leading to change in body fluids; a reduction in volume of the extracellular fluid (ECF) and intracellular fluid (ICF) takes place. The urine output is reduced, there is a rapid decrease in body weight and a state of dehydration of the cells occurs after a few days; a decrease in plasma volume (and also in blood volume) occurs, which will reduce cardiac output and lead to circulatory failure. An adult who has lost 5 liters of water from the body will be seriously ill; and death will occur when the water loss from the body is about 15 liters.

DISTRIBUTION OF BODY WATER

The distribution varies with age, sex and body composition. Percentage of body weight—water is about 80% in a full-term infant, 60% in a typical lean adult male and 45–50% for obese and elderly. This puts infants, elderly and obese individuals at greater risk for fluid-related problems. Body water is distributed as follows:

1. Inside the cells of tissue—intracellular (50%).
2. Outside the tissue cells—extracellular water (20%).

The extracellular water is further subdivided into:

1. Water in blood plasma (about 4%).
2. Interstitial water—the water in tissues space (9%).
3. Lymph in the lymphatic vessels (7%).

Additional minor divisions of extracellular water are cerebrospinal fluid and aqueous humor (in the anterior chamber of the eye). The gastrointestinal secretions amount about 7 L/day, but most of this is reabsorbed into the body. The cerebrospinal fluid is also secreted and absorbed daily, but the exact quantity is unknown. Eye fluids are small in amount, but there is a definite circulation of urine formed continuously and fluid is lost from the body. Sweat is also lost from the body; the amount varies with climate and work edema; when occurs, it is a symptom of some change in water metabolism in the body. Fluid spacing is a term used to classify the distribution of water in the body:

1. **First spacing:** It describes the excess accumulation of fluid in the body in both the intracellular and extracellular fluid compartments.
2. **Second spacing:** It describes the excess accumulation of fluid in the interstitial spaces, which is also called edema.
3. **Third spacing:** It occurs when fluid accumulates in areas that normally have no fluid or minimal amount of fluid, such as ascites and edema associated with burns. In extreme cases, third spacing can cause a relative hypovolemia.

4. **Fluid status:** About 1 liter of water weighs 2.2 pounds. A sudden weight gain or loss is the best indicator of fluid status. Patients who need to have their fluid status monitored, should not only have their intake and output measured but also daily bedside weights.

Fluid Compartments

There are two main fluid compartments separated by capillary walls and cell membranes (Figs 21.7 and 21.8A and B):

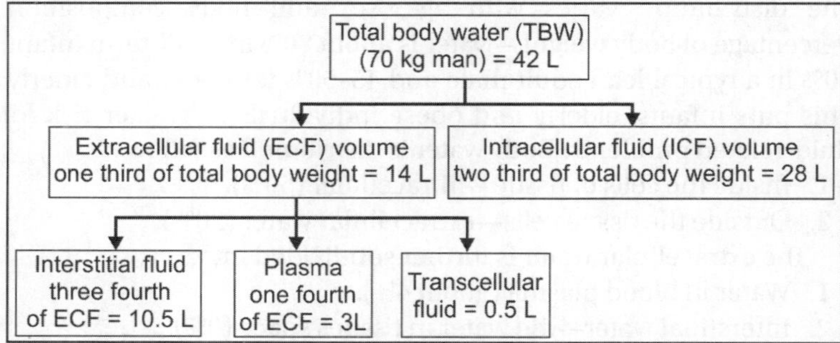

Figure 21.7: Distribution of water in fluid compartments

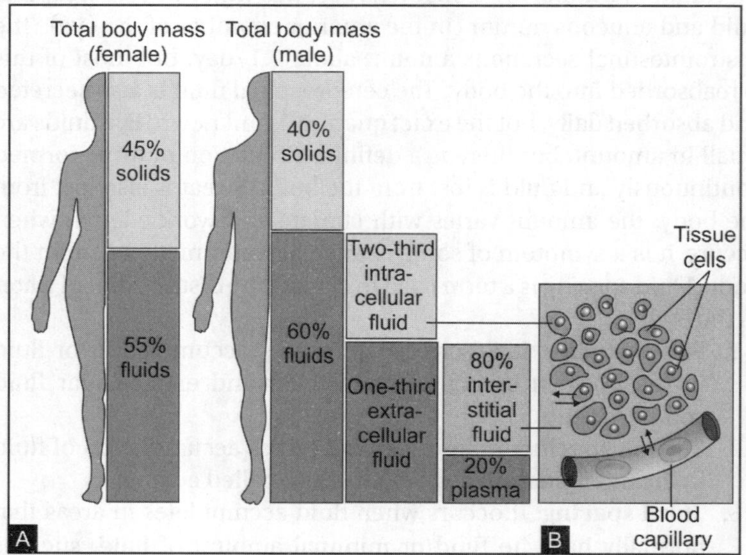

Figures 21.8A and B: Distribution of body water. **A.** In an average lean adult female and male; **B.** Exchange of water among body fluid compartments.

1. **Intracellular fluid:** The ICF within cells found in the body is 40% of body weight and 70% of total body water.
2. **Extracellular fluid:** It is found in outside body cells and is 20% of total body weight and 30% of total body water. It is comprised of:
   a. Interstitial fluid (ISF): Between cells (~ 2/3 ECF).
   b. Intravascular fluid (IVF): Plasma (~ 1/3 ECF); high-protein concentration.
   c. Transcellular fluid (TCF): Gastrointestinal tract, peritoneal, cerebrospinal, pleural and synovial fluid; small (~ 1L of ECF).

Chapter 22

Electrolytes and its Imbalances

ELECTROLYTES

Electrolyte is a substance that dissociates into ions in solution and acquires the capacity to conduct electricity. Sodium (Na), potassium (K), chloride (Cl), calcium (Ca) and phosphate (P) are the examples of electrolytes, informally known as lytes. Electrolytes replacement is needed when a patient has prolonged vomiting or diarrhea and as a response to strenuous athletic activity, electrolytes monitoring is important in treatment of anorexia and bulimia (Table 22.1 and 22.2).

Table 22.1: Electrolytes functions and sources

Electrolytes	Functions	Sources (mg)
Phosphate (PO_4): 1.8–2.6 mEq/L, 2.5–4.5 mg/dL	Forming bones and teeth Metabolizing carbohydrate, protein and fat Cellular metabolism; producing ATP* and DNA† Muscle, nerve and RBC‡ function Regulating acid-base balance Regulating calcium levels	Seeds: Sesame seeds, watermelon seeds Cheese: Goat cheese Fish: White fish and cod, carps Shellfish: Clams, shrimp, mollusks and crab
Bicarbonate (HCO_3^-): 22–26 meq/L	Major body buffer involved in acid base regulation	Fruits and fruit juices: Apples, bananas, grape juice, lemon juice Vegetables: Spinach broccoli, carrots, potatoes Milk, daily and eggs: Milk, eggs, cottage cheese Meat and meat products: Beef (lean only), chicken (meat only), liver sausage

Contd...

Contd...

Electrolytes	Functions	Sources (mg)
Magnesium (Mg^{2+}): 1.5–2.5 mEq/L, 1.6–2.5 mg/dL	Conservation and excretion by kidneys Intestinal absorption increased by vitamin D and parathyroid hormone	Bajra 137, jowar 171, rice 90, rice flakes 101, whole wheat 138, Bengal gram dal 130, black gram 154, cow pea 210, green gram 127, horse gram 156, soybean 238, spinach 24, drumstick leaves 42, amaranth 122, almonds 373, cashew nut 349, mango 270, custard apple 89
Chloride (Cl^-): 98–108 mmol/L	HCl production Regulating ECF[§] balance and vascular volume Regulating acid-base balance Buffer in oxygen-carbon dioxide exchange in RBCs	Table salt/Sea salt, seaweed, rye, tomatoes, lettuce, celery, olives

[‡]RBCs, red blood cells; *ATP, adenosine triphosphate; [†]DNA, deoxyribonucleic acid; [§]ECF, extracellular fluid.

Table 22.2: Laboratory values used in evaluating fluid and electrolyte status

Test	Usual reference guide	SI unit
Urinary sodium	50–200 mEq/day	50–220 mmol/day
Urinary potassium	40–80 mEq/day	40–80 mmol/day
Urinary chloride	110–250 mEq/day	110–250 mmol/day
Urinary specific gravity	1.025–1.035	1.025–1.035
Physiologic range after fluid restriction: 1.010–1.020 random specimen with normal intake		
Urine osmolality		
Extreme range	50–1,400 mOsm/L	40–1,400 mmol/kg
Typical urine	500–800 mOsm/L	500–800 mmol/kg
Urinary pH	4.5–8.0	4.5–8.0
Typical urine	< 6.6	< 6.6

Definition

Electrolytes (Fig. 22.1) are the substances found in extracellular and intracellular fluid dissociated into electrically charged particles

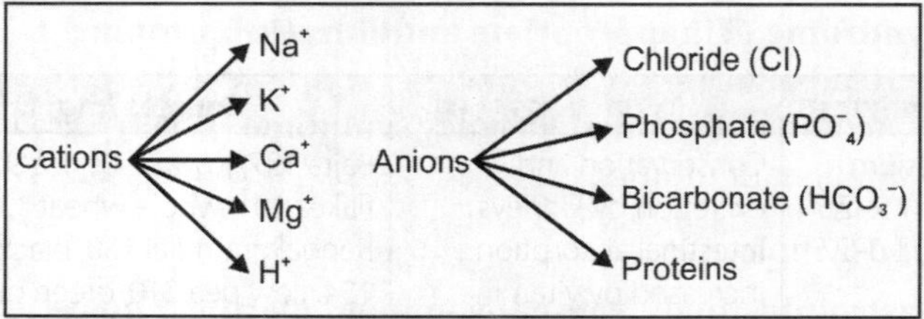

Figure 22.1: Electrolytes (cations and anions)

known as ions. Ions that carry positive charge are called and that carry negative charge are called anions.

ELECTROLYTE IMBALANCES

Hyponatremia

Definition

Electrolyte imbalance is a condition of Na deficiency in which the level of Na in blood plasma is less than 135 mEq/L.

Causes

- Severe burns, diabetic acidosis
- Large orchitis, urinary excretion, Cushing's disease
- Peritonitis
- Pleural effusion
- Severe vomiting
- Severe diarrhea
- Excess sweating and urination
- Dilution of plasma by taking a lot of plain water
- Addison's disease.

Risk Factors

1. **Loss of sodium:**
   - Gastrointestinal fluid loss
   - Sweating
   - Use of diuretics.
2. **Gain of water:**
   - Hypotonic tube feeding
   - Excessive drinking of water
   - Excess intravenous (IV) dextrose in water (D5W) administration.

3. **Syndrome of inappropriate antidiuretic hormone:**
    - Head injury
    - Acquired immunodeficiency syndrome (AIDS)
    - Malignant tumors.

Signs and Symptoms

1. **Gastrointestinal:** Nausea, vomiting, diarrhea, bowel sounds, abdominal cramps.
2. **Cardiovascular:** Decrease in diastolic pressure, tachycardia, orthostatic hypotension, weak pulse.
3. **Pulmonary:** Changes in respiration rate.
4. **Neurologic:** Headache, lethargy, confusion, slowed problem solving, diminished muscle tone on extremities, weakness and tremor.
5. **Integumentary:** Dry skin, pale, dry mucous membrane.
6. **Muscular:** Muscle twitching.

Medical Management

- Determine cause of hyponatremia and correct it
- Correct body water osmolarity
- If client has hyponatremia due to fluid volume excess, intake of fluids will be restricted to allow the sodium to regain balance
- If the serum sodium level falls below 125 mEq/L, sodium replacement is needed.

Laboratory Findings

- Serum sodium below 135 mEq/L
- Serum osmolality below 280 mOsm/kg.

Nursing Interventions

- Assess clinical manifestations
- Monitor fluid intake and output
- Assess client closely, if administering hypertonic saline solutions
- Encourage food and fluid high in sodium, if permitted (e.g. table salt, bacon, ham, processed cheese)
- Limit water intake as indicated.

Hypernatremia

Risk Factors

1. **Loss of water:**
    - Insensible water loss (hyperventilation or fever)

- Diarrhea
- Water deprivation.

2. **Gain of sodium:**
   - Parenteral administration of saline solutions
   - Hypertonic tube feeding without adequate water
   - Excessive use of table salt (1 tablespoon contains 2,300 mg of sodium).
3. **Conditions:**
   - Diabetes insipidus
   - Heat stroke.

Signs and Symptoms

1. **Thirst:**
   - Dry, sticky mucous membranes
   - Tongue is red, dry, swollen
   - Weakness.
2. **Severe hypernatremia:**
   - Fatigue, restlessness
   - Decreasing level of consciousness
   - Disorientation
   - Convulsions.

Laboratory Findings

- Serum sodium above 145 mEq/L
- Serum osmolality above 300 mOsm/kg.

Nursing Interventions

- Monitor fluid intake and output
- Monitor behavioral changes (e.g. restlessness, disorientation)
- Encourage fluids as ordered
- Monitor diet as ordered (e.g. restrict intake of salt and foods high in sodium).

Hypokalemia

Risk Factors

1. **Loss of potassium:**
   - Vomiting and/or gastric suction
   - Diarrhea
   - Heavy perspiration

- Use of potassium-wasting drugs (e.g. diuretics)
- Poor intake of potassium (as with debilitated clients, alcoholics, anorexia nervosa).

Signs and Symptoms

- Muscle weakness, leg cramps
- Fatigue, lethargy
- Anorexia, nausea, vomiting
- Decreased bowel sounds, decreased bowel motility
- Cardiac dysrhythmias
- Depressed deep tendon reflexes
- Weak, irregular pulses
- Laboratory findings
- Serum potassium below 3.5 mEq/L
- Arterial blood gases (ABGs) may show alkalosis
- T-wave flattening and ST-segment depression on the electrocardiogram (ECG).

Nursing Interventions

- Monitor heart rate and rhythm
- Monitor clients receiving digitalis (e.g. digoxin) closely, because hypokalemia increases risk of digitalis toxicity
- Administer oral potassium as ordered with food of fluid to prevent gastric irritation
- Administer IV potassium solutions at a rate no faster than 10–20 mEq/h; never administer undiluted potassium IV. For clients receiving IV potassium, monitor for pain and inflammation at the injection site
- Teach client about potassium-rich foods
- Teach clients how to prevent excessive loss of potassium (e.g. through abuse of diuretics and laxatives).

Hyperkalemia

Risk Factors

1. **Decreased potassium excretion:**
   - Renal failure
   - Hypoaldosteronism
   - Potassium-conserving diuretics.

2. **High-potassium intake:**
   - Excessive use of potassium-containing salt substitutes
   - Excessive or rapid IV infusion of potassium
   - Potassium shift out of the tissue cells into plasma (e.g. infections, burns, acidosis).

Signs and Symptoms

- Gastrointestinal hyperactivity, diarrhea, irritability, apathy and confusion
- Cardiac dysrhythmia or arrest
- Muscle weakness, a reflexia (absence of reflexes)
- Decreased heart rate
- Irregular pulse
- Paresthesias and numbness
- Laboratory findings
- Serum potassium above 5.0 mEq/L
- Peaked T wave, widened QRS on ECG.

Nursing Interventions

- Closely monitor cardiac status and ECG
- Administer diuretics and other medication such as glucose and insulin as ordered
- Hold potassium supplements and potassium-conserving diuretics
- Monitor serum potassium levels carefully, a rapid drop may occur as potassium shifts into the cells. Teach clients to avoid foods high in potassium and salt substitutes.

Hypocalcemia

Risk Factors

1. **Surgical removal of the parathyroid glands:** Results in the following:
   - Hypoparathyroidism
   - Acute pancreatitis
   - Hyperphosphatemia
   - Thyroid carcinoma.
2. **Inadequate vitamin D intake:** It results in:
   - Malabsorption
   - Hypomagnesemia

- Alkalosis
- Sepsis
- Alcohol abuse.

Signs and Symptoms

- Numbness, tingling of the extremities and around the mouth
- Muscle tremors, cramps; if severe, can progress to tetany and convulsions
- Cardiac dysrhythmias; decreased cardiac output
- Positive Trousseau's sign and Chvostek's sign
- Confusion, anxiety, possible psychoses
- Hyperactive deep tendon reflexes.

Laboratory Findings

- Serum calcium less than 8.5 mg/dL (total) or 4.5 mEq/L (ionized)
- Lengthened QT intervals
- Prolonged ST segments.

Nursing Interventions

- Closely monitor respiratory and cardiovascular status
- Take precautions to protect a confused client
- Administer oral or parenteral calcium supplements as ordered; when administering IV, closely monitor cardiac status and ECG during infusion
- Teach clients at high risk for osteoporosis dietary source rich in calcium
- Recommendation for 1,000–1,500 mg of calcium per day
- Calcium supplements
- Regular exercise
- Estrogen replacement therapy for postmenopausal women.

Hypercalcemia

Risk Factors

Prolong immobilization conditions such as:

- Hyperparathyroidism
- Malignancy of the bone
- Paget's disease.

Signs and Symptoms

- Lethargy, weakness
- Depressed deep tendon reflexes

- Bone pain
- Anorexia, nausea, vomiting
- Constipation
- Polyuria, hypercalcemia
- Flank pain secondary to urinary calculi
- Dysrhythmias, possible heart block.

Laboratory Findings

- Serum calcium greater than 10.5 mg/dL (total) or 5.5 mEq/L (ionized)
- Shortened QT intervals
- Shortened ST segments.

Nursing Interventions

- Increase client movement and exercise
- Encourage oral fluids as permitted to maintain dilute urine
- Teach clients to limit intake of food and fluid high in calcium
- Encourage ingestion of fiber to prevent constipation
- Protect a confused client; monitor for pathologic fractures in clients with long-term hypercalcemia
- Encourage intake of acid-ash fluids (e.g. prune or cranberry juice) to counteract deposits of calcium salts in the urine.

Hypomagnesemia

Risk Factors

- Excessive loss from the gastrointestinal tract (e.g. from nasogastric suction, diarrhea, fistula drainage)
- Long-term use of certain drugs (e.g. diuretics, aminoglycoside antibiotics)
- Condition such as:
  - Chronic alcoholism
  - Pancreatitis
  - Burns.

Signs and Symptoms

- Neuromuscular irritability with tremors increase reflexes, tremors, convulsions
- Positive Chvostek's sign and Trousseau's sign
- Tachycardia, elevated blood pressure, dysrhythmias
- Disorientation and confusion

- Vertigo
- Anorexia, dysphagia
- Respiratory difficulties.

Laboratory Findings

- Serum magnesium below 1.5 mEq/L
- Prolonged PR intervals, widened QRS complexes, prolonged QT intervals, depressed ST segments, broad-flattened waves, prominent U waves.

Nursing Interventions

- Assess client receiving digitalis for digitalis toxicity
- Hypomagnesemia increase the risk of toxicity
- Take protective measures when there is a possibility of seizures
- Assess the client's ability to swallow water prior to initiating oral feeding
- Initiate safety measures to prevent injury during seizure activity
- Carefully administer magnesium salts as ordered
- Encourage clients to eat magnesium-rich foods, if permitted (e.g. whole grains, meat, seafood and green leafy vegetables)
- Refer clients to alcohol treatment programs as indicated.

Hypermagnesemia

Risk Factors

- Abnormal retention of magnesium as in:
  - Renal failure
  - Adrenal insufficiency
  - Treatment with magnesium salts.

Signs and Symptoms

- Peripheral vasodilation, flushing
- Nausea, vomiting
- Muscle weakness, paralysis
- Hypotension, bradycardia
- Depressed deep tendon reflexes
- Lethargy, drowsiness
- Respiratory depression, coma
- Respiratory and cardiac arrest, if hypermagnesemia is severe.

Laboratory Findings

- Serum magnesium above 2.5 mEq/L
- Electrocardiogram showing prolonged QT interval, prolonged PR interval, widened QRS complexes, tall T waves.

Nursing Interventions

- Monitor vital signs and level of consciousness when clients are at risk
- If patellar reflexes are absent, notify the primary care provider
- Advise clients who have renal disease to contact their primary care provider before taking over-the-counter drugs.

Chapter 23

Fluid and Electrolyte Balance

MAINTENANCE OF FLUID AND ELECTROLYTE BALANCE

1. **Extracellular fluid (ECF):** Interstitial fluid, plasma, lymph, cerebrospinal fluid (CSF), synovial fluid, serous fluid, etc.
2. **Intracellular fluid (ICF):** Cytosol.
3. **Homeostasis:** It involves the regulation of composition and volume of both fluid divisions.

FOUR RULES AND REGULATIONS OF FLUIDS AND ELECTROLYTES

1. All homeostatic mechanisms for fluid composition respond to changes in the ECF:
   - Receptors monitor the composition of plasma and CSF, and trigger neural and endocrine mechanisms in response to change
   - Individual cells cannot be monitored and thus ICF has no direct impact.
2. No receptors directly monitor fluid or electrolyte balance:
   - Only plasma volume and osmotic concentration are monitored, which give an indirect measure of fluid or electrolyte levels.
3. Water follows salt:
   - Cells cannot move water by active transport
   - Water will always move by osmosis and this movement cannot be stopped.
4. The body's content of water or electrolytes rises and falls with gain and loss, to and from the environment:
   - Too much intake: High content in the body
   - Too much loss: Low content in the body.

FLUID, ELECTROLYTE AND PARTICLE MOVEMENT

Electrolytes move between ICF and ECF via concentration (toward lower concentration) and electric gradients (toward opposite charge):

1. **Diffusion:** Movement of molecules from an area of higher concentration to one of lower concentration.
2. **Facilitated diffusion:** Addition of specific carrier molecule to aid/accelerate diffusion (e.g. glucose transport into cell facilitated by insulin).
3. **Active transport:** Molecules move from the area of low to high concentration; external energy [adenosine triphosphate (ATP)] allows movement against concentration gradient (e.g. sodium pump, where potassium is moved into cell, sodium pumped out).

MOVEMENT OF FLUID ACCORDING TO PRESSURE FORCES

Hydrostatic Pressure

Pressure of blood fluid against capillary wall, if greater than pressure in interstitial space, fluids and solutes forced out of blood, if less, come back into blood.

Osmosis

Movement of water from area of higher to lower concentration ('diffusion of water') through membrane permeable to water, but not to solute; no energy needed, stops when solution concentrations equalize.

Osmotic Pressure

Movement of water by osmosis measured by osmolarity (mOsm/L) and osmolality (mOsm/kg), kidneys are mainly responsible for maintaining concentration of body fluids within normal range of osmolality through changes in antidiuretic hormone (ADH) secretion; normal osmolality is 275–295 mOsm/kg.

Tonicity and Intravenous Solutions

A solution's solute concentration (e.g. intravenous fluid) compared to another solution (e.g. blood), i.e. its effective osmolality; IV solution are categorized as follows:

1. **Isotonic:** Some effective osmolality as body fluids [e.g. 0.9% NaCl, dextrose 5% in water (D5W) prior to infusion, lactated ringers]causes intravascular expansion and possibly some interstitial edema, but no water shifts into or out of cells.

2. **Hypotonic solute concentration:** Less than 270 mOsm/kg [e.g. 0.2 or 0.4% NaCl, D5W (once in the body)] causes a shift of water out of vascular space. So, it can result in interstitial and cellular edema.
3. **Hypertonic higher solute concentration:** Less than 300 mOsm/kg [e.g. 3% NaCl, 5% dextrose in normal saline (D5NS), D5, 0.45% or D5 0.9% NaCl)] causes water to be pulled into vasculature from the interstitium and cells. So, it can result in cellular dehydration and vascular volume overload.

Plasma Colloid Osmotic Pressure

Osmotic or pulling force of albumin in the intravascular space opposes hydrostatic pressure to maintain equilibrium of fluid leaving and returning (if normal BP and plasma protein levels). Hypertension or hypoproteinemia (e.g. malnutrition, malabsorption, impaired albumin synthesis or protein loss) causes hydrostatic pressure to surpass colloid osmotic pressure (COP) resulting in edema.

PRIMARY REGULATORY HORMONES

1. **Antidiuretic hormone:**
   a. Osmoreceptors in the hypothalamus monitor the ECF and release ADH in response to high osmotic concentration (low water, high solute).
   b. Increased osmotic concentration: Increased ADH levels.
   c. Primary effects of ADH:
      i. Stimulate water conservation at kidneys.
      ii. Stimulate thirst center.
2. **Aldosterone:**
   a. Released by the adrenal cortex to regulate sodium absorption and potassium loss in the distal convoluted tubule (DCT) and collecting system in the kidney.
   b. Retention of sodium will result in H_2O conservation.
   c. Aldosterone is released in response to:
      i. High potassium or low sodium in ECF (e.g. renal circulation).
      ii. Activation of the renin-angiotensin system due to a drop in BP or blood volume.
      iii. Decline in kidney filtrate osmotic concentration at the DCT (more water less solutes).

Addison's disease = Hypoaldosteronism, which results in massive loss of NaCl and H_2O in the urine; must adjust diet to compensate.

3. **Natriuretic peptides:**
   a. Atrial natriuretic peptide (ANP) and brain natriuretic peptide (BNP) are released in response to stretching of the heart wall.
   b. They function to reduce thirst and block release of ADH and aldosterone resulting in diuresis (fluid loss in the kidney).

STABILIZING EXTRACELLULAR AND INTRACELLULAR FLUIDS

1. **Fluid balance:** Must have equal gain (food and metabolism) and loss (urine and perspiration) of water.
2. **Electrolyte balance:** Electrolytes are the ions from dissociated compounds that will conduct an electrical charge in solution; they must have an equal gain (absorption in FI) and loss (urine in kidney and perspiration in skin).
3. **Acid-base balance:** The production of hydrogen ions by metabolism must be matched by loss of these H^+ ions at the kidney (protons, H^+) and lungs (carbonic acid).

Fluid or Water Balance

The fluid or water balance exists when water intake equals water output.

Water Intake

1. The volume of water gained each day varies from one individual to other.
2. About 60% of daily water is gained from drinking, another 30% comes from moist foods and 10% from water metabolism.

Regulation of water intake

1. The thirst mechanism is the primary regulator of water intake.
2. The thirst mechanism from the osmotic pressure of extracellular fluids and a thirst center in the hypothalamus.
3. Once water is taken in, the resulting distention of the stomach will inhibit the thirst mechanism.

Water Output

1. Water is lost in urine, feces, perspiration, evaporation from skin (insensible perspiration) and from the lungs during breathing.
2. The route of water loss depends on temperature, relative humidity and physical exercise.

Regulation of water output

1. The distal convoluted tubules and collecting ducts of the nephrons regulate water output.
2. Antidiuretic hormone from the posterior pituitary causes a reduction in the amount of water lost in the urine.
3. When drinking adequate water, the ADH mechanism is inhibited and more water is expelled in urine.

Electrolyte Balance

An electrolyte balance exists when the quantities of electrolytes gained equal the amount lost.

Electrolyte Intake

1. The electrolytes of greatest importance to cellular metabolism are sodium, potassium, calcium, magnesium, chloride, sulfate, phosphate, bicarbonate and hydrogen ions.
2. Electrolytes may be obtained from food or drink, or produced as a byproduct of metabolism.

Regulation of electrolyte intake

1. A person ordinarily obtains the sufficient electrolytes from food eaten.
2. Salt craving may indicate an electrolyte deficiency.

Electrolyte Output

Losses of electrolytes occur through sweating, in the feces and in urine.

Regulation of electrolyte output

1. The concentrations of the cations, especially sodium, potassium and calcium are very important.
2. Sodium ions account for 90% of the positively charged ions in extracellular fluids, the action of aldosterone on the kidneys regulate sodium reabsorption.
3. Aldosterone also regulates potassium ions and these ions are excreted when sodium ions are conserved.

4. Calcium concentration is regulated, in part, by these hormone, which increases the concentrations of calcium and phosphate ions in extracellular fluids.
5. Generally, the regulatory mechanisms that control positively charged ions, secondarily control the concentrations of anions.

Acid-base Balance

Electrolytes that ionize in water and release hydrogen ions are acids, those that combine with hydrogen ions are bases. Maintenance of homeostasis depends on the control of acids and bases in body fluids.

Sources of Hydrogen Ions

Most hydrogen ions originate as byproducts of metabolic processes, including the aerobic and anaerobic respiration of glucose, incomplete oxidation of fatty acids, oxidation of amino acids containing sulfur, and the breakdown of phosphoproteins and nucleic acids.

Strengths of Acids and Bases

1. Acids that ionize more completely are strong acids, those that ionize less completely are weak acids.
2. Bases release hydroxyl and other ions, which can combine with hydrogen ions, thereby lowering their concentration.

Regulation of Hydrogen Ion Concentration

Acid-base buffer systems, the respiratory center in the brainstem and the kidneys regulate pH of body fluids:

1. **Acid-base buffer systems:**
   a. The chemical components of a buffer system can combine with a strong acid and convert it to a weaker one.
   b. The chemical buffer systems in body fluids include the bicarbonate buffer system, the phosphate buffer system and the protein buffer system.
2. **Respiratory center:**
   a. This center in the brainstem helps to regulate hydrogen ion concentration by controlling the rate and depth of breathing.
   b. During exercise, the carbon dioxide and the carbonic acid levels in the blood increase.

c. In response, the respiratory center increases the rate and depth of breathing, so the lungs excrete more carbon dioxide.

3. **Kidneys:** Nephrons secrete excess hydrogen ions in the urine.

Rates of Regulation

Chemical buffers are considered the body's first line of defense against shifts in pH, physiological buffer systems (respiratory and renal mechanisms) function more slowly and constitute secondary defenses.

Chapter 24

Overhydration, Dehydration and Diarrhea

OVERHYDRATION

Overhydration is less common than dehydration. Sometimes overhydration results from administering too much fluid intravenously, but may also occur when a person with impaired renal function drinks a large amount of fluid, which the kidneys are unable to excrete efficiently.

Definition

Overhydration is known as hypoosmolar imbalance or water intoxication; it occurs when water is gained in excess of electrolytes, resulting in low-serum osmolality and low-serum sodium levels.

Causes

- Renal disease
- Conditions that result in low blood flow to kidney (e.g. cardio insufficiency
- Too rapid infusion of IV fluids
- Steroid therapy or Cushing's syndrome
- Stress
- Overproduction of antidiuretic hormone (ADH).

Degrees of Overhydration

- **Mild:** 2% (2.4 lb gain in 120 lb person or 1 kg in a 54.5 kg person)
- **Moderate:** 5% (6 lb gain in 120 lb person or 2.7 kg in a 54.5 kg person)
- **Severe:** 8% or more (10 lb or more in a 120 lb person or 4.5 kg in a 54.5 kg person).

Types

The three types of overhydration are as follows:

1. **Isotonic overhydration:** Expansion of the extracellular fluid (ECF) only. It is also called hypervolemia (excess fluid in the ECF). In this type, fluid and electrolytes are gained in same proportions, so osmolarity is normal.
2. **Hypotonic overhydration:** Expansion of both the ECF and the intracellular fluid (ICF) compartments. Also called water intoxication. Here osmolarity decreases. The fluid shifts from the bloodstream into the cells (cellular swelling) causing an increased intracranial pressure (ICP) and neurological changes.
3. **Hypertonic overhydration:** Expansion of the ECF and contraction of the ICF. Cells are dehydrated as fluid is pulled out and into the vascular compartment (cells shrink). Increased serum osmolarity leads to fluid shifting from the cells into the bloodstream, causing cell shrinkage and fluid volume overload. Fluid volume overload leads to increased BP and increased cardiac workload can eventually lead to decreased cardiac output and congestive heart failure (CHF).

Signs and Symptoms

- Weight gain over short period
- Distended neck veins
- Distended peripheral veins
- Slow emptying peripheral veins
- Central venous pressure (CVP) over 12 cm H_2O in vena cava
- Peripheral edema
- Pulmonary edema, if severe
- Moist rales in lungs, shortness of breath (SOB), dyspnea
- Ascites, pleural effusion [when fluid volume excess (FVE) is severe, fluid shifts into body cavities]
- Decreased hematocrit value (due to plasma dilution)
- Bounding, full pulse, blood pressure (BP).

Treatment

1. Monitor intake and output, weight, vital signs and level of consciousness (LOC).
2. Elevate head of bed, place on the fall precautions.
3. Reduce stimuli, provide pain medications and apply ice or hyaluronic acid.
4. Restrict fluids as ordered.
5. Monitor serum sodium and osmolarity.
6. Osmotic diuretics are significantly useful.

7. Mild overhydration can generally be corrected by following a doctor's instructions to limit fluid intake. In more serious cases, diuretics may be prescribed to increase urination, although these drugs tend to be most effective in the treatment of excess blood volume.
8. Identifying and treating any underlying condition (such as impaired heart or kidney function) is a priority and fluid restrictions are a critical component of every treatment plan.
9. In patient with severe neurologic symptoms, fluid imbalances must be corrected without delay. A powerful diuretic and fluids to restore normal sodium concentrations are administered rapidly at first.
10. When the patient has taken in 50% of the therapeutic substances blood levels are measured. Therapy is continued at a more moderate pace in order to prevent brain damage as a result of sudden changes in blood chemistry.

Prevention

1. Avoid situations that provoke extreme or prolonged perspiration.
2. Drinking fluids that are specially balanced to replace lost electrolytes can also help to prevent intoxication.
3. Eating regularly can provide needed electrolytes, if only normal water is available for rehydration.
4. Sports drinks are popular among athletes, because they provide the necessary electrolytes to support extended exercise.

DEHYDRATION

Definition

Dehydration is defined as an excessive loss of body fluid. It occurs when more fluids are lost than taken in and the body does not have enough water and other fluids to carry out its normal functions.

Degrees of Dehydration

1. **Mild:** When the body has lost about 2% of its total fluid.
2. **Moderate:** When the total fluid loss reaches 5%.
3. **Severe:** When the body reaches 10% fluid loss, considered a emergency.

Types

1. **Hypotonic or hyponatremic:** When proportionally more sodium than water is lost, the sodium concentration of the

extracellular fluids falls, which therefore becomes hypotonic in comparison to intracellular fluid, so water moves from the extracellular fluid into the cells. This causes cell selling, possibly resulting in the brain swelling (cerebral edema).

2. **Hypertonic or hypernatremic:** When proportionally more water than sodium is lost from the body, the extracellular fluid has increased concentration of sodium and becomes hypertonic regarding the intracellular fluid, and therefore attracts water from the cells. This results in the cell shrinkage, which may cause brain shrinkage.
3. **Isotonic or isonatremic:** When proportionally the same amount of water and sodium is lost from the body, the sodium concentration of the extracellular fluid and hence its tonicity will not change—this is isotonic dehydration.

Causes

1. **External or stress-related causes:**
   - Prolonged physical activity without consuming adequate water especially in a hot and humid environment
   - Prolonged exposure to dry air, e.g. high-flying airplanes [5–15% relative humidity (rh)]
   - Blood loss or hypertension due to physical trauma
   - Diarrhea
   - Hyperthermia
   - Shock
   - Vomiting
   - Burns
   - Lacrimation
   - Use of methamphetamine
   - Drinking of alcohol.
2. **Infectious diseases:**
   - Cholera
   - Gastroenteritis
   - Yellow fever
   - Shigellosis.
3. **Malnutrition:**
   - Electrolyte disturbance, hypernatremia (caused by dehydration) and hyponatremia—especially from restricted salt

- Fasting and rapid loss may reflect progressive depletion of fluid volume.

4. **Other causes:**
    - Severe hyperglycemia, especially in diabetes mellitus
    - Glycosuria.

Signs and Symptoms

Mild-to-moderate dehydration is likely to cause:

1. Dry, sticky mouth.
2. Sleepiness or tiredness—children are likely to be less active than usual.
3. Thirst.
4. Decreased urine output—fewer than six wet diapers a day for infants, and 8 hours or more without urination for older children and teens.
5. Few or no tears when crying.
6. Muscle weakness.
7. Headache.
8. Dizziness or light headedness.

Diagnosis

Initial evaluation may include:

1. Mental status examination to evaluate whether the patient is awake, alert and oriented.
2. Vital signs may include postural readings (BP and respiration).
3. Temperature may be measured to assess fever.
4. Skin will be checked to see, if sweat is present and to assess the degree of elasticity. As dehydration progresses, the skin loses its water content and becomes elastic.
5. The purpose of blood tests is to assess potential electrolyte abnormalities associated with the dehydration.
6. Urine analysis may be done to determine urine concentration. The more concentrated the urine, the more dehydrated the patient.

Treatment

1. Correction of dehydrated state is accomplished by the replenishment of necessary water and electrolytes (rehydration, through oral rehydration therapy or intravenous therapy).

2. When dehydrated, unnecessary sweating should be avoided, as it adds to water loss.
3. If there is only dry food, it is better not to eat, as water is necessary for digestion.
4. The best treatment for minor dehydration is giving water, sports drinks and other fluids that are commercially sold for rehydration—should be used with care, as the balance of electrolytes, which they provide may or may not match the replacement requirements of the individual.
5. For severe cases of dehydration where fainting, unconsciousness or any other severely inhibiting symptom is present (the patient is incapable of standing or thinking clearly), emergency attention is required.
6. Fluids containing a proper balance of replacement electrolytes are given orally or intravenously with continuing assessment of electrolyte status, complete resolution is the norm in all, but the most extreme cases.

Prevention

1. Dehydration is best prevented by drinking plenty of water.
2. The greater the amount of water lost through perspiration, the more water must be consumed to replace it and prevent dehydration.
3. Since the body cannot tolerate large deficits or excesses in total body water, consumption of water must be roughly concurrent with the loss (in other words, if one is perspiring, he/she should also be drinking water frequently).
4. Drinking water slightly beyond the needs of the body entails no risk, since the kidneys will efficiently remove any excess water through the urine with a large margin of safety.

DIARRHEA

Definition

Diarrhea is a condition in which stools are passed more frequently and are looser or more watery than in usual for the person. Three or more loose or watery stools in a day can be considered as diarrhea.

Causes (Fig. 24.1)

- An infection of the bowel by very small germs passed out in the stools
- Lack of cleanliness
- Lack of sanitation
- Food poisoning.

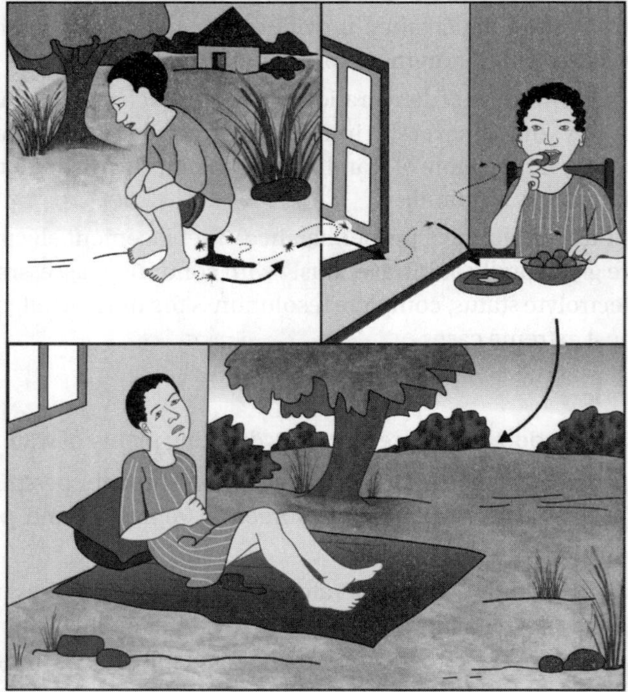

Figure 24.1: Causes of diarrhea

Feeding During and After Diarrhea

Many people think that all foods should be avoided during diarrhea. Foods are needed to replace what is lost during diarrhea. If a child with diarrhea is on breast milk, the mother should continue to breastfeed. Breast milk is safe, clean and nourishing. Breast milk should be given between drinks of oral rehydration solutions:

1. Breast milk supplies the body fluid, calories as well as nutrients and electrolytes such as potassium.

2. Discontinuation of breastfeeding and fasting may lead to decrease in breast milk, and this may make the baby more prone to malnutrition and infections. So-called 'resting the bowel' leads to diminished capacity to absorb glucose, salt, water and amino acids.
3. Small frequent meals should be given between drinks.
4. Feeding a child who is ill requires extra patience, time and care.

Simple Rules for Treating Diarrhea at Home

1. As soon as diarrhea starts, give the child more fluids than usual, such as rice water, fruit juices, coconut water, soup or salt and sugar solution, and breast milk or milk feeds mixed with digested foods for every 5–7 minutes a day, e.g. boiled rice, porridge, soup, egg, fish and well-cooked meat and food that contains potassium, such as banana, carrot and pineapple.
2. Provide sanitary latrines for use by the family. Wash hands thoroughly after using toilets.
3. Feed the child as far as possible.
4. Keep drinking water and food in clean and covered containers to keep off flies and dirt. Use safe drinking water only. Give enough fluids to drink to make up water loss.

Chapter 25

Water Intoxication

Water intoxication, also known as hyperhydration or water poisoning is a potentially fatal disturbance in brain function that results when normal balance of electrolytes in the body is pushed outside the safe limits by overconsumption of water.

RISK FACTORS

1. **Gastroenteritis, particularly in infants and children:** The severe diarrhea and vomiting associated with gastroenteritis can result in very large electrolyte losses. Management of gastroenteritis requires replacing water and electrolytes in proportions that avoid both dehydration and water intoxication. Water will replace lost water and avoid dehydration, but if the person is unable to take any other drink or food, then lost electrolytes will not be replaced, which can result in water intoxication.
2. **Endurance sports:** Marathon runners are susceptible to water intoxication, if they drink too much while running. This happens when sodium levels drop below 135 mmol/L when athletes consume large amounts of fluid.
3. **Overexertion and heat stress:** Any activity or situation that promotes heavy sweating can lead to water intoxication, when water is consumed to replace lost fluids. Persons working in extreme heat or humidity for long periods must take care to drink and eat in ways that help to maintain electrolyte balance.
4. **Iatrogenic:** When an unconscious person is being fed intravenously, the fluids given must be carefully balanced in composition to match fluids and electrolytes lost.

SIGNS AND SYMPTOMS

- Nausea
- Disorientation
- Confusion
- Gastrointestinal disturbances
- Edema
- Muscle cramps
- Slurred speech
- Hyponatremia
- Hydronephrosis.

Occasionally, other symptoms may also present themselves as symptoms of water intoxication, i.e. seizures, coma and death.

TREATMENT

Mild intoxication may remain asymptomatic and require only fluid restriction. In more severe cases, treatment consists of:

1. Diuretics to increase urination, which are most effective for excessive blood volume.
2. Normal saline given intravenously to restore sodium electrolyte levels.
3. Vasopressin receptor antagonists.

PREVENTION

1. The best way to prevent water intoxication is to drink liquids in moderation and to ensure that the daily diet includes sufficient electrolytes (specifically salt).
2. Sports drinks are popular among athletes because they provide the necessary electrolytes to support extended exercise.
3. They help to keep the body balanced and carrying the right amount of fluid, however, for those who do not prefer or want sports drinks. The recommended amount of sodium intake based on a 2,000 calorie diet is 2.5 g every 24 hours.
4. Note that a person's innate sense of thirst will not warn of an impending case of water intoxication. This is because, while the human thirst mechanism accurately detects the level of water in the blood, the human salt craving mechanism does not respond to an acute drop in blood sodium level. So the person does not realize he/she needs sodium, immediately.

Section VII

Balanced Diet

Chapter 26

Balanced Diet Elements

BALANCED DIET

A balanced diet may be defined as one which contains the various groups of foodstuffs such as energy-yielding foods, body-building foods and protective foods in the correct proportions, so that individual is assured of obtaining the minimum requirements of all the nutrients. The components of a balanced diet will differ according to age, sex, physical activity, economic status and the physiological state, viz. pregnancy, lactation and different age groups.

The proper nutrition depends on age and gender, but there are six basic nutrients to consider. Proper nutrition is complex, and exact recommendations depend on the individual. When determining the proper nutrition, one must consider the weight, height, age, gender and activity level. While the best nutritional plan is individualized, six major elements form the basis of all nutritional requirements.

Carbohydrates

Carbohydrates are the body's major source of energy. The fiber found in whole grains, fruits and vegetables also helps to reduce the risk of obesity, cardiovascular diseases and type 2 diabetes. The Food and Nutrition Board recommends getting 45–65% of the daily calories from carbohydrate. If a person follow a 2,000 calorie diet, this means he/she should consume 225–325 g of carbohydrate every day.

Fat

Fat has developed a bad reputation over the years, but it is actually a major nutritional element and a vital aspect of a healthy diet. Fat helps to insulate the body, allowing to maintain the body temperature. Fat also cushions the organs, which can help to protect them from trauma. Although fat is important, too much can be bad for the health. Limit the total fat intake to 20–35% of the daily calories. Aim to meet the fat requirements from unsaturated fats, such as nuts, nut butters, seeds, avocado and olive oil.

Protein

Protein has more physiological roles than any other major nutrient, according to the book *'Nutrition and You'* by Joan Salge Blake. Similar to carbohydrates and fat, protein can provide the body with energy when necessary, but it also helps to maintain water and pH balance. Protein keeps the immune system strong and allows the body to move and bend. Foods rich in protein include meat, poultry, fish, nuts, eggs, milk and milk products. Women should aim to consume 46 g of protein daily, while men should consume 56 g/day.

Vitamins Minerals

Similar to vitamins, minerals are substances that allow the body to grow and develop properly. Minerals are divided into two classes based on how much of each nutrients the body needs. Body needs the major minerals such as sodium, potassium, calcium, phosphorus, magnesium, sulfur and chloride in large amounts, while the trace minerals such as copper, fluoride, zinc, iron, chromium, selenium, iodine, molybdenum and manganese are needed in small amounts. The exact amount needed varies by mineral.

Water

Water is more than a thirst quencher. It is a major nutritional element that helps regulate body temperature, lubricate the joints and protect the major organs and tissues. Water also helps transport important substances such as oxygen, throughout the body. Aim to drink at least eight 8 oz glasses of water every day.

Elements (Essential Nutrients)

Food is made up of specific nutrients such as proteins, carbohydrates, fats, vitamins, minerals and water all of which are necessary for life, growth, body function and tissue repair. Any one food may contain several of these essential nutrients, together with the substances needed to assist their absorption. These essential nutrients can be broken into two main groups.

Macronutrients

Macronutrients include fats, carbohydrates and proteins. They produce energy and are required in quantities easily measurable by a common scale.

Micronutrients

Micronutrients include vitamins and minerals. They are essential for helping the bodies work properly and strengthening the immune system, so that we can resist infections. They are only required in very small or 'microscopic' amounts:

1. A balanced diet is the diet providing all the required nutrients in needed quantities and appropriate proportions. Proper combination of basic food groups makes it possible to formulate a balanced diet at affordable cost.
2. One needs to consider the differing nutrient requirements as per sex, occupation and physiological needs on one hand, and the local and seasonal availability, cost of the foods in the formulation of balanced diets on the other.
3. For guidance, the diet should be formulated in such a way that 60–70%, of total energy (kcal) required is met from carbohydrates, about 10–12% from proteins and the rest of energy from fat.
4. Apart from providing all the essential nutrients in desired amounts, balanced diet must also provide the necessary non-nutrients such as fiber, antioxidants, phytochemicals, which promote health.

Chapter 27

Food Groups

Body needs more than one nutrient to satisfy the body's needs. Food can therefore be divided in groups, so that selection of one or more foods from each group will result in a balanced diet (Fig. 27.1). These food groups are detailed below.

FOOD GROUPS/CATEGORIES

Protein Foods

- Milk and milk products, i.e. curds, butter milk
- Pulses, i.e. dal, gram, lentils, dried beans and peas
- Nuts and oil seeds
- Eggs
- Fish
- Meat, i.e. mutton, poultry, pork and beef.

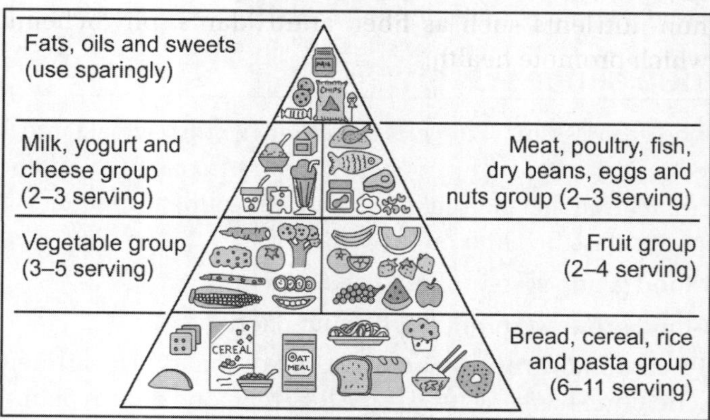

Figure 27.1: Food group system

Protective Foods (Vegetables and Fruits)

One or more from each of the following three groups:

1. **Leafy green vegetables:** Amaranth, radish tops, spinach, fenugreek, drumstick leaves, etc.
2. **Yellow or orange fruits and vegetables:** Carrot, pumpkin, papaya and mango.
3. **Vitamin C-rich fruits and vegetables:** Amla, guava, orange, grape fruit, sweet lime, pineapple and tomato.

Other Vegetables

Flowers, fruits and stems of plants, i.e. brinjal, ladies finger, beans and peas, cucumber, gourds and onions.

Cereals, Roots and Tubers

Rice, wheat, maize, jowar, bajra, ragi and others such as tapioca, potato, yam sweet potato, colocasia (cereals are more nutritious, if at least two different kinds are eaten at the same time).

Fats, Oils, Sugars and Jaggery

Vegetables, oils, vanaspati, ghee, butter, sugar, jaggery, honey fats and sugars are good sources of calories; condiments and spices contain some nutrients, but are used mostly to give flavor. Vegetarians who do not take flesh foods, more pulses and dal should be taken and an increased amount of milk must be used.

FOOD GROUP SYSTEMS

The food group system converts quantitative nutrient data into food-related information that can be used both by consumer and health professionals in diet planning to achieve nutritional adequacy. Food groups are classified into three types:

- **5-food group system:** Based on nutrients
- **3-food group system:** Based on function
- **Other food group system:** United States Department of Agriculture has suggested three different food groups plan:
  - 7-food group plan
  - 4-food group plan
  - 11-food group plan.

5-food Group System (Table 27.1)

Table 27.1: 5-food group system based on nutrients

Food groups	Main nutrients
Cereals, grains and products	
Rice, wheat, ragi, bajra, maize, jowar, barley, rice flakes, wheat flour	Energy, protein, invisible fat, vitamin B_1, B_2, folic acid, iron and fiber
Pulses and legumes	
Bengal gram, black gram, cowpea, peas, rajma, soybeans and beans	Energy, protein, invisible fat, vitamin B_1, B_2, folic acid, calcium, iron and fiber
Milk and meat products	
Milk products: Milk, curd, skimmed milk, cheese, butter, ghee **Meat products:** Chicken, liver, fish, egg, meat	Protein, fat, vitamin B_{12} and calcium Protein, fat and vitamin B_1
Fruits and vegetables	
Fruits: Mango, guava, tomato, papaya, orange, sweet lime, watermelon, pineapple, sapota, etc. **Vegetables:** • **Green leaves:** Amaranth, spinach, gogu, drumstick leaves, coriander leaves, mustard and fenugreek leaves • **Other vegetables:** Carrots, brinjal, ladies finger, capsicum, onion, drumstick, cauliflower, gourds, cucumber, etc.	Carotenoids, folic acid, calcium and fiber
Fats and sugars	
Fats: Butter, ghee, hydrogenated oils, cooking oils such as groundnut, mustard and coconut oil **Sugars:** Sugarcane jaggery, palm jaggery	Energy, fats, essential fatty acids Energy

3-food Group System (Table 27.2)

Table 27.2: 3-food group system based on function

Food groups	Main nutrients
Protective or regulatory foods: Vegetables and fruits	Carotene, vitamin C, mineral, fiber and carbohydrates
Body-building foods: Milk, meat, fish, egg	Protein, vitamins and rich in minerals
Pulses, nuts and oil seeds	Protein, vitamins, mineral and fiber
Energy-giving foods: Cereals, millets, roots and tubers	Carbohydrate
Sugar and jaggery	Only carbohydrate
Fats and oils	Energy, fat and essential fatty acids

Source: Gopalan C, Balasubramanian SC. Nutritive Value of Indian Foods. NIN, ICMR, Hyderabad; 2007.

Other Food Group Systems

7-food Group Plan (Table 27.3)

The 7-food group plan was developed by the United States Department of Agriculture in 1943.

Table 27.3: 7-food group plan

7-food groups	Main nutrients
Green and yellow vegetables	Vitamin C and iron
Oranges, grape fruits and tomato	Vitamin C
Potatoes, fruits and other vegetables	Vitamins and minerals
Milk and milk products	Calcium, phosphorus, protein and vitamins
Meat, poultry, fish and eggs	Proteins, phosphorus, vitamin B
Bread, flour and cereal	Vitamin B_1, B_3, iron and cellulose
Butter	Vitamin A and fat

4-food Group Plan (Table 27.4)

The 4-food group plan was developed by the United States Department of Agriculture in 1956.

Table 27.4: 4-food group plan

4-food groups	Main nutrients
Milk group: Milk, cheese and ice cream	Calcium, phosphorus, proteins and vitamins
Meat group: Beef, pork, lamb, poultry, fish and eggs	Protein, iron and B-complex vitamins
Vegetables, fruits group	Vitamins, minerals and cellulose
Bread, cereals group	Vitamin B_1, B_2, B_3, iron carbohydrates and cellulose

11-food Group Plan

Foods in each of the 11 group are given in Box 27.1.

Box 27.1: 11-food group plan

11-food groups
• Milk, cheese, ice cream • Milk, poultry, fish • Eggs • Dry beans, peas and nuts • Flour, cereals • Citrus fruits, tomatoes • Dark green and leafy vegetables • Potatoes • Other vegetables and fruits • Fats and oils • Sugar syrups and preservatives

Purposes of Food Group System

The food group system can be used by health professionals for the following purpose:

1. **Tool for nutritional assessment and screening:** A brief dietary history system can disclose inadequacies of nutrient from any of the five groups. This information can be the first clue for the possibility of the subject who may be at the risk of developing nutritional deficiency.
2. **Tool for nutritional counseling:** The dietary history based on the 5-food group system allows a health team to counsel or teach a patient about nutrition.
3. **Explaining therapeutic diets to a patient:** Therapeutic diets are scientifically based on nutrient composition and food groups, which can be used in menu planning.
4. **Food labeling and surveillance system:** Food groups can be used for food labeling and nutrition surveillance system.

Chapter 28

Nutritive Value of Common Food Articles

The food is classified on the basis of nutritive value into the following groups:

1. Cereals and millets:
   - Rice
   - Wheat
   - Maize
   - Jowar
   - Bajra
   - Ragi.
2. Pulses and legumes:
   - Grams
   - Peas
   - Beans.
3. Nuts and oil seeds.
4. Vegetables:
   - Green leafy vegetables
   - Roots and tubers
   - Other vegetables:
     - Cauliflower
     - Cabbage.
5. Fruits.
6. Fats and oils.
7. Foods of animal origin (meat, fish and eggs).
8. Milk and milk products.
9. Sugar and jaggery.
10. Spices and condiments.
11. Miscellaneous beverages.

Approximate nutritive value of some common food preparation and some common Indian recipes are given in Tables 28.1 and 28.2 respectively.

Table 28.1: Approximate nutritive value of some common food preparations

Food preparations	Quantity (per serving)	Weight (per serving in g)	Calories (kcal)	Protein (g)	Fat (g)	Carbohydrate (g)	Calcium (g)	Phosphorus (g)	Iron (mg)	Vitamin A value (IU)	Thiamine (mg)	Nicotinic acid (mg)	Riboflavin (mg)	Vitamin C (mg)
Cereal and millet preparations														
Rice preparations														
Plain rice	2 serving	504	595	11.9	0.9	134.8	0.02	0.20	4.8	–	0.20	3.0	0.09	–
"	–	100	118	2.4	0.2	26.8	0.004	0.04	1.0	–	0.04	0.60	0.02	–
Sambar rice	1 serving	485	405	13.5	5.1	76.2	0.08	0.16	3.4	132	0.20	1.70	0.10	5.1
"	–	100	84	2.8	1.05	15.7	0.02	0.03	0.7	27	0.04	0.35	0.02	1.1
Curd rice	1 serving	253	321	6.0	7.0	33.3	0.20	0.10	1.0	242	0.08	0.10	0.2.	2.3
"	–	100	87	2.4	2.8	13.2	0.08	0.04	0.4	96	0.03	0.04	0.08	0.9
Sweet rice	1 serving	177	432	3.6	12.0	77.4	0.01	0.06	0.6	265	0.04	0.50	0.04	–
"	–	100	244	2.0	6.8	43.7	0.006	0.03	0.3	150	0.02	0.28	0.02	–
Idli	2 pcs	136	130	4.6	0.2	27.6	0.03	0.08	0.8	8	0.10	1.2	0.05	–
"	–	100	96	3.4	0.15	20.2	0.02	0.06	0.6	6	0.07	0.9	0.04	–

Contd...

Contd...

Food preparations	Quantity (per serving)	Weight (per serving in g)	Calories (kcal)	Protein (g)	Fat (g)	Carbohydrate (g)	Calcium (g)	Phosphorus (g)	Iron (mg)	Vitamin A value (IU)	Thiamine (mg)	Nicotinic acid (mg)	Riboflavin (mg)	Vitamin C (mg)
Plain dosa	2 pcs	100	216	4.1	9.7	28.2	0.03	0.04	1.5	239	0.10	0.3	0.06	–
Masala dosa	1 pc	100	212	4.6	8.4	29.4	0.04	0.08	1.7	210	0.09	0.8	0.06	3.6
Pongal (hot)	1 serving	148	200	5.5	6.0	30.5	0.0.3	0.07	1.6	174	0.09	0.6	0.08	–
"	–	100	135	3.7	4.1	20.6	0.02	0.05	1.1	118	0.06		0.05	–
Adai (hot)	1 pc	96	193	6.6	4.4	31.8	0.03	0.09	2.2	152	0.10	0.8	0.10	2.5
"	–	100	203	6.9	4.6	33.1	0.03	0.09	2.3	158	0.10	0.8	0.10	2.6
Wheat preparations														
Wheat upma	1 serving	128	163	3.8	5.4	24.7	0.01	0.04	0.7	141	0.05	0.4	0.01	1.2
"	–	100	118	2.8	3.9	17.9	0.007	0.03	0.5	102	0.04	0.3	0.007	0.9
Chapatis	2 pcs	57	193	5.0	5.5	30.8	0.02	0.13	3.0	128	0.20	2.0	0.05	–

Contd...

Contd...

Food preparations	Quantity (per serving)	Weight (per serving in g)	Calories (kcal)	Protein (g)	Fat (g)	Carbohydrate (g)	Calcium (g)	Phosphorus (g)	Iron (mg)	Vitamin A value (IU)	Thiamine (mg)	Nicotinic acid (mg)	Riboflavin (mg)	Vitamin C (mg)
"	–	100	339	8.8	9.6	54.0	0.04	0.23	5.3	224	0.35	3.5	0.09	–
Puris	2 pcs	32	136	2.2	8.4	13.0	0.01	0.06	1.3	50	0.06	0.8	0.02	–
"	–	100	425	6.9	26.3	40.6	0.01	0.18	4.1	15	0.18	2.5	0.06	–
Plain parathas	1 pc	66	304	4.5	19.6	27.3	0.01	0.12	2.7	466	0.08	1.7	0.04	–
"	–	100	461	6.8	29.7	41.4	0.01	0.18	4.1	707	0.12	2.6	0.06	–
Rava idli	2 pcs	114	212	5.0	8.5	28.7	0.06	0.08	0.9	289	0.07	0.5	0.03	1.5
"	–	100	186	4.4	705	25.2	0.05	0.07	0.8	253	0.06	0.41	0.026	1.3
Kesari bath	1 serving	90	282	2.0	14.6	35.3	0.04	0.02	0.40	350	0.03	0.3	0.01	–
'	–	100	313	2.2	16.2	39.2	0.04	0.02	0.44	389	0.03	0.3	0.01	–
Luchi	2 pcs	71	346	4.0	24.0	28.0	0.01	0.03	0.4	583	0.05	0.3	0.02	–
"	–	100	487	5.6	33.8	39.4	0.01	0.04	0.56	821	0.07	0.4	0.03	–

Contd...

Contd...

Food preparations	Quantity (per serving)	Weight (per serving in g)	Calories (kcal)	Protein (g)	Fat (g)	Carbohydrate (g)	Calcium (g)	Phosphorus (g)	Iron (mg)	Vitamin A value (IU)	Thiamine (mg)	Nicotinic acid (mg)	Riboflavin (mg)	Vitamin C (mg)
Millet preparations														
Ragi ball	1 pc	336	446	8.0	7.6	86.8	0.40	0.30	6.0	230	0.50	4.2	0.13	–
"	–	100	133	2.4	2.3	25.8	0.10	0.09	1.8	68	0.15	0.36	0.04	–
Ragi roti	2 pcs	185	460	8.0	9.0	87.0	0.40	0.30	6.0	255	0.50	1.2	0.13	–
"	–	100	249	4.3	4.9	47.0	0.22	0.16	3.2	137	0.27	0.70	0.07	–
Maize roti	2 pcs	142	314	9.6	5.5	56.4	0.01	0.30	1.8	62	0.30	1.2	0.08	–
"	–	100	126	6.8	3.9	39.7	0.007	0.20	1.3	43	0.20	0.8	0.05	–
Jowar roti	2 pcs	150	252	7.5	1.3	52.5	0.02	0.20	4.5	90	0.24	1.3	0.08	–
"	–	100	138	5.0	0.87	35.0	0.01	0.13	3.0	60	0.16	0.87	0.05	–
Ragi puttu	1 plate	146	422	4.4	7.4	84.0	0.20	0.20	3.0	280	0.20	0.6	0.06	–
"	–	100	289	3.3	5.1	57.7	0.14	0.14	5.5	193	0.14	0.4	0.904	–

Contd...

Contd...

Food preparations	Quantity (per serving)	Weight (per serving in g)	Calories (kcal)	Protein (g)	Fat (g)	Carbohydrate (g)	Calcium (g)	Phosphorus (g)	Iron (mg)	Vitamin A value (IU)	Thiamine (mg)	Nicotinic acid (mg)	Riboflavin (mg)	Vitamin C (mg)
Pulse preparations														
Bengal gram dal, cooked	½ cup	151	284	9.0	16.4	25.2	0.07	0.13	3.8	366	0.14	2.4	0.10	2.0
"	–	100	188	6.0	10.9	16.7	0.05	0.09	2.5	242	0.10	1.6	0.07	1.2
Green gram dal, cooked	½ cup	142	171	7.0	7.7	18.4	0.08	0.09	2.7	33	0.14	2.4	0.11	1.6
"	–	100	120	4.9	5.4	12.9	0.06	0.06	1.9	23	0.10	1.7	0.08	1.1
Red gram dal, cooked	½ cup	96	110	6.4	2.0	16.4	0.05	0.07	2.6	64	0.13	0.7	0.7	–
"	–	100	115	6.7	2.1	17.1	0.05	0.07	2.7	65	0.14	0.73	0.73	–
Dal rasam	½ cup	196	29	1.5	0.9	3.8	0.03	0.05	0.9	72	0.03	0.2	0.2	1.5
"	–	100	15	0.8	0.5	1.9	0.02	0.02	0.5	37	0.02	0.1	0.1	0.8
Amaranth sambar	1½ cup	140	97	5.1	2.7	13.0	0.50	0.08	8.0	2009	0.07	0.2	0.03	53.0

Contd...

Food preparations	Quantity (per serving)	Weight (per serving in g)	Calories (kcal)	Protein (g)	Fat (g)	Carbohydrate (g)	Calcium (g)	Phosphorus (g)	Iron (mg)	Vitamin A value (IU)	Thiamine (mg)	Nicotinic acid (mg)	Riboflavin (mg)	Vitamin C (mg)
"	–	100	69	3.6	1.9	9.3	0.36	0.06	5.7	143.5	0.05	0.5	0.02	37.9
Radish sambar	1½ cup	196	101	4.1	3.6	13.1	0.04	0.07	2.2	73	0.07	0.5	0.03	3.0
"	–	100	52	2.1	1.8	6.7	0.02	0.04	1.1	37	0.04	0.26	0.02	1.5
Green gram sundal	1 plate	142	259	13.1	9.2	30.9	0.08	0.20	4.8	120	0.24	1.2	0.10	1.1
"	–	100	182	9.2	6.5	21.8	0.06	0.14	3.4	85	0.17	0.9	0.07	0.8
Bengal gram sundal	1 plate	142	272	13.2	11.1	29.7	0.11	0.15	5.5	198	0.16	1.4	0.08	1.1
"	–	100	192	9.2	7.8	20.1	0.08	0.11	3.9	140	0.11	0.98	0.06	0.8
Cowpea sundal	1 plate	142	255	13.5	8.8	30.3	0.05	0.20	2.5	71	0.30	0.9	0.15	1.1
"	–	100	180	9.5	6.2	21.4	0.03	0.14	1.8	50	0.21	0.6	0.11	0.8

Contd...

Contd...

Food preparations	Quantity (per serving)	Weight (per serving in g)	Calories (kcal)	Protein (g)	Fat (g)	Carbohydrate (g)	Calcium (g)	Phosphorus (g)	Iron (mg)	Vitamin A value (IU)	Thiamine (mg)	Nicotinic acid (mg)	Riboflavin (mg)	Vitamin C (mg)
Vegetable preparations														
Amaranth curry	½ plate	28	47	1.4	2.3	5.1	0.04	0.04	6.6	194.2	0.03	0.4	0.03	51.0
"	–	100	168	5.6	8.2	17.6	0.14	0.14	23.6	693.4	0.11	1.4	0.11	182.2
Brinjal curry	½ plate	45	122	1.4	10.7	4.9	0.02	0.05	0.9	9	0.03	0.5	0.06	10.1
"	–	100	266	3.1	23.8	10.9	0.04	0.11	2.0	20	0.07	1.1	0.13	22.5
Amaranth masala	½ plate	42	46	1.2	2.6	4.4	0.05	0.05	6.8	194.6	0.02	0.4	0.02	55.0
"	–	100	110	3.0	6.2	10.3	1.2	0.12	16.2	463.4	0.05	0.95	0.05	119.1
Cabbage and carrot curry	½ plate	56	81	1.5	5.6	6.1	0.04	0.12	0.9	102.8	0.04	0.3	0.03	38.0
"	–	100	145	2.7	10.0	10.9	0.07	0.21	1.6	183.5	0.07	0.05	0.05	67.9

Contd...

Contd...

Food preparations	Quantity (per serving)	Weight (per serving in g)	Calories (kcal)	Protein (g)	Fat (g)	Carbohydrate (g)	Calcium (g)	Phosphorus (g)	Iron (mg)	Vitamin A value (IU)	Thiamine (mg)	Nicotinic acid (mg)	Riboflavin (mg)	Vitamin C (mg)
Preparations containing milk														
Coffee	–	100	52	1.9	1.7	7.2	0.05	0.05	0.10	77	0.02	0.09	0.09	0.7
"	1 cup	200	104	3.8	3.4	14.4	0.10	0.10	1.20	154	0.04	0.18	0.18	1.4
Tea	–	100	36	0.7	0.8	6.5	0.03	0.02	–	38	0.01	0.05	0.05	0.3
"	1 cup	200	72	1.4	1.6	13.0	0.06	0.04	–	76	0.02	0.10	0.10	0.6
Cocoa	1 cup	200	174	7.5	7.0	20.2	0.20	0.15	0.30	306	0.08	0.2	0.34	2.7
"	–	100	87	3.8	3.5	10.1	0.10	0.08	0.15	153	0.04	0.1	0.17	1.35
Wheat payasam	1 cup	154	178	3.4	4.3	31.5	0.09	0.08	0.40	160	0.05	0.1	0.12	–
"	–	100	116	4.2	2.8	20.5	0.06	0.05	0.26	104	0.03	0.06	0.28	–
Rice payasam	1 cup	154	178	3.2	4.2	31.7	0.09	0.08	0.40	160	0.05	0.1	0.26	–
"	–	100	116	2.1	2.7	20.6	0.06	0.08	0.26	104	0.03	0.06	0.37	–

Contd...

Contd...

Food preparations	Quantity (per serving)	Weight (per serving in g)	Calories (kcal)	Protein (g)	Fat (g)	Carbohydrate (g)	Calcium (g)	Phosphorus (g)	Iron (mg)	Vitamin A value (IU)	Thiamine (mg)	Nicotinic acid (mg)	Riboflavin (mg)	Vitamin C (mg)
Bengal gram dal payasam	1 cup	140	121	7.7	5.1	35.9	0.07	0.14	4.7	197	0.05	0.2	0.40	–
"	–	100	158	5.5	3.6	25.5	0.05	0.10	3.4	141	0.04	0.14	0.28	–
Sago porridge	1 cup	266	227	3.7	4.0	44.0	0.14	0.10	0.70	204	0.60	–	0.23	2.0
"	–	100	85	1.4	1.5	16.5	0.05	0.04	0.26	77	0.02	–	0.09	0.8
Rice porridge	1 cup	280	263	7.6	6.2	44.3	0.30	0.20	0.7	306	0.10	0.3	0.34	2.0
"	–	100	94	2.7	2.2	11.8	0.11	0.07	0.25	109	0.04	0.11	0.12	0.8
Wheat porridge	1 cup	193	317	8.7	8.0	52.7	0.24	0.22	1.0	408	0.13	0.2	0.28	1.6
"	–	100	164	4.5	4.1	27.3	0.12	0.11	0.52	211	0.07	0.1	0.13	0.8
Ragi porridge	1 cup	280	263	6.9	6.3	44.7	0.39	0.20	1.7	321	0.20	0.2	0.34	2.0
"	–	100	94	2.5	2.2	15.8	0.11	0.07	1.61	115	0.07	0.07	0.12	0.7

Contd...

Contd...

Food preparations	Quantity (per serving)	Weight (per serving in g)	Calories (kcal)	Protein (g)	Fat (g)	Carbohydrate (g)	Calcium (g)	Phosphorus (g)	Iron (mg)	Vitamin A value (IU)	Thiamine (mg)	Nicotinic acid (mg)	Riboflavin (mg)	Vitamin C (mg)
Milk (cow)	1 cup	200	130	7.0	7.4	9.8	0.24	0.20	0.8	280	0.06	0.2	0.34	4.0
"	–	100	65	3.5	3.7	4.9	0.12	0.10	0.4	140	0..3	0.1	0.17	2.0
Milk (buffalo)	1 cup	200	216	8.4	16.0	9.2	0.42	0.30	0.8	368	0.06	0.2	0.42	3.4
"	–	100	108	4.2	8.0	4.6	0.21	0.15	0.4	184	0.03	0.1	0.21	1.7
Butter milk (curd from cow milk)	1 cup	200	36	1.8	2.8	2.0	0.07	0.07	0.2	102	0.03	0.10	0.11	0.9
"	–	100	18	0.9	1.4	1.4	0.04	0.04	0.1	51	0.02	0.05	0.06	0.45
Butter milk (curd from buffalo milk)	1 cup	200	66	2.4	5.4	2.8	0.07	0.07	0.2	92	0.02	0.10	0.10	0.9
"	–	100	33	1.2	2.5	1.4	0.04	0.04	0.1	46	0.01	0.05	0.05	0.45

Contd...

Contd...

Food preparations	Quantity (per serving)	Weight (per serving in g)	Calories (kcal)	Protein (g)	Fat (g)	Carbohydrate (g)	Calcium (g)	Phosphorus (g)	Iron (mg)	Vitamin A value (IU)	Thiamine (mg)	Nicotinic acid (mg)	Riboflavin (mg)	Vitamin C (mg)
Egg, fish and meat preparations														
Omelette	1 serving	39	77	5.8	5.7	0.5	0.03	0.10	1.0	140	0.06	0.1	0.15	–
"	–	100	197	14.9	14.6	1.3	0.08	0.26	2.6	210	0.15	2.26	0.38	–
Meat curry	1 serving	128	220	11.6	18.0	2.7	0.10	0.01	2.1	277	0.10	0.9	0.20	2.4
"	–	100	172	9.1	14.1	2.1	0.08	0.08	1.6	216	0.08	0.7	0.16	1.9
Meat fry	1 serving	142	339	21.8	26.0	4.5	0.23	0.20	3.3	294	0.23	7.8	0.30	7.8
"	–	100	239	15.4	18.3	3.2	0.16	0.14	2.3	207	0.16	5.5	0.21	5.4
Fish fry	1 serving	100	220	17.5	16.2	1.4	0.05	0.45	1.2	216	0.11	1.3	0.02	1.0
"	–													
Mutton pulav	2 serving	341	686	20.4	39.0	63.6	0.10	0.22	3.5	100	0.20	6.0	0.20	1.1
"	–	100	201	6.0	11.4	18.7	0.03	0.06	1.03	29	0.06	1.8	0.06	0.32

Table 28.2: Nutritive value of common Indian recipes (range of values per 100 g recipe)

Nutrients	Recipes			Based on pulses	Vegetables	Milk	Egg, meat and fish
	Rice	Wheat	Millets				
Calories (kcal)	84–244	118–487	133–289	15–192	110–266	18–164	172–220
Proteins (g)	2.0–6.9	2.2–8.8	2.4–6.8	0.8–9.5	1.2–5.6	0.35–5.5	6.0–17.5
Fat (g)	0.15–9.7	3.9–33.8	0.87–5.1	0.5–10.9	6.2–23.8	0.4–8.0	11.4–18.3
Carbohydrates (g)	13.2–43.7	17.9–54.0	25.8–57.5	1.9–23.4	8.1–14.6	1.4–27.3	1.3–18.7
Calcium (g)	0.004–0.08	0.007–0.05	0.007–0.22	0.02–0.15	0.04–0.50	0.04–0.21	0.03–0.16
Iron (mg)	0.3–2.3	0.44–5.3	1.3–5.5	0.5–5.7	1.6–23.6	0.05–3.4	1.03–2.6
Vitamin A value (IU)	6–239	15–821	43–193	230–1435	20–6934	19–211	29–2410
Thiamine (mg)	0.02–0.10	0.0–0.35	0.14–0.27	0.02–0.21	0.05–0.11	0.005–0.07	0.03–0.16
Nicotinic acid (mg)	0.04–1.3	0.3–3.5	0.36–0.87	0.1–1.7	0.21–1.4	0.05–0.14	0.26–5.5
Riboflavin (mg)	0.02–0.10	0.007–0.09	0.04–0.07	0.0–0.07	0.05–0.13	0.03–0.28	0.02–0.38
Vitamin C (mg)	0.9–3.6	0.9–1	–	0.8–37.9	22.5–182.2	0.15–4.1	0.32–5.4

CEREALS AND MILLETS

Cereals constitute the bulk of the daily diet. They include rice, wheat, maize, barley, oats and millets. Rice and wheat are called cereals. The term millets is used for smaller grains, which are ground and eaten without having the other layer being removed. They are jowar, maize and bajra, which have been grouped as major millets and ragi as minor millets.

Cereals and millets are the main sources of energy (carbohydrates). They also contribute 6–12% of proteins, minerals and B-group vitamins. In terms of energy, cereals provide about 350 kcal per 100 g. Cereals contribute 70–80% of the total energy intake and more than 50% of protein intake in typical Indian diets. If cereals are eaten with pulses, as in common in the traditional Indian diets, cereal and pulse proteins complement each other and provide a more balanced and 'complete' protein intake.

Rice

Rice is 'paddy' without husk. Rice grain consists of three parts:

- Outer pericarp
- Inner endosperm
- Germ or embryo.

The endosperm is composed of mostly of starch. The aleurone layer and the germ contain most of the essential nutrients. The milling process deprives the rice grain for its valuable nutritive elements (thiamine, riboflavin, protein). The losses may be up to 15% of protein, 75% of thiamine and 60% of riboflavin and niacin.

The white ones are polished rice, although attractive in appearance, is poor in nutritive value. People subsisting mainly on white or polished rice are prone to beriberi, the best known deficiency disease of rice eaters. It is advocated to use undermilled or 'parboiled' rice in place of white rice.

Washing and Cooking

Washing in large quantities of water would remove up to 60% of the water-soluble vitamins and minerals, and draining away the excess of water at the end of cooking leads to further loss of B-group vitamins. Thus the combined effect of washing and cooking may affect seriously the nutritive value of rice. It is therefore best to cook rice in just enough water (about 1 measure of rice for 2½ measures of water).

Parboiling

Parboiling (partial cooking in steam) is an ancient Indian technique of preserving the nutritive quality of rice. There are many techniques of parboiling. The technique recommended by the Central Food Technological Research Institute, Mysuru is known as the 'hot soaking process.'

The process starts with soaking the paddy (unhusked rice) in hot water at 65–70°C for 3–4 hours, which swells the grain. This is followed by draining of water and steaming the soaked paddy in the same container for 5–10 minutes. The paddy is then dried and later home pounded or milled.

During the steaming process, a greater part of the vitamins and minerals are present in the outer layer of the rice grain are driven into the inner endosperm. During drying process, the germ gets attached more firmly to the grain. In addition, the heat used in drying hardens the rice grain. The starch also gets gelatinized, which improve the keeping quality of rice. The serious disadvantage of parboiling is the development of a peculiar 'smell or off flavor,' which some consumers do not relish.

Wheat

Next to rice, wheat is the most important cereal. Wheat contains more protein than rice. In India, wheat is consumed mostly as 'atta,' which is whole grain wheat flour. The other products of wheat are maida and suji.

Maize

Corn ranks next to rice and wheat in world consumption. In certain areas, it is the principal source for proteins and energy. It is also used as a food for cattle and poultry.

Jowar

Jowar is an important cereal crop in India. It is a stable diet for several population groups.

Bajra

Bajra is grown in the dry belts of Northern peninsular India, e.g. Rajasthan, Gujarat and Maharashtra, where it forms the stable food of large sections of the population.

Ragi

Ragi is the cheapest among millets. Ragi flour is cooked and eaten as porridge. Ragi is rich in calcium. Ragi is popular millet in Andhra Pradesh and Karnataka.

PULSES AND LEGUMES

Pulses comprise a variety of grams, also known as 'dal.' Most commonly eaten pulses are Bengal gram (chana), red gram dal (tuvar or arhar), green gram (moong) and black gram (urad). Other includes 'lentils (masur), peas and beans including soybean.' Khesari dal (*Lathyrus sativus*) is consumed in parts of Madhya Pradesh, Uttar Pradesh and Bihar, excessive consumption of which is associated with lathyrism.

Pulses contain 20–25% of proteins. In fact, pulses contain more protein than eggs, fish or flesh foods. But in regard to quality, pulse proteins are inferior to animal proteins. Pulse proteins are poor in 'methionine' and to lesser extent in 'cystine.' In addition, pulses are rich in minerals and B-group vitamins such as 'riboflavin' and 'thiamine.' In dry state, pulses do not contain vitamin C. Germinating pulses, however, contain higher concentration of vitamins, especially vitamin C and B. Fermentation also enhances vitamin content, particularly that of 'riboflavin, thiamine and niacin.'

Antinutritional Factors

In the raw state, pulses have some antinutritional factors such as phytates and tannins, which adversely affect the availability to the body of some nutrients. However, most of the antinutritional factors are destroyed by heat. Presence of high amounts of certain sugars known as 'oligosaccharides' is known to be associated with flatulence.

Soybean

Soybean is the richest among pulses. It contains about 40% of protein, 20% of fat and 4% of minerals. Soybean is exceptionally rich in protein, containing up to 40%. Soybean can be cooked and eaten as dal. It can be tried in other forms such as mixing its powder with atta for chapatis; soybean milk and curd, and in baby foods. Soybean is yet to become popular in this country despite more than 50 years of publicity.

VEGETABLES

Vegetables are grouped as 'protective foods'; their value resides in their high vitamin and mineral content. Vegetables usually have a large water content, low energy and protein content, and varying amounts of 'dietary fiber.' Some vegetables, e.g. green peas and beans are also good sources of protein. Vegetables are divided into three groups namely green leaves, roots and tubers, and others.

Green Leaves

The term 'green leaves' designates a number of indigenous leafy vegetables consumed by the people. They include palak (spinach), amaranth, cabbage, fenugreek (methi), etc. The darker the green leaves, the greater their nutritive value. Green leaves are rich sources of carotenes, calcium, iron and vitamin C. They are also fair sources of riboflavin, folic acid and many other nutrients. Leafy vegetables are high in water content and dietary fiber.

Note: 100 g leafy vegetables give 25–50 kcal of energy. Because of their low calorie value and large bulk, they have an important place in the dietaries of obese people who wish to cut down their calorie intake. The recommended daily intake of green leafy vegetables is about 40 g for an adult.

Roots and Tubers

- Included in this group are potato, sweet potato, tapioca, yam, carrots, onion, radish and colocasia
- Potatoes and tapioca are good sources of carbohydrate; carrots, are exceptionally high in beta carotene
- The recommended daily intake of roots and tubers is 50–60 g for an adult.

Other Vegetables

There is a wide range of 'other' vegetables such as brinjal, tomatoes, cauliflower, etc. Many of them are fair sources of minerals and vitamins. The daily recommended intake is 60–70 g.

NUTS AND OILS SEEDS

Included in this group are groundnut (also called peanut), cashew nut, coconut, walnut, almonds, pistachio, mustard seeds, sesame seeds, cotton seeds, sunflower seeds, maize germ and many others from which cooking oils are extracted. Nuts and oil seeds contain good amounts of fat and good quality protein in small quantity.

Regarding the fat content, walnuts contain 64.5%, almonds 58.7%, cashew nuts 46.9% and groundnut 40%. Regarding protein content, groundnut tops the list with 26.7%. Nuts are good sources of vitamins of the B group. They contribute minerals such as calcium, phosphorus and iron. Cashew nuts and almonds are good sources of iron, but pistachio is the richest containing 14 mg of iron per 100 g.

Most of the vegetable oils are rich in essential fatty acids. After oil extraction in the case of some, the residue (oilseed cake can be formulated into acceptable foods rich in protein). However, nuts eaten in mixed diet are extremely valuable source of protein. Peanuts for human consumption should be thoroughly dried and properly stored to avoid the growth of *Aspergillus flavus,* which produces 'aflatoxin.'

FRUITS

Fruits are invaluable in human nutrition. They are prized for their vitamins, e.g. vitamin C, carotene and minerals. Some fruits such as banana and mango have a high caloric value because of their sugar content. Fruits can be eaten raw and fresh.

Dried fruits such as raisins, dates and apricots are good sources of calcium and iron. Fruits furnish dietary fiber, which assists in normal bowel function. Nutrition experts recommend a daily intake of 85 g or more of fresh fruit for maintenance of good health.

ANIMAL FOODS

Foods of animal origin include meat, poultry, fish, eggs, milk and dairy products (Table 28.3). They provide high-quality protein (containing all the essential amino acids) and good amount of fats, besides some vitamins and minerals.

Vitamin B_{12} is one of the rare nutrients found only in animal foods. Since animal foods are expensive, consumed in small amounts in

Table 28.3: Nutritive value of meat, fish and eggs (g/100 g)

Food items	Proteins	Fat	Minerals
Meat (goat)	21.4	3.6	1.1
Fish	19.5	2.4	1.5
Egg (hen)	13.3	13.3	1.0
Liver	20.0	3.0	1.3

most developing countries. Among the animal foods, cow's milk and hen's egg are perhaps nature's two most nearly perfect foods.

Egg

Egg contains all the nutrients except carbohydrate and vitamin C. About 12% of egg is made of shell, 58% of egg white and 30% of egg yolk. An egg weighing 60 g contains 6 g of protein, 6 g of fat, 30 mg of calcium and 1.5 mg of iron and supplies about 70 kcal of energy.

Except for vitamin C, egg contain all the fat-soluble and water-soluble vitamins in appreciable amount. Boiled egg is nutritionally superior to raw egg. The cholesterol content of egg is 250 mg/egg. A reduction in intake of eggs is advised for those at risk of coronary heart disease (CHD). Two large eggs without shell weigh about 100 g.

Fish

Fish is a nutritious food rich in protein (15–25%) with a good biological value and a satisfactory amino acid balance. Fish liver oils are the richest source of vitamins A and D. Fish bones when eaten are an excellent source of calcium, phosphorus and fluorides. Sea fish contain iodine. Of all the sea foods, oysters and lobsters are the richest in iodine. The fish proteins are easily digested. The nutritive value of diet is greatly enhanced by inclusion of fish.

Meat

The term 'meat' is applied to the flesh of cattle, sheep and goats. Meat contain 15–20% of protein, which is less than that found in pulse. Meat proteins are a 'good source of essential amino acids'. The iron content in per 100 g meat is 2–4 mg. Besides iron, meat provides minerals such as zinc and B-group vitamins. It is poor in calcium and phosphorus.

MILK

Milk is the best and most complete of all foods. It is a fine blend of all the nutrients necessary for growth and development of the young ones. Thus, milk is good source of proteins, fats, sugars, vitamins and minerals (Table 28.4). It is so created by animals to serve as the sole and wholesome food for their suckling young ones.

Table 28.4: Comparison of nutritive value of milk (values per 100 g)

Content	Buffalo	Cow	Goat	Human
Fat (g)	8.8	4.1	4.5	3.4
Protein (g)	4.3	3.2	3.3	1.1
Lactose (g)	5.1	4.4	4.6	7.4
Calcium (mg)	210	120	170	28
Vitamin (mg)	1	2	1	3
Minerals (g)	0.8	0.8	0.8	0.1
Water (g)	83.00	87.25	87.50	88.20
Energy (kcal)	117	67	72	65

Proteins

The chief protein of milk is casein. It occurs in combination with calcium as calcium caseinate. The other proteins present in the milk are 'lactalbumin and lactoglobulin.' Milk proteins contain all the essential amino acids. Animal milks contain nearly three times such protein as human milk. The human milk proteins contain greater amounts of tryptophan and sulfur-containing amino acids (especially cysteine) than the animal proteins.

Fat

The fat content of milk varies from 3.4% (human milk) to 8.8% (buffalo milk). Milk fat is a good source of retinol and vitamin D.

Sugar

The carbohydrate content in all sources of milk is lactose or milk sugar. It is less sweet than cane sugar and is readily fermented by lactic acid bacilli. Human milk contains more sugar than animal milks.

Minerals

Milk contains calcium, phosphorus, sodium, potassium, magnesium, cobalt, copper and iodine. Milk is particularly rich in calcium. It is a poor source of iron. Milk is a good source of all vitamins except vitamin C.

MILK PRODUCTS

We consume milk in variety of forms as whole milk, butter, ghee, cheese, dried and condensed milk, khoa, ice cream, etc. Milk from which fat has been removed, is known as 'skimmed milk.' It is devoid of fat and fat-soluble vitamins, but a good source of milk protein (35%) and calcium.

Toned Milk

Toned milk is a blend of natural milk and made-up milk. Toned milk contains one part of water, one part of natural milk and one-eighth part of skim milk powder. The mixture is stirred, pasteurized and supplied in bottles. Toned milk has a composition nearly equivalent to cow's milk. It is much cheaper and yet a wholesome product.

Vegetable Milk

Milk prepared from certain vegetable foods (groundnut, soybean) is termed vegetable milk. It may be used as a substitute for animal milk.

FATS AND OILS

Fats, which are liquid at room temperature are called oils. Fats and oils are good sources of energy and fat-soluble vitamins. Fats of animal origin are poor sources of essential fatty acids. Those of vegetable origin are rich in polyunsaturated fatty acids, except coconut and palm oils. The vegetable oils contain no vitamin A and D. The vegetable oils of red palm oil is extremely rich in carotene.

SUGAR AND JAGGERY

Sugar is produced from sugarcane in India and from sugar beet elsewhere. Jaggery is prepared from sugarcane in India and is consumed in place of sugar. It contains useful amounts of carotene and iron derived from cooking pans. Honey consists of about 75% sugars, mostly fructose and glucose.

CONDIMENTS AND SPICES

Condiments and spices includes asafetida, cardamom, chilies, garlic, cloves, ginger, mustard, pepper, tamarind, turmeric, etc. They are used to enhance the palatability of foods and stimulating appetite. The essential oils present in them have carminative properties and may aid in digestion. Excessive consumption of condiments is associated with peptic ulcer.

MISCELLANEOUS

Beverages

Beverages include drinks, which are appreciated for their flavor or their stimulating properties. They are classified as follows:

1. Coffee, tea, cocoa.
2. Soft drinks: Aerated water, lemonade, Pepsi, Cola, fruit juices, etc.
3. Alcoholic beverages: Wine, beer, whisky and traditional preparations. Alcoholic beverages are rich in calories.

Coffee, Tea and Cocoa

Coffee: It contains caffeine, volatile oils (caffeol) and tannic acid. When coffee seeds are roasted, tannin is destroyed, protein are coagulated and the pleasant aroma is liberated.

Tea: There are two main varieties of tea, the green and the black varieties. Green tea is more astringent than the black variety. The chemical composition of tea is as follows:

- **Caffeine:** 2–6%
- **Tannic acid:** 6–12%
- **Theophylline:** Traces
- **Essential volatile oils:** 5%.

Tea is prepared by adding leaves to boiling water. When milk is added, the casein of milk combines with tannin and forms a harmless complex.

Cocoa: It is obtained from cocoa beans. It is rich in fat and contains theobromine, which has stimulating properties. The caloric value of coffee tea and cocoa in kilocalorie value (per cup or 75 mL) is coffee 98.0 kcal, tea 79.0 kcal and cocoa 213.0 kcal.

Soft Drinks

The principal ingredients of soft drinks are carbon dioxide, sugars, acids such as citric acid or tartaric acid, and also coloring and flavoring agents. Some are carbonated and others noncarbonated, e.g. fruit juices. Fruit beverages comprise fruit juices, squashes, etc.

Alcoholic Beverages

Alcoholic beverages are beer, whisky, rum, gin, arrack, etc. Alcohol supplies about 7 kcal per gram. The alcohol content in beers is 4.5–6%, 40–45% in whisky, rum, gin and brandy.

Vinegar

Natural vinegar is made from fermentation of fruits, malt and molasses. It contains a minimum of 3.7% acetic acid. Synthetic vinegar should not be harmful, if it is free from lead, copper, arsenic or mineral acids. Synthetic vinegar should be distinctly labeled 'synthetic' according to Prevention of Food Adulteration Act rules.

Chapter 29

Recommended Daily Allowances

NUTRIENT REQUIREMENT

For using balanced diet, recommended daily allowances (RDAs) are the professional tools, which are very essential to know the daily requirements for different nutrients for different age groups. The RDAs take into account individual variation in nutrient needs and also the availability of nutrients, which may vary from diet to diet. RDAs are considered daily food guide for meal planning, as it provides guidelines regarding amount of nutrients to be actually consumed in order to meet the requirements of the body. RDAs are based on gender, age, body size, type of activity and physiological state. Diseases and drugs prescribed for treatment can alter the requirement for one or more nutrients.

Man requires a wide range of nutrients to keep himself healthy and active. The information on physiological requirement of nutrients to be practical, values must be translated in terms of foods consumed in habitual diets. The science of human nutrition is mainly concerned with defining the nutritional requirements for the promotion, protection and maintenance of health in all groups of population. A variety of terms have been used to define the amount of nutrients needed by the body such as:

- Optimum requirements
- Minimum requirements
- Recommended daily allowances or intakes
- Safe level intake.

Out of these, the term RDA has been widely accepted. International organizations such as Food and Agriculture Organization (FAO) and World Health Organization (WHO) have also undertaken this exercise on a global scale. Expert committees of different countries examine the available information on nutrient requirement and the national food habit arrive at what is normally called recommended dietary or daily allowances, or recommended dietary intakes (RDIs).

DEFINITION OF RDA

1. The RDA is defined as the intake of nutrient derived from diet, which keeps nearly all people in good health (according to ICMR).
2. The RDA is defined as the amount of nutrient present in diet, which satisfies the daily requirement of nearly all normal individuals in a population.
3. The term RDA is defined as the amount of nutrients sufficient for the maintenance of health in all people. They are reference standards of nutritional intake. The value will meet the requirements of 97.5% of the population. In fact, for many individuals, this level will be in excess of their needs.
4. The RDAs as the levels of intake of essential nutrients considered in the judgment of the committee on dietary allowances of the Food and Nutrition Board, on the basis of available scientific knowledge, to be adequate to meet the nutritional needs of practically all healthy persons.
5. The word 'allowances' should not be confused with the word 'requirement'. An individual's requirement for nutrients is influenced by numerous physical, environmental and social factors, and dietary habits, which are interdependent on one another. The allowances are the amounts of nutrients to be actually consumed.

REFERENCE RANGE (TABLE 29.1)

For Man and Woman

There is a need to define the characteristics of reference person for whom the RDA is being prescribed. For this purpose, normal Indian adult man, woman, infant and children are considered. In case of children, body weight and height of well-nourished healthy children published by WHO for children under 5 years and adolescents drawn from several developing countries are used.

For Man

Man is between 20–30 years of age and weighs 60 kg. He is free from diseases and physically fit for active work. On each working day, he

Table 29.1: Characteristics of reference person

Characteristics	Adult (man)	Adult (woman)
Age (year)	20–39	20–39
Weight (kg)	60	50
Height (cm)	163	151

is employed for 8 hours in occupation that usually involves moderate activity. While not at work, he spends 8 hours in bed, 4–6 hours sitting and moving around, and 2 hours in walking and in active recreation.

For Woman

Woman is between 20 and 39 years of age, healthy and weighs 50 kg. She may be engaged for 8 hours in general household work, in light industry or in other moderately active work. Apart from 8 hours in bed, she spends 4–6 hours sitting or moving around only through light activity and 2 hours in walking or in household duties.

FACTORS AFFECTING RDA

The nutritional requirements are affected by several factors:

1. **Age (infants, adolescents, aged):** An infant requires more protein per kilogram of body weight than an adolescent, since their metabolic rate is much faster than that of adolescents.
2. **Sex (male or female):** Adolescent girls require more iron than adolescent boys, in order to replace the iron lost during menstruation every month.
3. **Body size (height, weight, stature):** A tall heavily built man needs more calories than small statured man, since his body surface area is more than that of the latter.
4. **Physiological state (pregnancy, lactation):** Pregnant woman requires more nutritious food than an ordinary adult woman, since she has to meet the additional nutritional requirements of the growing fetus.
5. **Type of work (sedentary, moderate, heavy work):** A sedentary worker requires less calories than a heavy worker, since the former expands less energy than the latter during work.

RECOMMENDING AUTHORITIES

The dietary allowances for Indians were first recommended by nutritional advisory group in 1944. These were revised in 1958, 1978 and last in 1988 by expert group constituted by Indian Council of Medical Research (ICMR, 1990). Recommended dietary allowances for specific nutrients are:

1. Protein allowance recommended is about 1 g/kg body weight per day. S0ince Indians are predominantly vegetarians, this protein is derived from a mixture of vegetable foods. Proteins of animal origin have superior biological value as compared to vegetable proteins.
2. The intake of fat should be limited, not more than 15% of the calories in the diet. At least 15 g of vegetable oils should be included in the diet, to meet the requirements of essential fatty acids.
3. About 70% of the total caloric requirement may be met through intake of carbohydrates.
4. Allowance of phosphorus is not mentioned, since most of the dietary ingredients are rich in phosphorus.
5. A normal well-balanced diet generally meets the requirements for trace elements such as Mg, Cu, I_2, etc. Hence no RDA is mentioned.
6. Vitamin A is found either as retinol or beta carotene in the diet.
7. Vitamin D is formed in the body by conversion of its precursor by the action of sunlight.
8. The requirements for B_1, B_2 and B_3 are related to the calorie intake of the person.

USES OF RDA

1. The RDAs are very useful to evaluate the adequacy of the national food supply and setting goal for food production.
2. For setting the standards for menu planning, for the funds and various nutritional programs [Mission Mode Projects (MMP), Integrated Child Development Service (ICDS)].
3. To evaluate the nutritional policy for public assistance, nurseries and homes, and to establish guidelines for food assistance program.
4. To interpret the adequacy of diet in food consumption, studies and surveillance.
5. Used to develop materials for nutritional education.
6. Used for setting the patterns for diet in hospitals.
7. For setting guidelines for formation of new products and location of specific food.

8. To develop food guides and evaluate new food products.
9. To evaluate the adequacy of food supplies in relation to nutritional needs.
10. To establish guidelines for labeling of food from the nutritional stand point of view.

CONDITIONS FOR OPERATING RDAS

The RDAs are operative under following conditions:

1. While defining RDA for a particular nutrient, the intakes of all the other nutrients are considered to be at a safe level, since utilization of any nutrient is influenced by adequacy of other nutrient.
2. The RDA suggested for individuals are for well-nourished healthy individuals.
3. Allowances for undernourished or malnourished individuals and affected by diseases or infection may be higher.

LIMITATIONS OF RDA

1. These are very complex for direct use by the consumers. Only health personnel, dieticians and others who have studied this subject can only use.
2. They do not state ideal for optimal levels of intake. These are only concepts, which cannot be realized.
3. Data on food contents of some nutrients is limited.
4. The RDAs do not evaluate nutritional status because the allowances are higher than the requirements.
5. The RDAs do not apply to the sick people. They require increased or decreased level of nutrients.
6. Calculation of RDAs is time-consuming process.
7. The RDAs cannot be used at Nutrition Educational Programs, because it is very difficult to calculate RDA and more number of people may attend these programs.
8. The RDAs do not apply to Public Food Assistance Programs, because people are having different needs and it is not a easy way to fulfill their needs.

RECOMMENDED DIETARY INTAKE

1. Each day our body needs a number of nutrients to carry out its activities efficiently. A lot of research has been carried out to determine the nature and quantity of nutrients, which a healthy person needs each day.

2. The nutritional requirements of Indian people have been worked out and presented as RDI for Indians. These have been set up by an advisory committee of the Indian Council of Medical Research (ICMR).
3. In a number of studies, the harmful effects of nutrient deficiencies on the human body and its function were observed. These were so revealing that it is necessary to set up a committee to review available experimental data and RDA for each of the nutrients that were known at that time.
4. During the Second World War (1939–1945), the military recruiting officers had to reject a number of young men, who wanted to enlist because they were underweight. Another related problem was the need to estimate the amount of food to be sent to various army units. This led to the setting up of RDA in a number of countries between 1940 and 1944.
5. India was one of the first countries to set up RDA in 1944. On the basis of new research findings, these recommendations have been revised in 1958, 1968, 1981 and 2010.
6. The word 'recommended' is used to emphasize that values need to be revised periodically on the basis of new research data.

The RDIs of nutrients for an adult reference woman and man are given in Table 29.2.

Table 29.2: Recommended dietary intakes of nutrients (Indians)

Nutrient	Reference (man)	Reference (woman)
Energy (kcal)	2,400	1,900
Proteins (g)	55	45
Calcium (mg)	400–500	400–500
Iron (mg)	24	32
Water-soluble vitamins		
Vitamin C (mg)	40	40
B vitamins—B_1 (mg)	1.2	1.0
Niacin (mg)	16	13
Fat-soluble vitamins		
Vitamin A—retinol (µg)	750	750
Beta carotene	3,000	3,000
Vitamin D (IU) (1 IU = 0.025 µg)	200	200

Uses of RDIs

The recommended dietary intakes for nutrients have a number of practical uses. These are:

- To enable government to predict food needs of the people
- To provide basis for food distribution quota
- To guide agricultural planning policy
- To guide policy of food export and import
- To guide planning of nutritionally adequate diets for inmates of large catering establishments such as hospitals, hostels, hotels, army canteens, etc.
- To evaluate the findings of food consumption and surveys of various population groups
- Nutrient needs vary with age, activity and physiological status such as pregnancy and lactation. Our physical activity is normally depended on our occupation.

Chapter 30

Calculation of Balanced Diet for Different Categories

BALANCED DIET

Based on the RDA, balanced diets for various groups of individuals were suggested and updated by the 1979 Committee of Indian Council of Medical Research (ICMR). A new set of balanced diets based on the latest recommended dietary allowances have been formulated. The constraints used in developing the balanced diets are given below (Table 30.1):

- Energy derived from cereals should be not more than 75% of total requirement
- Ratio of cereal protein to pulse protein should be between 4:1 and 5:1
- Minimum level of leafy vegetables has been kept to 80 g or less and all vegetables put together to be not more than 150 g
- A minimum milk intake of 100 mL is required
- Energy derived from fat or oil not to exceed 15% of total calories.

Table 30.1: Balanced diets (the quantities are given in grams)

Food items		Adult man			Adult woman		Children		Boys	Girls
	Sedentary	Moderate work	Heavy work	Sedentary	Moderate work	Heavy work	1–3 year	4–6 year	10–12 year	10–12 year
Cereals	460	520	670	410	440	575	175	270	420	380
Pulses	40	50	60	40	45	50	35	35	45	45
Leafy vegetables	40	40	40	100	100	50	40	50	50	50
Other vegetables	60	70	80	40	40	100	20	30	50	50
Roots and tubers	50	60	80	50	50	60	10	20	30	30
Milk	150	200	250	100	150	200	300	250	250	250
Oil and fat	40	45	65	20	25	40	15	25	40	35
Sugar/Jaggery	30	35	55	20	20	40	30	40	45	45

SUBSTITUTION FOR NONVEGETARIANS (TABLE 30.2)

Table 30.2: Suggested substitution for nonvegetarians

Food item, which can be elected from non-vegetarian diets	Substitution that can be suggested for deleted item
50% of pulses (20–30 g)	One egg or 30 g of fish, additional 5 g of fat or oil
100% of pulses (40–60 g)	Two eggs or 50 g of meat or fish, 10 g of fat or oil

DURING PREGNANCY AND LACTATION (TABLE 30.3)

Table 30.3: Additional allowances during pregnancy and lactation

Food items	During pregnancy (g)	Calories (kcal)	During lactation (g)	Calories (kcal)
Cereals	35	118	60	203
Pulses	15	52	30	105
Milk	100	83	100	83
Fat	–	–	10	90
Sugar	10	40	10	40
Total		293		521

PRESCHOOL CHILDREN (TABLE 30.4 AND 30.5)

Table 30.4: Recommended nutrient allowances for preschool children (ICMR, 1968)

Nutrients	1–3 year	4–6 year
Calories (kcal)	1,200	1,500
Proteins (g)	17–20	22
Calcium (g)	0.4–0.5	0.4–0.5
Iron (mg)	15–20	15–20
Vitamin A (µg)	250	300
Ascorbic acid (mg)	30–50	30–50
Thiamine (mg)	0.6	0.8
Riboflavin (mg)	0.7	0.8
Nicotinic acid (mg)	8	10
Folic acid (µg)	50–100	50–100
Vitamin B_{12} (µg)	0.5–1.0	0.5–1.0
Vitamin D (IU)	200	200

Table 30.5: Balanced diets at high, moderate and low costs for preschool children

Foodstuffs	High cost				Moderate cost				Low cost			
	1–3 year		4–6 year		1–3 year		4–6 year		1–3 year		4–6 year	
	V* (g)	NV† (g)	V (g)	NV (g)	V (g)	NV (g)	V (g)	NV (g)	V (g)	NV (g)	V (g)	NV (g)
Cereals	100	100	140	140	120	120	170	170	150	150	200	200
Pulses	30	20	40	30	50	40	60	50	50	40	60	50
Green leafy vegetables	50	50	75	75	50	50	75	75	50	50	75	75
Other vegetables (e.g. roots and tubers)	30	30	30	30	30	30	50	50	30	30	50	50
Fruits	100	100	100	100	100	100	100	100	50	50	50	50
Milk	1,000	700	1,000	700	600	400	600	400	300	200	250	200
Fats and oils	20	20	25	25	20	20	25	25	20	20	25	25
Meat, fish and eggs	–	30	–	30	–	40	–	50	–	30	30	–
Sugar and jaggery	30	30	40	40	30	30	40	40	30	30	40	40

*V, vegetarian; †NV, nonvegetarian.

NUTRITIONAL REQUIREMENTS OF SCHOOL CHILDREN AND ADOLESCENTS

Data regarding the mean daily nutritional requirements of school children suggested by the ICMR. Balanced diet for this category at different levels of cost are detailed in Tables 30.6 to 30.9.

Table 30.6: Dietary requirements of school children and adolescents (ICMR Nutrition Expert Group, 1968)

Nutrients	School children		Adolescents (13–18 year)	
	7–9 year	10–12 year	Boys	Girls
Calories (kcal)	1,800	2,100	2,500–3,000	2,200
Protein (g)	33	41	55–60	50
Calcium (g)	0.4–0.5	0.4–0.5	0.5–0.7	0.5–0.7
Iron (mg)	15–20	15–20	25–35	25–35
Vitamin A (retinol) (µg)	400	600	750	750
Carotene (µg)	1,600	2,400	3,000	3,000
Thiamine (mg)	0.9	1.0	1.3–1.5	1.1
Riboflavin (mg)	1.0	1.2	1.4–1.7	1.2
Nicotinic acid (mg)	10	14	17–21	14
Ascorbic acid (mg)	30–50	30–50	30–50	30–50
Folic acid (µg)	50–100	50–100	50–100	50–100
Vitamin B_{12} (µg)	0.5–1.0	1.0	1.0	1.0
Vitamin D (IU)	200	200	200	200

Table 30.7: Balanced diets (g) at high cost for school children and adolescents

Foodstuffs	School children						Adolescents			
							Boys		Girls	
	7–9 year		10–12 year		13–15 year		16–18 year		13–18 year	
	V*	NV†	V	NV	V	NV	V	NV	V	NV
Cereals	200	200	260	260	370	370	390	390	290	290
Pulses	40	30	40	30	50	30	50	30	50	30
Green leafy vegetables	75	75	100	100	100	100	100	100	150	150
Other vegetables	50	50	75	75	75	75	100	100	75	75
Fruits	100	100	100	100	100	100	100	100	100	100
Milk	1,000	700	1,000	700	1,000	700	1,000	700	1,000	700
Fats and oils	30	30	35	35	35	40	45	50	35	40
Meat, fish and eggs	–	90	–	90	–	120	–	120	–	120
Sugar and jaggery	50	50	50	50	30	30	40	40	30	30
Peanut (roasted)	30	20	40	30	40	30	50	30	50	30

*V, vegetarian; †NV, nonvegetarian.

Table 30.8: Balanced diets (g) at moderate cost for school children and adolescents

Foodstuffs	School children						Adolescents			
							Boys		Girls	
	7–9 year		10–12 year		13–15 year		16–18 year		13–18 year	
	V*	NV†	V	NV	V	NV	V	NV	V	NV
Cereals	220	220	290	290	400	400	420	420	320	320
Pulses	70	60	70	60	70	50	70	50	70	50
Green leafy vegetables	75	75	100	100	100	100	100	100	150	150
Other vegetables (roots and tubers)	50	50	75	75	150	150	175	175	150	150
Fruits	100	100	100	100	100	100	100	100	100	100
Milk	600	400	600	400	600	400	600	400	600	400
Fats and oils	30	30	30	30	30	30	40	40	30	30
Meat, fish and eggs	–	60	–	60	–	80	–	80	–	80
Sugar and jaggery	30	30	30	30	30	30	30	30	30	30
Peanut (roasted)	30	20	40	30	40	30	50	30	50	30

*V, vegetarian; †NV, nonvegetarian.

Table 30.9: Balanced diets (g) at low cost for children and adolescents (ICMR Nutrition Expert Group, 1968)

Foodstuffs	School children						Adolescents			
							Boys		Girls	
	7–9 year		10–12 year		13–15 year		16–18 year		13–18 year	
	V*	NV†	V	NV	V	NV	V	NV	V	NV
Cereals	250	250	320	320	430	430	450	450	350	350
Pulses	70	60	70	60	70	50	70	50	70	50
Green leafy vegetables	75	75	100	100	100	100	100	100	150	150
Other vegetables (roots and tubers)	50	50	75	75	150	150	175	175	150	150
Fruits	50	50	50	50	30	30	30	30	30	30
Milk	250	200	250	200	250	150	250	150	250	150
Fats and oils	30	30	35	35	35	40	45	50	35	40
Meat, fish and eggs	–	30	–	30	–	30	–	30	–	30
Sugar and jaggery	50	50	50	50	30	30	40	40	30	30
Peanut (roasted)	–	–	–	–	–	–	50	50	–	–

*V, vegetarian; †NV, nonvegetarian.

DIETS FOR PREGNANT AND NURSING MOTHERS

Balanced diets at low cost suggested by the ICMR Nutrition Expert Group for pregnant and lactating women are given below. It will be observed that the diets contain minimal amounts of milk and other animal foods, which are costly. The diets include fair amounts of legumes and green leafy vegetables. Balanced diets at moderate and high costs are also given in Tables 30.10 to 30.12. The recommended daily nutrients allowance for this group is given in Table 30.13.

Table 30.10: Balanced diets for normal, pregnant and lactating women (low cost) (ICMR Expert Group, 1968)

	Normal women						Additional allowances during	
	Sedentary work		Moderate work		Heavy work		Pregnancy	Lactation
Foodstuffs	V*	NV†	V	NV	V	NV	V	NV
Cereals	300	300	350	350	475	475	50	100
Pulses	60	45	70	55	70	55	–	10
Green leafy vegetables	125	125	125	125	125	125	125	125
Other vegetables	75	75	75	75	100	100	–	–
Roots and tubers	50	50	75	75	100	100	–	–
Fruits	30	30	30	30	30	30	–	–
Milk	200	100	200	100	200	100	125	125
Fats and oils	30	35	35	40	40	45	–	15
Sugar and jaggery	30	30	30	30	40	40	10	20
Meat and fish	–	30	–	30	–	30	–	–
Eggs	–	30	–	30	–	30	–	–
Peanut (roasted)	–	–	–	–	40	40	–	–

*V, vegetarian; †NV, nonvegetarian.

Table 30.11: Balanced diets (g) for normal, pregnant and lactating women (moderate cost)

Foodstuffs	Normal women						Additional allowances during			
	Sedentary work		Moderate work		Heavy work		Pregnancy		Lactation	
	V*	NV†	V	NV	V	NV	V	NV	V	NV
Cereals	260	250	310	300	440	425	–	–	110	110
Pulses	60	50	60	50	60	50	20	–	40	–
Green leafy vegetables	100	100	100	100	100	100	–	–	–	–
Other vegetables	75	75	75	75	100	100	–	–	–	–
Roots and tubers	50	50	75	75	100	100	–	–	–	–
Fruits	60	60	60	60	60	60	50	50	50	50
Milk	400	250	400	250	400	250	400	200	600	300
Fats and oils	30	35	35	40	40	45	–	–	20	20
Sugar and jaggery	30	30	30	30	40	40	–	–	20	20
Meat and fish	–	60	–	60	–	60	–	25	–	40
Eggs	–	30	–	30	–	30	–	–	–	–
Groundnuts	40	40	40	40	40	40	–	–	–	–

*V, vegetarian; †NV, nonvegetarian.

Table 30.12: Balanced diets (g) for normal, pregnant and lactating women (high cost)

Foodstuffs	Normal women						Additional allowances during			
	Sedentary work		Moderate work		Heavy work		Pregnancy		Lactation	
	V* (g)	NV† (g)	V (g)	NV (g)	V (g)	NV (g)	V (g)	NV (g)	V (g)	NV (g)
Cereals	230	220	280	270	410	400	–	–	70	70
Pulses	60	50	60	50	60	50	–	–	–	–
Green leafy vegetables	100	100	100	100	100	100	–	–	–	–
Other vegetables	75	75	75	75	100	100	–	–	–	–
Roots and tubers	50	50	75	75	100	100	–	–	–	–
Fruits	100	100	100	100	100	100	50	50	50	50
Milk	600	400	600	400	600	400	500	200	700	300
Cheese	40	–	40	–	40	–	30	–	40	–
Fats and oils	30	35	35	40	40	40	–	–	20	20
Sugar and jaggery	30	30	30	30	40	40	–	–	20	20
Meat and fish	–	100	–	100	–	100	–	25	–	40
Eggs	–	60	–	60	–	60	–	–	–	–
Groundnuts	40	40	40	40	40	40	–	–	–	–

*V, vegetarian; †NV, nonvegetarian.

Table 30.13: Daily allowances for nutrients for expectant and nursing mothers (ICMR nutrition expert group, 1968)

Nutrients	Normal women				
	Sedentary work	Moderate work	Heavy work	Pregnancy	Lactation
Calories (kcal)	1,900	2,200	3,000	+ 300	+ 700
Protien (g)	45	45	45	45	45
Calcium (g)	0.4–0.5	0.4–0.5	0.4–0.5	1.0	1.0
Iron (mg)	30	30	30	40	30
Vitamin A (retinol) (µg)	750	750	750	750	750
Carotene (µg)	3,000	3,000	3,000	3,000	4,600
Thiamine (mg)	1.0	1.1	1.5	+ 0.2	+ 0.4
Riboflavin (mg)	1.0	1.2	1.7	+ 0.2	+ 0.4
Nicotinic acid (mg)	13	15	20	+ 2	+ 5
Ascorbic acid (mg)	50	50	50	50	80
Folic acid (µg)	100	100	100	150–300	150
Vitamin B_{12} (µg)	1.0	1.0	1.0	1.5	1.5
Vitamin D (IU)	200	200	200	200	200

Low-cost Balanced Diets

The diets that are poor, can be improved nutritionally by:

- Replacing a single cereal with mixed cereals; one of them being a millet
- Inclusion of at least 50 g green leafy vegetables to improve the intake of vitamin A, iron and calcium
- Inclusion of inexpensive yellow fruits such as papaya or mango and greens to increase vitamins A and C intake
- Inclusion of at least 150 mL of milk improves intake of riboflavin, calcium besides improving protein quality of the diet
- Another extra 10 g of oil increases energy and EFA intake.

NUTRITIONAL REQUIREMENTS FOR OLD AGE PEOPLE

Data regarding the nutritional requirements of old people is briefly discussed in Table 30.14. Balanced diets for old age people at different cost is given in Tables 30.15 and 30.16.

Table 30.14: Daily allowance of nutrients for old people

Parameters	NRC*, USA†		UK‡ expert panel		ICMR§ India	
	Male	Female	Male	Female	Male	Female
Age (year)	55–75		65-75	55–75	–	–
Body weight (kg)	70	58	63	53	55	45
Calories (kcal)	2,400	1,700	2,350	2,050	2,100	1,700
Protein (g)	65	55	59	51	55	45
Calcium (g)	0.8	0.8	0.5	0.5	0.5	0.5
Iron (g)	10.0	10.0	10.0	10.0	–	–
Vitamin A (IU)	5,000	5,000	2,500	2,500	2,500	2,500
Thiamine (mg)	1.2	1.1	0.9	0.8	1.2	1.0
Riboflavin (mg)	1.7	1.5	1.7	1.3	1.3	1.0
Nicotinic acid (mg)	14.0	13.0	18.0	15.0	16.0	13.0
Ascorbic acid (mg)	60	55	30	30	50	50
Vitamin D (IU)	400	400	200	200	200	200
Folic acid (µg)	400	400	–	–	100	100
Vitamin B_{12} (µg)	6.0	6.0	–	–	1.0	1.0

*NRC, Nutrition Resource Center; †USA, United States of America; ‡UK, United Kingdom, §ICMR, Indian Council of Medical Research.

Table 30.15: Balanced diets(g) at high cost, moderate cost and low cost for old people over 60 years

Foodstuffs	High cost				Moderate cost				Low cost			
	Sedentary work				Sedentary work				Sedentary work			
	Male		Female		Male		Female		Male		Female	
	V*	NV†	V	NV	V	NV	V	NV	V	NV	V	NV
Cereals	320	320	220	200	320	320	220	220	350	350	250	250
Pulses	70	50	70	50	70	55	60	45	70	55	70	55
Green leafy vegetables	100	100	125	125	100	100	125	125	100	100	125	125
Other vegetables	75	75	75	75	75	75	75	75	75	75	75	75
Roots and tubers	75	75	50	50	75	75	50	50	75	75	50	50
Fruits	150	150	150	150	75	75	75	75	30	30	30	30
Milk	800	600	800	600	600	400	600	400	300	200	300	200
Fats and oils	30	30	30	30	30	30	30	30	35	40	30	35
Cheese	50	–	50	–	–	–	–	–	–	–	–	–
Meat and fish	–	100	–	100	–	60	–	60	–	–	–	–
Eggs	–	40	–	40	–	30	–	30	–	–	–	–
Meat and eggs	–	–	–	–	–	–	–	–	–	30	–	30
Sugar and jaggery	30	30	30	30	30	30	30	30	30	30	30	30
Multivitamin mineral tablet	–	–	–	–	1	1	1	1	1	1	1	1

*V, vegetarian; †NV, nonvegetarian.

Dietary Guidelines to Reduce the Cost of a Meal

Table 30.16: Balanced diet

Ingredients	Amount (g)
Cereals	460
Pulses	40
Green leafy vegetables	50
Other vegetables	60
Roots and tubers	50
Milk	150

1. Foodstuffs that are distributed through public distribution system (ration shops) can be used.
2. Inclusion of millets such as ragi, jowar and bajra can reduce the cost of a meal.
3. Cereals, since they are less expensive, can be increased to more than the normal amount present in a balanced diet.
4. Big and thick rotis can be prepared.
5. Unbranded foods can be included.
6. Broken rice, broken eggs, leftover vegetables and fruits, and cheaper cuts of meat can be bought.
7. Greens particularly from trees such as drumstick are cheaper and locally available or kitchen garden produce can be used.
8. Fermenting, matting and sprouting can be done at home, which enhance the nutritive value without increasing the processing cost.
9. Inclusion of dry fish may supply good amount of nutrients without increasing the cost.
10. Leaves of cauliflower, carrots, knol khol and beetroot, which are highly nutritious, can become part of a meal. Curry leaves can be used in consumable forms such as chutneys, powders or pulao.
11. Recipes made at home are cheaper than bought. Homemade food can be carried to the workplace instead of buying from the canteen.
12. Natural foods are less expensive compared to processed and preserved food.
13. Low-priced biscuits or buns can be used as snacks in the diet.
14. Pulses such as horse gram can be included to reduce the cost of a meal.
15. Steamed foods are less expensive than fried foods.
16. Jaggery can be used instead of sugar.
17. Inclusion of locally available ingredients and seasonal foods reduce the cost of a meal.

NUTRITIONAL REQUIREMENTS FOR INDUSTRIAL WORKERS

The recommended allowances of various dietary essentials for men and women doing light, moderate and heavy work, and their balanced diet at various costs suggested by ICMR Nutrition Expert Group are given in Tables 30.17 to 30.19.

Table 30.17: Daily allowances of nutrients for industrial workers (ICMR Nutrition Expert Group, 1968)

Nutrients	Men			Women		
	Light work	Moderate work	Heavy work	Light work	Moderate work	Heavy work
Calories (kcal)	2,400	2,800	3,900	1,900	2,200	3,000
Proteins (g)	55	55	55	45	45	45
Calcium (g)	0.4–0.5	0.4–0.5	0.4–0.5	0.4–0.5	0.4–0.5	0.4–0.5
Iron (mg)	20	20	20	20	20	20
Vitamin A as retinol (μg)	750	750	750	750	750	750
Vitamin A as carotene (IU)	3,000	3,000	3,000	3,000	3,000	3,000
Thiamine (mg)	1.2	1.4	2.0	1.0	1.1	1.5
Riboflavin (mg)	1.3	1.5	2.0	1.0	1.1	1.5
Nicotinic acid (mg)	16	19	26	13	15	20
Ascorbic acid (mg)	50	50	50	50	50	50
Folic acid (μg)	100	100	100	100	100	100
Vitamin B_{12} (μg)	1	1	1	1	1	1
Vitamin D (IU)	200	200	200	200	200	200

Table 30.18: Balanced diet for adult male and female workers (moderate cost) (g/caput/day)

Foodstuffs	Male workers						Female workers						Additional allowance during			
	Sedentary work		Moderate cost		Heavy work		Sedentary work		Moderate cost		Heavy work		P*		L†	
	V‡	NV§	V	NV	V	NV	V	NV			V	NV	V	NV	V	NV
Cereals	380	380	450	450	630	630	260	260	310	310	440	440	–	–	100	100
Pulses	70	55	80	65	80	65	60	50	60	50	60	50	20	–	40	–
Green leafy vegetables	100	100	125	125	125	100	100	100	100	100	100	100	–	–	–	–
Other vegetables	75	75	75	75	100	100	75	75	75	75	100	100	–	–	–	–
Roots and tubers	75	75	100	100	100	100	50	50	75	75	100	100	–	–	–	–
Fruits	60	60	60	60	60	60	60	60	60	60	60	60	–	–	–	–
Milk	400	250	400	250	400	250	400	250	400	250	400	250	400	200	600	300
Fats and oils	35	40	40	40	50	50	30	35	35	40	40	45	–	–	20	20
Sugar and jaggery	30	30	40	40	55	55	30	30	30	30	40	40	–	–	20	20
Meat and fish	–	60	–	60	–	60	–	60	–	60	–	60	–	25	–	40
Eggs	–	30	–	30	–	30	–	30	–	30	–	30	–	30	–	30
Groundnuts (roasted)	50	50	50	50	50	50	40	40	40	40	40	40	–	–	–	–

*P, pregnancy; †L, lactation, ‡V, vegetarian, §NV, nonvegetarian.

Table 30.19: Balanced diets for adult male and female workers (low cost)—Nutrition Expert Group, ICMR (1968) (g/caput/day)

Foodstuffs	Male workers						Female workers						Additional allowance during	
	Sedentary work		Moderate cost		Heavy work		Sedentary work		Moderate cost		Heavy work			
	V*	NV†	V	NV	V	NV	V	NV	V	NV	V	NV	P‡	L§
Cereals	400	400	475	475	650	650	300	300	350	350	475	475	50	100
Pulses	70	55	80	65	80	65	60	45	70	55	70	55	–	10
Green leafy vegetables	100	100	125	125	125	125	125	125	125	125	125	125	25	25
Other vegetables	75	75	75	75	100	100	75	75	75	75	100	100	–	–
Roots and tubers	75	75	100	100	100	100	50	50	75	75	100	100	–	–
Fruits	30	30	30	30	30	30	30	30	30	30	30	30	–	–
Milk	200	100	200	100	200	100	200	100	200	100	200	100	125	125
Fats and oils	35	40	40	40	50	50	30	35	35	40	40	45	–	15
Sugar and jaggery	30	30	40	40	55	55	30	30	30	30	40	30	10	20
Meat and fish	–	30	–	30	–	30	–	30	–	30	–	30	–	–
Eggs	–	30	–	30	–	30	–	30	–	30	–	30	–	–
Groundnuts (roasted)	–	–	–	50†	50†	–	–	–	–	–	40†	40†	–	–

*V, vegetarian; †NV, nonvegetarian; ‡P, pregnancy; §L, lactation. *Note:* Additional 25 g of fats and oils can be included in the diet in place of groundnut.

Chapter 31

Planning Menu

PRINCIPLES OF BALANCED DIET

In constructing balanced diet, the following principles should be kept in mind:

1. First and foremost, the daily requirement of protein should be met. This amounts 15–20% of the daily energy intake.
2. Next comes the fat requirement, which should be limited to 20–30% of the daily energy intake.
3. Carbohydrate rich in the natural fiber should constitute the remaining food energy.
4. The requirements of micronutrients should be met.

Balanced Diets at High Cost

Balanced diets at high cost will include liberal amounts of costly foods such as milk, eggs, meat, fish and fruits, and moderate quantities of cereals, pulses, nuts and fats.

Balanced Diets at Moderate Cost

Balanced diets at moderate cost will include moderate amounts of milk, eggs, meat, fish, fruits and fats, and liberal amounts of cereals, pulses, nuts and green leafy vegetables.

Balanced Diet at Low Cost

Balanced diets at low cost will include small amounts of milk, eggs, meat, fish and fats, and liberal amounts of cereals, pulses, nuts, and green leafy vegetables. To plan a balanced or adequate diet, it is necessary to know the requirements of the body for the different nutrients. Total calories vary with the degree of activity, but it should be noted that for adults, the requirements of many nutrients are the same, whatever the activity, although there may be slight variations with differences in weight.

There are much greater variations when the body has some special requirement, as for growth in children and adolescents, and for the nourishment of both child and mother during pregnancy and lactation. The dietary pattern varies widely in different parts of the world. It is generally developed around the kinds of food produced or imported depending upon the climatic conditions of the region, economic capacity, religion, customs, taboos, tastes and habits of the people.

NORMAL DIET

Dietary Goals

All countries should follow a national nutrition and food policy that sets 'dietary goals' for achievement. The dietary goals ('prudent diet') recommended by the various expert committees of World Health Organization (WHO) are as follows:

1. Dietary fat should be limited to approximately 20–30% of total daily intake.
2. Saturated fats should contribute no more than 10% of the total energy intake. Unsaturated vegetable oils should be substituted for the remaining saturated fats.
3. Excessive consumption of refined carbohydrate should be avoided; some amount of carbohydrates rich in natural fiber should be taken.
4. Sources rich in energy such as fats and alcohol should be restricted.
5. Salt intake should be reduced to an average of not more than 5 g/day (salt intake is more in tropical countries; in India, it averages 15 g/day).
6. Junk foods such as colas, ketchups and other foods that supply empty calories should be reduced.

There may be conditions under which the above recommendations for daily food intake do not apply. For example, diet should be adapted to the special needs of growth, pregnancy, lactation, physical activity and medical disorders, e.g. diabetes.

MENU PLANNING

Meal or menu planning is the process whereby family resources, both material and human are used to obtain the family goal. Menu planning means planning for adequate nutrition. Adequate nutrition is a vital need for every person in all stages. Meal planning is both an art and science. Art is the skillful blending of color, texture and flavor. Science is the wise choice of food for optimum nutrition and digestion.

A well-planned meal is always appealing to the eye. Meal planning is a pleasant and satisfying task when the family shares together the happy experiences on the family table. In the hospital, it becomes one of the important responsibilities of the nurse and dietetics department to plan the meal for the patients according to their disease condition, i.e. cardiovascular disease (CVD), renal disease, etc.

Definition

Menu planning is defined as a simple process, which involves application of the knowledge of food, nutrients, food habits, likes and dislikes to plan wholesome and attractive meal. It is a simple practical exercise, which involves applying the knowledge of food, preparation of foods, nutritional requirements, individual preferences to plan adequate acceptable meals.

Aims

Aims of meal planning in hospital is to meet the nutritional needs of the patients to:

- Fasten the recovery of the patient
- Plan meals within the food cost
- Provide variety of foods
- Save money, time and energy
- Improve the quality of food
- Improve the appetite, so that maximum diet is consumed and waste is minimized.

Objectives

The objectives of menu planning are to:

- Simplify purchase, preparation and storage of meals
- Provide attractive, appetizing meals with no monotony.

Other Objectives of Menu Planning

1. To satisfy the nutritional needs of the family members according to their age and occupation.
2. Keep expenditure within family's food budget.
3. To decide amounts of food to be purchased from each food group.

4. To consider family size and composition.
5. To consider food storage space and condition of storage, to decide how often they need to purchase various foods.
6. Prepare a food purchase list, taking the food preferences of all members.
7. Use methods of preparation, which retain nutrients without sacrificing palatability.
8. Serve meals that are appetizing and attractive, and fit in the schedule of the members.
9. Manage the time, energy and available materials efficiently with the help of the family members.
10. Maintain and plan a budget for each food item.

Importance of Meal Planning

1. Proper meal planning fulfills the nutritional request of all family members. If the meal planning is not properly done, it may satisfy the request of an adult, but children may not grow as they have to. So, this is very essential to keep them strong, healthy, free from disease and any deficiency.
2. It saves time, energy and money. The foods can be selected and stored when they are in abundance. Proper cooking of foods from proper place saves money as well as time.
3. Properly planned food is palatable and appealing to the eyes. If the food is not good to look at, nobody will prefer it, even though it has excellent nutritive value.
4. Planning of meals should always be done according to the budget of the family. So, it saves money spent on costly food, instead of that money, cheap and nutritious foods are selected. Thus, it encourages one to plan within the family's means.
5. If the food is planned, then it can look after the customs and traditions of the family.
6. The food planning before cooking can improve the quality of the food by enriching the nutritive value of foods, e.g. by sprouting, fermentation, etc.
7. It is economizing, if the leftover foods can be used up and the planning of next meal is improved.

Basic Consideration in Menu Planning

A major consideration in meal planning for most families is the cost of food and the amount of money that is available for food purchase.

Food expenditures are controlled by the best available purchase information, by menu adjustment, by adequate storage facilities, by appropriate preparation techniques and by control of waste from the point of purchase to the plate at the table. There are three steps in this process:

1. This includes menu, market order, details of preparing and serving the meal, and aftercare.
2. To put this plan into action or operation under constant direction or homemaker.
3. To evaluate the outcome in terms of satisfaction achieved or recovery of the patient, if in hospital.

Nutritional Adequacy in Menu Planning

The first prerequisite of a good meal plan is that it should meet the nutritional needs of the whole family. Thus, each meal should include cereals and their products such as:

1. **Dal, milk, egg, fish, meat:** To provide energy and proteins; to supply proteins, vitamin B and some other minerals.
2. **Protective vegetables and fruits:** To provide vitamins A and C, minerals and fiber.
3. **Sugars, oils and fats:** To provide energy, satisfy and improve palatability.

Nutritional adequacy in meal planning includes the suggested number of units from each group; it can reasonably be assured of meeting needs for proteins, vitamins and minerals. The variety chosen within a group will be determined by the taste preferences of the family.

Energy foods: Grains as well as starchy roots are economical sources of food energy. Grains supply proteins in addition to energy. Fats, oils, sugar and jaggery, which are used to make food palatable and also sources of energy, but these are expensive. Butter, ghee and vanaspati are good sources of vitamin A.

Protein foods: Whole beans and peas are the cheapest protein foods. Dehydrated fish may be another inexpensive source. Less expensive cuts of meat can be used as protein. In the rural areas, eggs and poultry are produced at home by some ensuring economy. Milk is an important source of protein, but expensive one.

Vegetables and fruits: These are important sources of minerals and vitamins. Green leafy vegetables (GLV) are a rich source of the vitamins A, C and the minerals such as calcium, iron. The fruits amla, guava, citrus fruits, pineapple and tomatoes are a good source of vitamin C. Some vegetables and fruits are seasonal, while others are available throughout the year at a competitive cost. Various greens are available throughout the year at very little cost. Vegetables and fruits at the peak of the season are not only inexpensive but are of high quality in terms of acceptability and nutrient content.

The food budget of rural agricultural families is different from that of the city dwellers. The staple foods are normally available from the farms; with a little planning they can produce the dal, vegetables, fruits for home consumption, so that the quality of their diets may improve. In estimating food cost, it is good to note that a number of non-food items are purchased at the food store, i.e. soap, hair oil, cleaning agents, equipment, etc. These may appear on the bill and must be subtracted from the total money spent for food.

MENU PLANNING PROCESS

It is necessary to plan the menu on a monthly basis. There are five main steps in meal planning:

1. Make a list of food from each food group that are available in the market.
2. Check the prices and decide, which of the foods from each group fit in the food budget on the basis of the number of family members.
3. Estimate the day's needs for all the family members on the basis of the daily food guide and calculate the month's food needs from it.
4. Make list of foods to be purchased monthly, fortnightly, weekly and daily.
5. Plan menu to meet the daily needs of the family.

Steps Followed in Planning Process

While planning a menu, the following steps have to be considered:

1. Collect information regarding the individual with respect to age, gender, activity, level, religion, socioeconomic background and food habits.
2. Decide number of meals the individual takes per day.
3. Determine the number of portions of various food groups by using Indian Council of Medical Research (ICMR) table.

Table 31.1: Sample for each meal

Food group	Number of portions	Portions per meal			
		Breakfast	Lunch	Snacks	Dinner

Table 31.2: Sample for menu based on food group

Meal time	Cooked recipe	Ingredients	Amount	Number of portions

4. Distribute portion for each meal (Table 31.1).
5. Select food items for each food group and plan the menu for a day (Table 31.2).

Changing Food Habits

Each of us have food habits, which are our favorites. They are served on special occasions such as birthday parties or other celebrations. Though one should take the likes and dislikes of family members into account in meal planning, allowing people to develop a restricted food pattern may lead to a poorly balanced diet and could be a social disadvantage. Trying to prefer new food enlarges one's food enjoyment, social experience as well as diet.

Food Selection

The selection of foods is made according to the daily food guide. The amount of foods included from the various groups will depend on the body size and activity of the individual. The foods selected, need to be used in the day's meals, which fit into the daily schedule of the person, e.g. labors may need more cereals, oils and fat to meet their energy needs as compared to a sedentary person.

Planning Each Time Menu (Table 31.3)

Breakfast—Important Meal

The first meal in the day is important, as it is about 12 hours between dinner and breakfast. About one fourth to one third of the day's food should be taken for breakfast. But in the cities, the pattern

Table 31.3: Model menu planning for a day

Meal time	Cooked recipe	Ingredients	Amount	Number of portions
Morning breakfast	Chapati: 2	Wheat flour	60 g	2
	Potato curry: 1 cup	Potato	5 g	1
		Onion	75 g	1
		Oil	25 g	1
	Milk	Milk	100 mL	1
		Sugar	5 g	1
Lunch	Rice	Rice (raw)	120 g	4
	Dal: 1 cup	Red gram dal	30 g	1
	Papad: 1	Black gram dal	15 g	½
	Cabbage fry	Cabbage	100 g	1
		Oil	5 g	1
	Curd	Milk	50 mL	½
	Banana	–	100 mL	1
Snacks	Biscuits	Refined flour	60 g	2
		Butter	10 g	2
		Sugar	15 g	3
	Milk	Milk	100 mL	1
		Sugar	5 g	1
Dinner	Rice	Rice (raw)	90 g	3
	Jowar	–	30 g	1
	Sambar	Red gram dal	30 g	1
		Beans	25 g	¼
	Brinjal curry	Brinjal	75 g	¾
		Oil	5 g	1
	Curd	Milk	50 mL	½

varies from region to region. Some regions have a certain definite pattern of breakfast and some preparations are clearly associated with breakfast, e.g. Idli-chutney, upma are considered as breakfast foods in Tamil Nadu and Kerala. But it is known that a person, who eats a good breakfast, performs better at work and is likely to eat less during the day. A person who skips breakfast has a tendency to take snacks or eat more at lunch and dinner, thus increasing the total food intake.

Lunch, Often a Poor Meal

1. About one third of day's food intake should be contributed by lunch or the noon meal. Lunch should be counted as a part of

food plan for the day and not just a snack to starve off hunger at dinner time.

2. A good lunch should provide proteins and health-protecting foods; selection of vegetables or fruits may help to meet part of the needed protective foods.
3. Lunch, whether served at home or packed and carried to work, or purchased at the place of work, should be planned or chosen with care. A missed meal is not easily made up.
4. Consistent neglect of this important meal may affect the individual's performance at work, behavior with colleagues and attitude to life.
5. The lunch should be planned in relation to the other needs, so that it supplies a fair share of the day's nutrients through the foods selected.

Snacks

1. Snacks have become an accepted practice in most offices and factories for workers to have a tea break. Most of the canteens and cafes, which serve tea and coffee, also serve snacks, most of which are shallow or deep fat-fried preparations.
2. The choice of snack may decide if it will provide only energy or other nutrients, e.g. dishes such as pakodas, idli-sambar, lassi, ice cream and fruits may provide some nutrients in addition to energy.

Dinner

1. Dinner is the main meal of the day, which may be served at noon or night depending on the family's schedule custom.
2. It is good to plan a menu for dinner, which helps to balance the total intake in terms of energy, protein as well as other nutrients for the day.
3. One may prepare an additional vegetable salad; one may add a sweet, to add a variety. As this is a leisurely meal, which is eaten by the family together, it contributes much of the feeding of belonging, enjoyment of the company and relaxation.

PRINCIPLES OF MEAL PLANNING

1. **Meeting nutritional requirements:** A good menu is one which will not only provide adequate calories, fat and proteins but also minerals and vitamins, which are essential for the physical well-being of each member of a family by keeping them strong, healthy, free from diseases.

2. **Meal pattern must fulfill family needs:** A family meal should cater to the needs of the different members. A growing adolescent boy and girl may need nutrient-rich food to satisfy their appetite, where a young child may require soft and balanced diet. Pregnant women require more greens in the diet. A heavy worker requires more calories and B-complex group vitamins than other members of the family, whereas preschool- and school-going children require more proteins, vitamins and minerals diet. Old-aged people require soft diet.
3. **Meal planning should save time and energy:** The meal planning should be done according to the metabolic changes of the members. Planning of meals should be done in such a way that the recipe should be simple and nutritious. By using pressure cooker, time and energy can be saved.
4. **Economic consideration:** Any meals that are planned, but if they do not satisfy the budget of the family, suit cannot be put into practice. The cost of the meals can be reduced by:
   - Seasonal foods
   - Bulk purchasing
   - Substituting greens for fruits
   - Combination of foods such as cereals and pulses making it equivalent to good quality animal protein
   - Locally available foods.
5. **Meal plan should be given maximum nutrients:** Loss of nutrients during processing and cooking should be minimized. Sprouted grams, malted cereals, fermented foods enhance the nutritive value. Good quality protein should be distributed in all meals.
6. **Consideration for individual likes and dislikes:** The meal planned should not only to meet RDA but also individual preferences, particularly vegetarian or non-vegetarian preferences. If a person does not prefer greens, it can be tried in a different form or substitute by equally nourishing food.
7. **Planned meals should provide variety:** If the meals are monotonous, they cannot be consumed. Variety can be introduced in color, texture and taste.
8. **Meal should give satiety:** Each meal should have some amount of fat, protein and fiber, and the variety can be introduced in color, texture and taste.
9. **Religion, traditions and customs:** Food habits and person's preferences about foods must be kept in mind, while planning,

preparing and serving of meals for family members. From all these factors, meal planning should differ from person to person, individual, family members, religion to religion and country to country.

PLANNING MEALS FOR A FAMILY

According to WHO, 'health is a state of complete physical, mental, and social well-being, not merely an absence of disease or infirmity. So, to maintain good health, ingesting a diet containing the essential nutrients in correct amounts is very important:

1. **Nutritional requirements:** Each diet should meet the nutritional requirements of the family members. A balanced diet is one, which contains different types of foods in such quantities and proportion that the need for calories, proteins, fats, minerals, vitamins and other nutrients is adequately met, and a small provision is made for extra nutrients to withstand short duration of leanness.
2. **Recommended dietary allowances:** These imply addition of safety factor, amount to the estimated requirement to cover both the variation among individuals and the lack of precision inherent in the estimated requirement. To calculate balanced diet, there is a need to know recommended dietary allowances for different age groups prescribed by Nutrition Expert Committee of ICMR (1991).
3. **Explaining therapeutic diets to the patient:** These diets are scientifically based on nutritional composition and groups, which can be used in menu planning.
4. **Food labeling and surveillance system:** Food groups can be used for food labeling and for nutritional surveillance system.

POINTS TO BE CONSIDERED IN PLANNING A DIET

The next step would be to distribute the foods in food list to different meals such as breakfast, lunch and evening tea and dinner. For planning the menu, the following points should be considered:

1. Energy derived from cereals should be not more than 75%.
2. Whole grain cereals, parboiled or malted grains give higher nutritive value.
3. It is better to include two cereals in one meal such as rice and wheat.
4. Flour should not be sieved for chapati, as it will reduce nutrient content.

5. One serving of cereal is 25 g (one chapati, one katori rice two phulkas). A day's menu may require servings.
6. Minimum ratio of cereal protein to pulse protein should be 4:1. In terms of the grains, it will be 4 parts of cereals and 1 part of pulses.
7. One serving of pulse is 25 g (1 calorie of dal); 2–3 servings should be taken.
8. One serving of vegetables is 75 g. The GLV can be taken more than 1 serving, if fruit is not included in the diet.
9. It is better to serve the fruit raw without much cooking or taking juice out of it. Every day diet should contain at least one medium-sized fruit.
10. There should be a minimum milk of 100 mL/day, 1–2 glasses of milk or curd should be included in the balanced diet.
11. Energy derived from fats or oils is 15–20% of total calories and 5% from sugar and jaggery.
12. One egg weighs around 40 g. This can be served along with cereals or pulses to improve the quality of protein. Instead, serving of poultry or fish can also be included in the diet.
13. Inclusion of salads or raita not only helps in meeting the vitamin requirements but also the meals should be attractive and have high satiety value due to the fiber content.
14. Fried foods cannot be planned, if oil allowance is less or in low-calorie diet.
15. One third of nutritional requirements, at least calories, proteins should be met by lunch and dinner.
16. If possible, meals should be planned for several days.
17. Usually the number of meal servings would be four and for very young children and diseased persons, number of meals can be more.
18. Ideally, each meal should consist of all the five food groups.
19. For quick calculations, average value of calories and protein from the same group can be taken.

FACTORS AFFECTING/INFLUENCING THE SELECTION OF FOOD AND PLANNING OF MEAL

Factors Influencing Food Selection

The factors, which influence food selection, may be summarized as follows:

1. Requirements of the family group, taking into consideration.
2. Composition of the family.

3. Occupation of the adults.
4. Special requirements for children, adolescents, and pregnant and nursing mothers.

The nutrition of infant and young children needs special consideration and adjustment according to their needs in growth and development activities, and ability to digest. Pregnancy and lactation are normal conditions, which, however, make greater demands upon the body. The woman receiving an adequate diet during pregnancy is more likely to deliver an infant in good physical condition. While inadequate and improper diet may have a harmful effect on the growing fetus; complications such as prematurity, congenital defects and still births may occur. Toxemia of pregnancy may also occur in the mother.

Weight of the infant at birth is a reflection of the weight gained by the woman during pregnancy. This weight gain should be 8–10 kg. Most of this should occur during the last trimester when the growth of the fetus is most rapid. During the latter half of pregnancy, calorie intake should be increased by 300 calories and protein by 14 g/day. Good quality protein, calcium/phosphorus, iron and vitamin are all important in the diet of a pregnant woman. Milk is a good source of most of these nutrients.

Factors Affecting Food Selection

1. **Food acceptance:** Each one of us has certain foods we prefer and which we do not, as we move from one place to another. It helps us to enjoy our new environment in the way of bringing variety in meal planning.
2. **Tradition:** Most of our food selection is influenced by tradition. It may be national, regional or family traditions. A lot of traditional selection is based on experience. It is a good practice to evaluate traditional food.
3. **Food misinformation:** Food is an important topic of conversation in articles, newspapers, magazines and books. People see and hear about it in advertisements too. Some of this information may be useful, but a large part may not be. False ideas about food are common and also prove to be wrong information. But many of these originate in ignorance. Those people who learn about food composition will be able to use this knowledge to guide food selection.
4. **Other factors affecting meal planning:** Skill in food preparation is an essential part of an acceptable, enhancing meal. Skill in food

preparation is acquired by practice. Indigenous combinations improve acceptability of foods; add to variety and thus make food enjoyable. One can develop skill by observing people who perform well and practice, e.g. addition of grated coconut or jaggery also makes the flavor of the finished vegetable acceptable.

5. **Variety:** The enjoyment of food can be enhanced by learning ways to prepare dishes from other regions of India and foreign countries.
6. **Availability of foods:** It is important to study the seasonal variation in availability of food. In each season, one can find some foods from each group. Using seasonal foods reduces cost. Some vegetables and fruits can be grown in the kitchen garden. Some foods such as beans, rice, wheat can be purchased soon after the time of harvest, when the price is reasonable and stored for the whole year.
7. **Home production:** If some of the vegetables and fruits are grown at home, these need to be used in meal planning. Some of the fresh condiments such as coriander leaves, curry leaves, green chilies, mint and different leafy vegetables can easily be grown at home. In rural areas, where most of the staples are produced at home, meal planning helps to decide realistically the amount of food the family should retain for home use, so that the needs of the family are met. It also helps to decide what vegetables and fruits can be grown economically to improve the family's meal pattern, without adding to the food cost. When fruits and vegetables are produced in excess of the family needs, the surplus can be sold.
8. **Schedules of family members:** When planning a meal pattern, one needs to think of the schedules (time table of the family member's meal time and number of meals eaten at home and those that are eaten away from home).
9. **Time:** The time available for meal preparation and the individual who is preparing food, be it children or elders, may affect the menu and choice of foods bought.
10. **Family size and composition:**
    a. Family size: This affects the foods that can be served. It is known that the money spent for food per person decreases as the family size increases. When the family does not

change with the size of it, a large part of it has to be spent to meet the nutritional needs. Staples such as wheat, rice, jowar are bought in larger amounts, but the amount of milk, vegetables, fruits bought may decrease. Thus, the quality of the diet is lowered. In extreme cases, it may not be possible to meet the food needs of the family members resulting in partial starvation. As this happens to a large number of families, who migrate to cities in hope of improved living condition, it is important to emphasize the relation of family size to family's food intake and health, and promote small family norms in the interest of better health and survival.

b. Family composition: It affects the kinds and amounts of food needed and the pattern of meals served. For example, as the child grows, the meal pattern changes to accommodate the school hours and the need to pack lunch. When children are below 5 years of age, more milk is needed and the number of meals is more, as the child cannot take large amounts at a time. Adolescents in the family need more food than adults, as they need large quantities of food to support growth and their activities. The food needs of the adult members will depend on how active they are.

Factors Affecting Meal Planning

Nutritional/Social/Religious Factors

The planning of an adequate diet has been mainly based on nutritional requirements, but there are some social, religious and other factors, which influence selection and planning of meals. They are:

1. **Development:** People in rapid period of growth (infancy and adolescence) have increased needs for nutrients. During pregnancy and lactation also, the dietary pattern differs from that of others. Older people need few calories than adults.
2. **Gender:** Nutritional requirements are different for men and women because of body composition and reproductive functions. The large muscle mass of men means a greater need for calories and proteins. Because of menstruation, women require more iron than men.
3. **Occupation:** According to the energy expenditure for the work, the amount and type of food will vary. Laborious adults need extra energy and proteins than the adults who do white collar jobs.

4. **Health status:** A good appetite is a sign of health, while anorexia is an almost universal symptom of disease. The disease process disturbs absorption, metabolism and excretion of essential nutrients. Depending upon the disease condition, the amount and pattern of the diet will be modified.
5. **Culture and religion:** This practice also affects diet. In different religions, there are different laws regarding food restriction. For example, Hindus do not eat beef. Muslims do not eat pork. Cultural patterns should be considered in planning diet. Some people will not take non-vegetarian foods on certain days. Some will keep fasting on special occasions.
6. **Socioeconomic status:** The amount of family income available for buying food varies. Food expenses are not always a fixed amount. When money is tight, many people spend less on food.
7. **Personal preference:** Individual likes and dislikes have perhaps the strongest influence on diet, e.g. some people may prefer sweet and sour tastes. Some may not prefer milk smell; So, will avoid to take milk. All individual preferences must be considered when planning diet.
8. **Beliefs about food:** This can affect food choice. Many people acquire their beliefs about food through television, magazines and others practices.
9. **Psychological factors:** Some people do not take any food or take very little food in their stress and depression. Others eat more food under the same conditions.
10. **Drugs and alcohol:** Ingestion of alcohol and other drugs affect nutritional status either directly or indirectly by affecting dietary patterns. Alcohol may depress the appetite by replacing part of the diet, thus reducing the intake of food. According to the therapy of the patient, diet needs to be changed. Because many drugs may produce anorexia, nausea, vomiting and diarrhea-like side effects.
11. **Emotional attitude:** This attitude of the homemaker is an important factor, i.e. if she is concerned about nutritious meals, the family is more likely to be well fed.
12. **Composition of the family:** The number of persons in the family table makes a difference in planning and preparing a simple meal. The amount and types of food to be served, as well as the preparation needed, will influence meal planning.

13. **Nutritional needs:** Some family members may require modifications of the diet due to certain illnesses. Certain food requirements may increase the food budget and special attention must be given to planning, so that individual's nutritive needs are met.
14. **Work and activities:** The work and other activities of the family must be taken into consideration. A working mother, who must leave earlier in the morning, faces a real problem in planning. The other activities of family members such as club meeting, business appointments and community activities, etc. also influence the planning.
15. **Values of family members:** The values, which people place upon food cannot be overlooked, e.g. the kind of food served for holidays.
16. **Entertainment:** The amount of entertaining a family must also be viewed in family meal planning, e.g. if family member bring friends into the home, at that moment, preparing excess meals may be required.

Other Factors Influencing Menu Planning

While planning a meal, the factors need to be considered are as detailed below:

1. **Nutritional adequacy:** Foods from all basic groups should be included in each meal, so that the meal is balanced and nutritionally adequate. Nutritional needs may be modified for hospital diets.
2. **Economic status:** The spending power of the client has to be kept in mind and meals have to be planned within the budget. Low-cost nutritious substitutes should be included in the menu to keep the costs low.
3. **Type of food service:** Menus should be planned in relation to the type of food service, whether it is cafeteria, seated service, buffet, etc.
4. **Equipment and workspace:** The menu should be planned keeping the available equipment and workspace in mind, e.g. Deep freezers, refrigerators, grinders, boilers, etc. Adequate storage space and hygienic standards should be ensured to minimize the risk of communication and spoilage of food.
5. **Food habits:** Food served to an individual should be acceptable. Special attention should be paid when a particular type of community is catered.

6. **Availability:** Seasonal fruits and vegetables should be given preference. During the season, the cost is reasonable and quality is better. Regional availability influences menu planning, e.g. fish and sea foods are cheaper in coastal areas.
7. **Meal pattern:** The meal timings and number of meals consumed in a day, whether meals are packed or served at the table, also influence the selection of food items on the menu.
8. **Variety:** A variety of foods from the different food groups should be included. The term 'variety' means:
   - Variety in food ingredients
   - Method of cooking
   - Variety in presentation and garnish
   - Meal should look attractive and be appetizing
   - Variety in recipe
   - Color, texture and flavor.

Factors Affecting Food Acceptance

We spend a number of hours each day to plan, purchase, prepare and enjoy food. A large part of our income is utilized to purchase food for the family. Therefore, it is important to understand personal preferences in food without giving attention to the sensory aspects of food, there can be no true enjoyment of it.

Color in Food

1. Color affects our acceptance of food. First impression of food is formed by its appearance, which includes color, shape and aroma. It is added to food products during processing to improve its acceptance. Fruit preserves, cheese, butter, ice cream, cakes and confections are some of the food products that have such addition of color. When one buys these products, it is important to select appropriate delicate color to ensure attractive, acceptable appearance.
2. The initial attraction or rejection of food depends on its looks. Most of our traditional color concepts affect our reaction to food, e.g. orange-yellow color with ripe mangoes, red color with ripe tomatoes and green color with leafy vegetables; light-colored tomato looks unripe and does not attract us.
3. The color of food is one way to judge its quality, e.g. green color is associated with unripe fruit such as mango or orange, a brown banana is thought to be spoilt.

4. Coloring materials used in foods belong to two groups, i.e. natural-coloring materials and synthetic coal tar dyes. After extensive testing, it has been found that only some of the coal tar dyes can be safely used in foods and these have been certified. Some of these are used in carbonated beverages and fruit preserves.
5. Some of the natural-coloring matters, which we use in food preparation are turmeric and saffron. In addition to these, other natural substances used in food preparations are betaine, caramel, carotene and chlorophyll.
6. In food purchase, color is used as an important criterion of quality:
   a. Mature ripe mangoes have orange-yellow color. If the color is pale or darkened, the fruit is immature. But color is not always a true indicator of quality.
   b. Some varieties of oranges have a green color, even when these are mature.
   c. Fruit preserves and vegetable pickles darken during storage. Such darkening is caused by oxidative changes. These changes can be minimized by reducing the oxygen in the top of the container by heat before sealing it. The presence of traces of metals such as iron, tin and copper in foods also causes darkening and it should be avoided.

Texture in Foods

1. Each food has a particular texture. Thus, well-cooked rice is soft, potato wafers are crisp and cucumber slice has a crunchy texture.
2. A variety of qualities are included in texture, such as crisp, soft, hard, sticky, elastic, tough and gummy.
3. If there is change in the accepted characteristic texture, we find the food unacceptable.
4. The textural qualities of food depend on the ingredients, their proportion, the manner in which these are combined and the method of preparation such as:
   a. Cereals: In preparation of chapati, we knead the dough and set it aside for a few minutes to obtain a soft velvet-textured chapati.
   b. Fruits and vegetables:
      i. The texture of fruits and vegetables is determined by the cell wall. The is composed of polysaccharides.

ii. During maturation, ripening and preparation, there are changes in the amount and kinds of polysaccharides, which result in changes in the texture of vegetables and fruits. For example, when a bean gets matured it toughens, its texture becomes very hard and it needs more time to cook than the immature bean. Thus, the texture of the food affects the time taken to cook or process it. It also affects its acceptability.

c. Meat: The texture of meat depends on the part of the animal from which the cut is taken, the age of the animal and the method of preparation and the duration.

Flavor in Food

1. Flavor is the sum total of the sensory impression formed, when we eat food. It includes aroma, taste and the texture, and thus involves all our senses.
2. Food flavor is related to food preparation practices. We prefer flavor of foods made in our home because these are familiar to us. Thus, food flavor acceptance is related to our dietary pattern.

Odor

The odor or smell of food influences our food acceptance. The odor affects our acceptance of food, depending on whether it is liked or not. The primary odors are sweet, sour and burnt. Therefore, anything that affects its function, impairs our enjoyment of food. For example, if person suffers from cold, sense of smell gets impaired and the person finds that the food does not taste as good as when the person is well. Similarly, the functions of sensory organs impaired with age, results in decreased enjoyment of food by the aged persons.

Touch

1. The sense of touch contributes to our perception of food. It identifies the textural qualities of the food such as softness and hardness.
2. Similarly, we perceive the crisp, sticky texture by touching food.

Taste

1. Taste sensations are the sum total of the sensations created by food, when it is put in the mouth. The sensation of taste is perceived when the taste receptors (tastebuds) are stimulated.

The tastebuds are located on the surface of the tongue. The food must be dissolved in liquid to enable us to perceive its taste. Hence, we have to masticate dry foods such as roasted groundnuts to mix with saliva, so that we can taste their senses.

2. There are four primary taste sensations—sweet, sour, salt and bitter. The taste of the food is determined by its chemical composition.
3. Sugars added to foods are responsible for sweet taste. While salty taste is due to salts present in foods. Sour or acid taste is contributed mainly by organic acids found in foods (i.e. citric acid in limes, tamarind extract added to dal, lactic acid formed when milk is made into curd). Certain foods such as coffee beans and fenugreek have bitter taste.
4. The primary tastes can be modified by combination of the compounds responsible for these, for example, the sourness of lime can be reduced by addition of sugar. The bitterness of fenugreek is reduced by adding coconut and jaggery.
5. We can use flavoring substances, naturally present in foods/ those synthesized in the factory, during food preparation and processing to improve acceptability and add variety to our diet.

Flavoring substances

1. A variety of materials are used in food preparation and processing to enhance, blend and alter the natural flavors. Appropriate use of these can make a dish into a highly palatable product.
2. A large variety of flavoring substances are used in Indian homes. These include salt and spices.

Salt

1. Salt is the most widely used condiment. It is one of the few pure chemicals used in food preparation.
2. It is obtained by evaporation of sea water. It is used to season all food preparations except sweets.
3. It is used in food preservation to make pickles, chutneys and sauces.
4. Salt has the unique property of enhancing the flavor of herbs and spices in food preparation.

Acids

1. Lemon juice, tamarind and vinegar are the acid substances very commonly used in Indian homes.

2. Lemon juice is used in salads and savory preparations such as upma, etc.
3. Tamarind is soaked and the acid extract obtained is used in sambar, rasam, tamarind rice and many other vegetable preparations in the southern parts of India.
4. Vinegar is dilute acetic acid. It is used to flavor salads, pickles and sauces. Amchur made from raw mangoes, is also used in some preparations to impart acidic taste.

Herbs and spices

1. India is known as the home of spices. The spices and herbs form an indispensable part of our cultural food pattern. These impart substantial flavor to foods.
2. Spices and herbs come from various parts of plants such as the fruits, seeds, berries, roots, rhizomes, leaves, bark and the floral parts.
3. The flavor is due to small amounts of essential oils and organic acids present in the specific part of the plant.
4. Each one of these has a characteristic component, which is responsible for its individual flavor.
5. These are available as whole dried spices and ground powders also.
6. One problem associated with spices is adulteration. These are expensive products. Ground hulls, saw dust and other waste materials are added to increase the bulk and profit margin. Microscopic and chemical tests can help to identify adulterants.

STEPS INVOLVED IN PLANNING A DIET

There are three steps involved in planning a menu.

Step I

Recommended dietary allowance (RDA): To calculate balanced diet as a first step, there is a need to know RDA for different age groups prescribed by Nutrition Expert Committee of ICMR.

Step II

Food list: The list can be prepared either by using ICMR data (Table 31.4) or exchange lists (Table 31.5).

Using ICMR Tables

As a second step, while planning the daily diets, the foods are chosen from all five food groups. To make menu planning more convenient,

ICMR has suggested the portion size and balanced diets for adults and for different age groups. The balanced diets for adults and different age groups are given as multiples of these portion sizes for menu plan.

Table 31.4: Planning a menu (ICMR)

Food groups	Portions	Energy (kcal)	Protein (g)	Carbohydrates (g)	Fat (g)
Cereals and millets	30	100	3.0	20	0.8
Pulses	30	100	6.0	15	0.7
Egg	50	85	7.0	–	7.0
Meat, chicken/fish	50	100	9	–	7.0
Milk	100	70	3.0	5	3.0
Roots and tubers	100	80	1.3	19	–
Green leafy vegetables	100	45	3.6	–	0.4
Other vegetables	100	30	1.7	–	0.2
Fruits	100	40	–	10	–
Sugar	5	20	–	5	–
Fats and oils*	5	45	–	–	5

*Energy value of fat and oil are included in the exchange list. *Source:* Dietary guidelines for Indians—A manual, NIN, ICMR, Hyderabad; 1999.

Table 31.5: Menu plan based on exchange lists

Name of exchange	No. of exchange	Name of recipe	Quantity for serving	Energy (kcal)	Protein (g)
Breakfast					
Cereal exchange	3	Rava upma	1½ kg	300	7.5
Pulse exchange	1	Roasted Bengal gram	½ kg	100	4.0

Contd...

Contd...

Name of exchange	No. of exchange	Name of recipe	Quantity for serving	Energy (kcal)	Protein (g)
Milk exchange	1	Chutney			
Sugar	–	Milk	1 cup	100	4.5
Fruit exchange	–	Banana	1 pc	100	–
Lunch					
Cereal exchange	2	Vegetables pulav	1 kg	200	5.0
Cereal exchange	1	Chapati	1	200	5.0
Vegetable exchange	1	Palak gravy	1 kg	100	–
Milk exchange	1	Curd	1½ cup	100	4.5
Meat exchange	1	Scrambled egg	1	100	5.0
Evening tea					
Pulse exchange	1	Sundal	1 kg	100	4.0
Milk exchange	1	Tea	1 cup	100	4.5
Sugar exchange	1	Sugar	2 tsp	40	–
Fruit exchange	1	Orange	2 ½	100	–
Dinner					
Cereal exchange	3	Rice	2 ¼ kg	300	7.5
Cereal exchange	1	Chapati	1 pc	100	2.5
Pulse exchange	1	Sambar	1 ½ kg	100	4.0
Roots and tubers	2	Potato fry	1 kg	200	–
Milk exchange	1	Milk	1 cup	100	4.5
Sugar	–	Sugar	5 g	20	–

Total energy—2,380 kcal; total protein—62.5 g.

Chapter 32

Budgeting of Food

NEED FOR FOOD BUDGET

The expenditure on food is an important and often largest part of the family's budget and is influenced by the family size, number of children, their age group, activity and special needs of pregnancy, lactation and disease condition. It is a proven fact that although the absolute amount of money spent on food increases with increase in family's total income, the proportion of expenditure on food decreases. On the other hand, the proportionate expenditure on food increases with a decrease in total income.

Moreover, in such cases, a higher proportion of the food budget goes in for staple as compared to protective foods such as milk, vegetables and fruits. The type of food consumed by a family depends to a large extent on the amount of money available. Hence, it is necessary that one must plan meals and buy food wisely, so as to achieve maximum nutrition from the money spent.

Knowledge of prevailing prices of food items is essential in planning meals for various age groups in different income levels. The relationships between economy and quality of food are multidimensional. Economy in food purchasing can be exercised in good measure by bulk purchase of foods, especially staples such as cereals and pulses. The prices of vegetables and fruits are much lower when they are in season and therefore available in plenty.

Majority of the incomes earned earlier were spent on food. As the earning capacities are increasing, literacy levels are raising, awareness in nutrition is increasing; there is a need to spend money wisely on food to formulate balanced diets for all the members in the family. Selection of seasonal vegetables and fruits for daily needs purchases and proper storing of staples, pulses and items consumed in bulk at harvest times will form an important step in the budgeting for nutrition.

MEANING OF FOOD BUDGET

Budgeting the food means, to provide budget for the nutritional requirements of an individual, a family or a community. The practice of family budget in India is almost nonexistent, because of lack of education and tradition. Budgeting of food is becoming important in view of the greater literacy percentage of women. Food budgeting is becoming an important factor in family budgeting in the service class or in fixed income group families.

IMPORTANCE OF FOOD BUDGET

1. To decide the expenditure of food in relation to income.
2. To receive subsidy in food planning. Fulfillment of special nutrition for vulnerable groups (children, pregnant women, lactating mother and old age).
3. Prebudgeting for contingencies such as guests and parties.
4. Possibility of changes in diet, keeping in mind the nutritional requirements as per budget.
5. To raise the health status of the individual or the family by food budgeting, so as to minimize the spending on disease and treatment.

ADVANTAGES OF FOOD BUDGET

1. The food budget gives the picture of approximate expenditure to be incurred in family.
2. Unnecessary expenditure is controlled.
3. Long-term goals can be achieved with the help of family budget.
4. Acts as a reminder of various purchases and commitment.
5. It helps the family to maintain an even standard of living.
6. Budget gives more confidence in emergencies.
7. It fulfills the needs and desires of all the family members.

FACTORS AFFECTING FOOD BUDGET

1. Lack of nutrition education or less literacy.
2. Poverty or unemployment.
3. Less individual income or low per capita income.
4. Fluctuation in market prices of food.
5. Lack or tradition of family and food budgeting.
6. Disturbances of family budget due to tradition of entertaining guests and arranging parties.

FACTORS TO BE CONSIDERED WHILE BUDGET PLANNING

1. **Number of family members:** Number of members, their age, sex, occupation, and increased meal during pregnancy, lactation and adolescence has to be kept in mind.
2. **Family's income:** The proportion of money spent on the food depends upon the income of the family. Budget is increased if income is more.
3. **Location of market:** Although supermarkets generally provide food at low cost than small neighborhood market, transportation is again problem for some people.
4. **Alternative marketing choice:** Such as ration stores, selling the food products at low cost or to buy from the wholesale market; although these products may not be graded for quality, but the nutritive value of these foods is good.
5. **Home-prepared and convenient foods:** Some convenient foods come favorably in cost with home-prepared products such as canned soups, pickles, juices and ice cream. Some convenient foods are more expensive, as they have very less shelf-life such as pastries, frozen vegetables, etc.
6. **Snack items and beverage:** This category can substantially increase the food expenditure without adding appreciably to the nutritive value of food.
7. **Availability of supplementary programs where income is limited:** Food in the school (mid-day meal), supplementary feeding for pregnant and lactating mothers increases the available food supply.

USEFUL TIPS FOR FOOD PURCHASE

Following are some useful tips, which help to stock the rupee in purchase of food items:

1. Prepare shopping list, so as to know what is needed and avoid extra tips for forgotten items.
2. Use gift coupons to refund offers, etc. only for food items that are actually needed.
3. Buy quantity that is best suited for needs and storage space. Avoid impulsive and expensive extra purchases.
4. Buy perishable foods only in amounts that can be used before they spoil. Check expiry date on perishable packaged foods.

5. Buy seasonal foods, as they are cheaper and at their peak in quality. Shop at times, when fruits and vegetables are fresh and plentiful. Avoid foods in fancy packages, as they are tentative, but expensive.
6. Read labels carefully to know ingredients used, nutrients content, cost and date of manufacture in case of packaged foods.
7. Avoid foods packaged in individual servings, as the extra packing usually increases the price. At the same time, buy bigger packs keeping in mind the quantity needed.
8. Try low-priced brands. They may be similar in quality to more expensive ones.
9. Do not shop when hungry, tired or in a hurry and shop without the pressure of children asking for snack foods.

Chapter 33

Diet as a Therapeutic Agent

The chapter discusses about:

1. Diet in the treatment of disease.
2. Methods of modifying diet in relation to:
   - Calorific value
   - Increasing and decreasing of constituents by cooking.

TYPES OF DIET USED IN HOSPITALS

Regular or Full Diet

Vegetarian or non-vegetarian foods should be well balanced and adequate for normal nutrition. This is for patients who do not need any special modifications.

Soft or Light Diet

Soft or light diet is the step between the full liquid and the regular diet. This is an easily digest able diet for patients with moderate fever, after surgery and in many medical conditions. Congee, bread, milk, eggs, fish, chicken may be served, and coffee, fruit juice and other fluids can be given; fried foods, mutton, nuts and excess of condiments are omitted from the diet.

Bland Diet

Bland diet is soft and easily digestible food with no condiments. It is often ordered in gastrointestinal (GI) conditions.

Fluid Diet or Liquid Diet

Fluid diet is given to the patients with high fever, those who are unable to take or tolerate solid food, and those being fed by tube. Patients on fluid diet should be offered drinks at least every 2 hours during the day time, and take a total of about 2,000 mL or 4 pints.

Every four hourly feeds should have milk as a basis, fortified with egg, wheat flour or skimmed milk powder and sugar or glucose. In between these feeds, sweetened fruit juice or barley water may be given.

Types of Liquid Diet

Liquid diet is for those who are unable to take solid food. A liquid diet may be either a clear liquid or a full liquid diet.

Clear liquid diet: It is used when an acute illness or surgical procedure produces a marked intolerance to food and it is advisable to restrict the intake of nutrients. The only foods permitted on this diet are clear tea, weak black coffee, fat-free broth, clear soup, meat and yeast extracts, soda water and other aerated beverages, clear fruit juice, barley water, gelatin (jelly), sugar and glucose. Such fluids have practically no food value other than calories. The calories may be increased by the use of glucose. This diet is usually continued for only 1 or 2 days.

Full liquid diet: It is given when the total nutrition of the patients must be maintained by fluids for a long period of time. This is necessary when the patient is unable to swallow solid food or if the patient must be fed by intragastric or gastrostomy tubes. This diet includes all foods that are liquid at room temperature and at body temperature. It is free from cellulose and irritating condiments. Milk usually forms the basis of such diets, because it provides adequate protein and calcium. When giving a full liquid diet, six or more feedings must be given daily. The protein content of the diet can be increased by adding whole egg or skimmed milk broth or soup. The calorie value of the diet may be increased by:

1. Adding cream to milk
2. Adding butter or oil to the cereal gruel (congee) and soup,
3. Including glucose or lactose or corn syrup in beverages (these are expensive, but less sweet and can be used in larger quantities than sugar).
4. Using ice cream.

If a decreased volume of fluid is desired, skimmed milk powder can be given instead of part of the fluid milk. If protein must be restricted, starches such as arrow root, sago and cornflour can be used to increase the calories. When the patient cannot tolerate food by mouth, a tube feeding may be used. The liquids, which can pass through the tube will provide adequate nourishment.

Modified Diet

Modified diet is for those requiring modification of the regular diet in order to supply various needs of the body in disease. Modifications of the regular diet may be made by:

1. Changing the methods of preparation, e.g. soft diet.
2. Changing the consistency, e.g. liquid diet.
3. Increasing/Decreasing the total amount of energy (calories).
4. Adding/Reducing one/more nutrients, e.g. high protein, low sodium.
5. Increasing/Decreasing bulk, e.g. high- /low-fiber diets.
6. Including/Excluding specific foods, e.g. for allergy conditions.

High-protein Diet

High-protein diet is ordered for patients with burns, protein deficiency disease, preeclamptic toxemia, and in one type of chronic kidney disease. Extra protein can be supplied by adding skimmed milk powder or egg to the milk, and by eating wheat instead of rice. Nonvegetarians can be given meat and fish. Vegetarians should include curds and dal in the diet.

Low-fat Diet

Fats are restricted in liver and gallbladder conditions such as cirrhosis, jaundice, gallstone. Bile is necessary for the digestion of fat and in these conditions, bile does not reach the duodenum in sufficient quantity. Whole milk is not allowed, but skimmed milk can also be given. Tea, coffee, sugar or jaggery, bread, rice, dal, vegetables and greens, plantains and fruits can be given. Care must be taken that no fat is used in cooking; nuts, egg yolk, biscuits and eatables fried in oil are not allowed.

Salt-free Diet

Salt is closely connected with the fluid balance of the body and a salt-free diet is ordered whenever there is edema or collections of fluid, including ascites. Edema occurs in diseases such as acute nephritis, anemia, chronic heart failures and preeclamptic toxemia. Salt is present in many foods in small quantities, but it can be restricted if no salt is added in the preparation and cooking of food, while eating. Food can be made palatable by squeezing a few drops of lime juice onto the food or by adding sugar.

Low-calorie Diet

Low-calorie diet is ordered for patients with obesity or heart conditions in which it is necessary to reduce the weight. When calories are reduced in the diet, the body takes and uses fat from its storehouses for fuel. A low-calorie diet may also be ordered for a patient with mild diabetes:

1. Sugar and jaggery are not allowed, and saccharine tablets may be used for sweetening.
2. Only a very little fat or oil may be used in cooking.
3. Cereals are allowed only in very small quantities. Wheat and ragi are preferred to rice, which contains more starch.
4. Potatoes and yams are not allowed, but other vegetables and greens may be eaten in greater quantities.
5. Fruits are allowed, but not more than one plantain a day.
6. Protein foods including milk, curds, eggs, cheese, fish, chicken, mutton, dal, etc. may be given liberally.

Low-residue Diet

Low-residue diet is a diet without roughage or anything, which would stimulate bowel action. It is given in cases such as colitis, colostomy, and may be ordered for a few days after perineal suturing. Arrowroot congee, milk and eggs, tea, toast, strained fruit juices are allowed; also vegetables and fruits, which have been softened and pressed through a sieve (puree), rough cereals, green vegetables, skins, pips, nuts, dal, peas, beans, etc. are not allowed.

Diabetic Diet

In the disease called diabetes mellitus, there is a deficiency of the hormone insulin, normally secreted by the pancreas. Insulin is needed for the proper use of carbohydrate in the body. Diet in this disease must be strictly regulated according to the amount of sugar found in specimens of urine and the amount of insulin ordered by the doctor. When an injection of soluble insulin has been given, food should follow within half-an-hour. The doctor's instruction regarding diet must be strictly followed. The patient must be helped to understand the importance of diet in his/her disease and about the dangers of coma. The nurse must be observant and prevent the patient from taking forbidden foods such as sweets and deep oil-fried eatables, sweetened coffee, etc. A diet as outlined in low-calorie diet is usually ordered.

Chapter 34

Diet and the Patient

ENVIRONMENTAL/PSYCHOLOGICAL/ CULTURAL FACTORS IN ACCEPTING DIET

To answer psychological as well as physical needs of the patient, the nurse must be aware of the important role played by the attractiveness of the patients' room. Although esthetic factors may not be accepted as being essential to good physical health, they are nevertheless of great value in establishing the desired psychological reaction.

The arrangement of furniture in the room will help to produce a harmonious effect, if it is orderly and pleasing to the patient. Color used to good advantage will help to make almost any room appear brighter and more interesting—color may be added by carefully selected drapes or bedspread, by very pretty gowns and bed jackets worn by woman patients, and by plants or flowers sent by thoughtful friends and relatives. Flowers have a definite therapeutic value for the patients. Knowing where to place flowers in a room is just as important as knowing how to arrange them. To create a pleasant environment for the patient, room should be well-ventilated, quiet, decorated and in order during meals.

Religious Practices

In different religion, there are different laws regarding foods, which may be forbidden, e.g. Hindus to not eat beef; Muslims and Jews do not eat pork. Therefore, apart from radical customs, adequate diets must be planned to meet the needs of nonvegetarians, vegetarians who eat eggs and who do not eat eggs.

Racial Habits

Choice of food varies with the custom of different groups, communities and races, and may partly be determined by the availability of food. This, in turn, is dependent to a large extent upon soil and climate.

Satiety Value

Food must also be satisfying. Physical and mental fatigue should be avoided. Physical exhaustion can be relieved by resting before a meal. Mental fatigue can be overcome by arousing a pleasant thought or ideals. If the nurse is engaged in the conversation that will impress the patient, it makes the meal a pleasure experience for him/her.

Attractive surroundings and a cheerful atmosphere add greatly to the enjoyment and hence to the digestion of a meal. The environment should be free from anything offensive to the senses such as noise, disorder, confusion, dirt, unpleasant odors, excessive heat or cold, all unappetizing objects such as sputum cups, bedpans, all equipment used for carrying out medical treatment or nursing procedure, etc.

The patient should be undisturbed by treatments, dressings, visitors, doctors' rounds and loud cries of other patients during their meal times. Visitors who demand attention from the patient, should be excluded; an agreeable and understanding companion should be encouraged to visit. Provision should be made to wash hands and the face of the patient before and after the meals.

POINTS TO BE CONSIDERED IN SERVING FOOD TO PATIENTS

1. Food must be properly cooked in order to render it digestible, and although this may not be one's duty, it is nevertheless within one's province to see that the food is invitingly served.
2. It is usually considered inadvisable to discuss food with patients except in so far as to consult their wishes, and likes and dislikes with regard to it in a purely general way, as far as they have settled down in hospital.
3. Care should be taken to avoid monotony in diet and although this may not be altogether within the scope of the nurses in hospital; it is possible in many instances to make little alterations.
4. With regard to breakfast, lunch and evening meal, there is a need to variety in the diet to give pleasure to patients. In case of a patient on milk diet, small variations can be made—a little fruit juice and sugar will serve to make milk pudding more appetizing to some.

5. Punctuality:
   a. Punctuality in serving meals is important, and absolute regularity must be observed in the administration of fluid feeding and special diets.
   b. The patient carefully observes the time; it is due, if he/she watches the nurse leave ward for the kitchen and thinks he/she will get it in next diet; if it does not come, the patient is disappointed, and perhaps by the time it arrives, the pleasurable anticipation has given place to painful and irritable anxiety; in which case the digestion of the meal may be seriously impaired.

FEEDING HELPLESS PATIENT/ PREPARATION OF PATIENT

The ward should be quiet and orderly; all unpleasant sights should be removed; any seriously ill patients should have screens placed round their beds; no visitors should be permitted, so that the patients may eat undisturbed and unobserved. Nurse should concentrate on meal time, i.e. serving the patient's meal.

The bed table should be placed where it will be comfortable. The table napkin or diet cloth should be placed within the reach of patient; or if he/she is helpless, it should be arranged in the most convenient position for the patient to reach conveniently. As far as possible, a meal should not be given immediately after a distressing treatment or painful dressing. When a helpless patient requires to be entirely fed with food and drink a diet, cloth or table napkin should be tucked underneath the chin to avoid spilling over patient's personal clothing and bed clothes in case of accident. Patients with poor appetite and a distaste for food should be gently persuaded to take food, yet they should never be forced.

A little change of dish, an alternative diet if possible, or a simple measure such as taking the patient's plate away and rearranging the food upon it, may secure the eating of the food. In giving a drink to a very helpless patient, the head should be raised by the nurse placing arm underneath the patients' pillow and elevating the head and shoulders; the drink is then put to the patient's lips and small mouthfuls given at a time. A patient should be allowed time to breathe between mouthfuls, as he/she cannot both breathe and swallow at the same time.

Longer rest should be given at intervals in all cases; and most particularly when swallowing is difficult or painful, and whenever dyspnea present. Small helpings should always be given and food placed very nearly on the plate; the patient's wishes ought to be consulted, as to whether he/she prefer gravy with meat, sauce with fish and so on. Cold food should be served on a cold plate, hot food on a really hot plate. One course is served at a time, and the soiled articles from the previous course should be removed before the next is delivered. The tray should be removed the moment patient has finished, so that he/she can be made comfortable in bed and rest, and so fulfill the requirements necessary for perfect digestion of the meal.

Food Chart

When food chart is kept, it is used to indicate the amount of food taken. A nurse should always report on the amount of food a patient has eaten.

Waste Food

The waste food has to be burnt in the incinerator.

OPPORTUNITIES FOR NUTRITION EDUCATION

Methods

By Incidental Teaching

- During patient care
- Meeting relatives.

By Organized Teaching

Toward groups: For example in a medical ward, there may be several patients suffering from anemia, group teaching can be given by discussing with them the various causes of anemia and how this condition can be prevented.

At clinics: Health teaching of interest and value to certain groups can be given at special clinics such as antenatal child welfare, leprosy and other clinics.

In the community: In every community, there are different groups—mothers, fathers, school children and teachers, occupational groups, religious groups or those living is a certain neighborhood. If there are already organized groups, contact should be made with the group leaders to try to get their interest in health problems of community.

What to Consider in Health Teaching?

1. **It should be purposeful:** It includes:
   a. Contribute towards the patients' recovery.
   b. Prevent recurrence of disease.
   c. Explain nursing procedures.
   d. Promote healthier living.
   e. Develop a desire to take action.
2. **It should be acceptable:** For instance, vegetarians, must not be advised to eat animal foods. Some practices are harmful, and much in fact, patience and understanding will be needed to get people to accept changes. Other customs may need only to be slightly modified to make them healthful.
3. **It should be practicable:** When teaching about nutrition, think of the cost of foods, which is to be recommend, and of what is in season. It is more better to call foods by name such as wheat, milk, fruit, etc. and not refer to 'vitamins,' 'proteins,' unless we are sure of the bearer's understanding level.
4. **Approach:** It includes the following:
   a. Friendly and courteous.
   b. Understanding from their point of view.
   c. Encouraging with praises for even the smallest sign of effort.
   d. Enthusiastic approach must continue until the goal is reached.

Chapter 35

Therapeutic Diets

PRINCIPLES OF DIET THERAPY

The general principles of nutrition relating to health apply also to the treatment of patients suffering from various diseases. Diet in disease must be planned as part of the complete care of the patient. Many modifications may have to be made according to the disease and the condition of the patient, but there are certain general principles, which may be used for guidance.

Diet therapy deals with modifications necessary in the diet in the treatment of different diseases. This is necessary, as the metabolism of the individual changes in different diseases with respect to one or more nutrients. The types of changes required in the diets in different diseases are briefly discussed below.

MODIFICATIONS OF NUTRIENTS IN THERAPEUTIC DIETS

Modifications of quantities of some of the nutrients may be necessary, but the following points should be noted:

1. **Carbohydrates:** These are usually well tolerated and are necessary to maintain the stores of liver glycogen. Sugars and well-cooked starches are easily digested and absorbed, and are not held for long in the intestine. High-carbohydrate diet may be indicated in Addison's disease, various diseases of the liver and in preoperative conditions. Hypoglycemia may be present in Addison's disease, while in the other two conditions, adequate glycogen storage is of considerable value in the therapy of these conditions. Restricted carbohydrate diet is essential in the treatment of diabetes mellitus.
2. **Fats:** Tolerance of fats varies in different individuals and this nutrient should not be forced if there is nausea and vomiting. During diseased conditions, if food taken by the patient is not

adequate for the body needs, then the fat stored in adipose tissue will be used for energy. Fatty acids coming from these fats are broken down to ketone bodies in the liver. The ketone bodies are then sent to the peripheral tissues for completion of oxidation to carbon dioxide and water. In the absence of carbohydrate, ketone bodies are produced more rapidly in the liver and then they are oxidized in the tissues, and so they accumulate in the blood, resulting in the condition known as ketosis. Moderately high-fat diet is used in the treatment of severe undernutrition. Restricted or low-fat diet may be necessary in the treatment of steatorrhea, malabsorption syndrome and diseases of the liver.

3. **Proteins:** In illness, there is usually an increased demand for proteins, due to wasting and this should be given in easily digestible forms such as milk, egg, chicken and fish. However, if the level of urea in the blood is greater than normal, the amount of protein in the diet must be restricted. High-protein diets, i.e. about twice the actual requirements with restriction in other nutrients are prescribed in a variety of diseases such as protein-calorie malnutrition (PCM), cirrhosis of liver, peptic ulcer, malnutrition, nephrosis and celiac diseases. Low protein or complete withdrawal of proteins may be necessary in hepatic coma, acute uratemia, etc.
4. **Inorganic elements:** The requirements of calcium and iron must be maintained during illness and it is therefore necessary to check these elements, if a patient is on restricted diet for a long time. Sodium and potassium may sometimes need to be restricted, especially if there is edema and ascites.
5. **Vitamins:** These must always be adequate to maintain the balance of a diet. Fat-soluble vitamins often need to be added as concentrates, if a patient has to be on a fat-restricted diet for a long time. Vitamin B complex are often deficient in Indian diets and may not be adequately absorbed in pathological conditions of the gastrointestinal (GI) tract. The demand for vitamin C is greatly increased in fevers, and is especially necessary for the healing of wound after surgery. Increase in the content of vitamins can be easily achieved by the addition of synthetic vitamins. This is essential, as most of the therapeutic diets may be partially lacking in one or more vitamins. Modifications in diets rich in fiber are prescribed for the treatment of constipation, while low-fiber diets are essential in the treatment of several GI

disorders such as peptic ulcer, ulcerative colitis, celiac diseases, diarrhea and dysentery.

6. **Roughage:** Excessive bulk hinders the penetration of the digestive juices, but it may be necessary to include foods with a moderately high-residue content to produce daily bowel action.
7. **Fluids:** These are every important to prevent dehydration, which is common in conditions of fevers, diarrhea and vomiting. In such condition, 2,500–3,000 mL of fluids must be given in 24 hours with as much variety as possible, both in appearance and in taste. If adequate fluids cannot be given by mouth, they must be given intravenously. Fluids with added protein are necessary for patients who must be fed on liquid diets for a long time.

In almost all diseases, milk is one of the best foods; except for its deficiency in iron, histamine and ascorbic acid, it can be modified and flavored in different ways to prevent monotony.

Calorie content

Diets with increased calorie value are used for the treatment of patients who are markedly underweight and also for patients with increased calorie requirements as in fever, infections, malabsorption and hyperthyroidism. Low-calorie diets are used for the treatment of obesity, cardiovascular disease, acute uremia and hepatic coma.

Mineral content

High-calcium diet is essential in the treatment of rickets and osteomalacia, where a diet restricted in calcium and phosphate is desirable in renal calculi. Sodium-restricted diets are essential in the treatment of cardiac failure and hypertension. Restriction in NaCl intake is essential in diseases of the kidney.

Other Constituents

Diets low in purine content are prescribed in the treatment of gout, while diets low in oxalic acid and purines are prescribed in renal calculi. The most important are the liquid diets used in oral feeding and nasogastric feeding. The basis of such diets is milk to which soluble carbohydrates such as sucrose, glucose and Dextri-Maltose and emulsified fats are added to increase their calorific value. The changes in the diet pattern required in some common diseases are inefficient utilization of carbohydrates in diabetes mellitus, inability of the kidney to excrete sodium chloride in nephritis, increased production and inefficient elimination of uric acid in gout, and increase in energy metabolism and in catabolism of tissue proteins in fever. The simplest modification of diets is the treatment of allergy where the food(s) responsible for the allergic reactions are eliminated. Modifications in diets in other diseases may involve changes in different constituents such as:

1. Bland diets omitting condiments and spices.
2. Low- or high-fiber diets.
3. High- or low-protein diets.
4. High- or low-fat diets.
5. High- or low-carbohydrate diets.
6. High- or low-calorie diets.
7. Low-sodium and low-purine diets.

In case the patient is unable to consume food orally, then administration of nutrients through parental route or through nasogastric tube is essential to avoid starvation, and loss of protein and other nutrients from the tissues.

MANAGEMENT OF SPECIAL DIETS

Consideration of the Patient's Food Habits

When a special diet is advised by a doctor, the management of that diet is as important as any other part of a patient is treatment. It must be carefully noted what type of diet is being given and whether there are any restrictions or addition needed, e.g. fat, protein, carbohydrate, salt. The patient must then be questioned about his/her food habits as follows:

1. Does he/she take non-vegetarian or vegetarian food?
2. If nonvegetarian, does he/she take all foods such as egg, mutton, fish, liver, beef, pork?
3. If vegetarian, does he/she take egg?
4. What type of cereal does he/she take for breakfast, lunch and dinner? For example, congee, bread, rice (parboiled or raw) chapati, wheat, rice products that are common in his/her community.
5. Does he/she take coffee or tea or both? At what time?
6. How much milk does he/she normally take, and can this be increased if necessary? Does the patient take it plain or with sugar or flavoring?
7. What types of dal and green vegetables are taken?

8. How much seasoning is generally used in food preparation?
9. Is there any food, which the patient cannot or will not take?

Methods of Calculation

Based on the patient's food habits and the doctor's diet prescription, the diet must be calculated as follows:

1. The minimum requirement of protein per day, i.e. the grams per kilogram body weight for an adult should be met, unless the doctor advice any restriction.
2. Foods containing carbohydrate and fat must be added in the diet to make up the remainder of the required calories.
3. If an increased amount of any nutrient is required, the foods, which the patient will not have difficulty in taking, should be added.
4. Check the diet qualitatively for mineral and vitamin content.
5. Adjust the special requirements accurately, if necessary.

Methods of Cooking

Ordinary methods of cooking may be used unless there is restriction of salt, fat, seasonings in the diet order. The quantity of fat or oil used, need to be reduced in diets of low-calorie value, and seasonings and spices must be reduced in bland diets, especially for gastric ulcer cases. Further preparation may be necessary after cooking, e.g. straining of vegetables in low-residue diets.

Educating the Patient

It is often necessary for a patient to continue on special diet after he/she is discharged from hospital and must, therefore, know details of the diet before leaving. The reason for this special diet should be explained clearly and simply, with stress on foods, which must be increased or decreased. If any food is forbidden, the reason should be made quite clear. Alternative foods, which may be allowed to provide variety, should be given, and if possible, the patients should be instructed regarding the length of time for which the special diet must be continued. The quantities of food allowed should be weighed in hospital and shown to the patient in a common measures with which he/she is familiar, so that the patient can estimate the right amount at home.

MODIFICATIONS IN DIET CONSISTENCY

Diets will have to be modified with regard to consistency to suit the needs of the patient. These include:

- Soft diet
- Clear fluid diet
- Full fluid diet.

Further, for patients who cannot consume diets or fluids orally, tube feeding will have to be resorted; the diets suitable for tube feeding are also discussed in this section.

Soft Diet

The soft diet is used in acute infection, some GI disorders and in postoperative cases. The diet soft in consistency, easily digested and contains very little fiber, spices and condiments is called soft diet. The composition of soft diet for an adult and a simple menu are given in Tables 35.1 and 35.2.

Table 35.1: Composition of soft diet for an adult (g/caput/day)*

Foodstuffs	Vegetarian	Nonvegetarian
Milled cereals and cereal products (cooked rice, idli, bread)	300	300
Dal	50	30
Milk	1,000	600
Meat and fish sausages	–	100
Egg	–	30
Cheese	80	30
Tender vegetables	50	50
Potato	100	100
Tender leafy vegetables	100	100
Fruits (banana, apples, oranges)	100	100
Fats and oils (butter and vegetable oil)	30	30
Sugar	80	80

*Calorie 2,000–2,200 kcal; proteins 60–70 g.

Table 35.2: Sample menu based on soft diet

Vegetarian	Nonvegetarian
Morning	
Milk with sugar 1 cup	Milk with sugar 1 cup
Breakfast	
Corn flakes with milk or	Corn flakes with milk or
Bread 4 slices with butter or	Bread 4 slices with butter or
Idli 2	Idli 2
Cheese 2 slices	Egg, half boiled 1
Fruits 1 serving	Fruits 1 serving
Milk or milk beverage 1 cup	Milk or milk beverage 1 cup
Lunch	
Cooked rice	Cooked rice
Cooked macaroni 1 serving	Cooked macaroni 1 serving
Vegetable soup 1 serving	Mutton soup 1 serving
Mashed dal 1 serving	Meat or fish sausages 1 serving
Curds 1 cup	Curds 1 cup
Fruits 1 serving	Fruits 1 serving
Milk pudding 1 serving	Milk pudding 1 serving
Evening (tea time)	
Bread 2	Bread 2
Cheese 2 slices	Cheese 2 slices
Milk 1 cup	Milk 1 cup
Dinner	
Same as lunch	Same as lunch

Clear Fluid Diet

Clear fluid diets are prescribed for patients with marked intolerance to foods as manifested by nausea, vomiting, loss of appetite, etc. These consist of tea with lemon and sugar, fat-free broth, carbonated beverages, fruit juices, glucose water, cereal water and plain gelatin. The clear fluid diets are usually used for 1 or 2 days, till the patient is able to retain and digest a more liberal liquid diet. At the beginning, the amount of fluid given to patient is restricted to about 40-80 mL/h; the quantity is gradually being increased to 100–120 mL, as the patient improves. Clear fluid diets are meant to provide some calories and to make up the water loss in the body. The composition of clear fluid diet is detailed in Table 35.3.

Table 35.3: Composition of clear fluid diet

Fluid diet	Composition (mL)
Orange juice	1,000
Glucose water (10%)	1,000
Barley water (with glucose) or	1,000
Tender coconut water	1,000
Total	4,000

Full Fluid Diets

Full fluid diets are prescribed when the patient is unable to chew and swallow solid foods. These consist of milk, eggs, cereal porridge, soup, fruit juices and gelatin dessert. The diet will provide the minimum requirements of proteins, calories, vitamins and minerals. The composition of the full fluid diet for an adult and sample menu plan is given in Tables 35.4 and 35.5.

Table 35.4: Composition of full fluid diet for an adult (g/caput/day)*

Foodstuffs	Vegetarian	Nonvegetarian
Semolina and corn flour	50	50
Dal flour	30	–
Milk	1,500	1,000
Sugar	100	100
Meat	–	100
Egg	–	50
Fruit juice	–	One
Cream	4 tablespoon	4tablespoon

*Calories 1,820 kcal; proteins 50–55 g.

Table 35.5: Daily menu based on full fluid diet

Vegetarian	Nonvegetarian
Morning	
Milk 1 cup	Milk 1 cup
Breakfast	
Cereals porridge with cream, sugar and milk 2 cups	Cereals porridge with butter, sugar and milk 2 cups
Milk or coffee 1 cup	Milk or coffee 1 cup
Midmorning	
Fruit juice 1 glass	Fruit juice 1 glass
Breakfast	
Dal soup 1 cup with cream	Strained meat soup 1 cup
Tomato juice 1 cup	Tomato juice 1 cup
Custard pudding 1 serving	Eggnog 1 serving
Milk 1 cup	Milk 1 cup
Midafternoon	
Fruit juice 1 glass	Fruit juice 1 glass
Evening (tea time)	
Milk beverage 2 cups	Milk beverage 2 cups
Dinner	
Same as lunch	Same as lunch

SPECIAL FEEDING METHODS

Patients suffering from severe illnesses are unable to consume foods and fluids orally. Hence, special feeding methods have been used for feeding such patients. These include:

1. Tube feeding (nasogastric feeding).
2. Gastrostomy (tube feeding directly into the stomach).
3. Jejunostomy (tube feeding directly into the jejunum).
4. Intravenous feeding.

Diets for Tube Feeding

The diets used in tube feeding (Table 35.6) may be of three types:

1. High-carbohydrate diet.
2. High-carbohydrate and normal protein diet.
3. High-protein and high-calorie diet.

Calories

An average adult patient will require 1,500–2,000 kcal. After surgical operation, injury, burns, in severe PCM, provision of 3,000 kcal may be necessary. If adequate calories are not supplied, wasting of body muscle will take place.

Proteins

In the case of hepatic coma, protein should be given, while an average patient suffering from other diseases will need 60–70 g of proteins. In the case of injury, burns after surgery and in severe malnutrition, large quantities of proteins (100–200 g) should be administered.

Table 35.6: Composition of tube feeds (g/caput/day)

Type of feed	Composition
1. High-carbohydrate feed (no proteins)	
• Water	1.5
• Glucose	300 g
• Sucrose	100 g
• Orange juice	1 L
• Electrolytes	as required
• Vitamins	as required
Total	> 2.5 L
2. High-carbohydrate, moderate fat and protein feed	
• Milk (cow's)	1.5 L
• Barley water	1.0 L
• Glucose	300 g
• Sucrose	100 g
Total	> 2.5 L
3. High-calorie and high-protein feed	
• Milk (cow's)	1.5 L
• Evaporated milk	100 g
• Glucose	200 g
• Maltodextrin	100 g
• Cane sugar	100 g
Total	> 2.5 L

Fat

Fat should be in the form of emulsion.

Carbohydrates

Glucose, cane sugar and Dextri-Maltose can be used as source of carbohydrates. About 300–500 g will have to be administered daily depending on the calorie needs of the patient.

Fluid

The daily fluid requirements of an adult are about 2,500–3,000 mL and can be easily provided.

Electrolytes

Electrolytes such as sodium chloride, potassium chloride, etc. can be easily added to the food depending on the needs of the patient.

Vitamins

The daily requirements for all essential vitamins can be given in the food.

Gastrostomy Feeding

It may be necessary to feed a patient with carcinoma of the esophagus through gastrostomy. The tube is inserted directly into the stomach at the time of operation. The composition of tube feeds table can be used depending on the condition of the patient.

Jejunostomy Feeding

Feeding through jejunum, i.e. through a tube introduced directly into the jejunum will be necessary in the case of patients with extensive inflammation and malignancy of the esophagus and stomach or after esophageal resection or total gastrostomy. The tube is inserted into the jejunum at the time of operation. Since salivary and gastric digestion are completely eliminated and the stomach, which serves as a reservoir of food is absent, the patients should be given small quantities of feed (100 mL) every 30 minutes by using homogenized milk to which glucose and vitamins have been added. Hollander and co-workers (1945) have recommended a special formula of cream with predigested proteins and carbohydrates together with vitamin and mineral supplements.

Intravenous Feeding

The main objectives in intravenous feeding are:

1. To provide water and electrolytes—to prevent dehydration and correct electrolyte imbalance.

2. To make up the loss of tissue proteins.
3. To provide energy to meet the daily needs of the patients.

Intravenous feeding will have to be resorted to, in the following diseases:

1. In the surgery of GI tract, extensive burns, etc.
2. In cancer of the mouth, pharynx and esophagus, which obstructs the passage of food.
3. Patients who are unconscious due to hepatic failure, diabetic coma, acute uratemia, injury of the brain, etc.

Techniques used in Intravenous Feeding

The techniques employed are:

- Peripheral venous infusion
- Infusion through a polyethylene tube into the deep veins.

Peripheral venous infusion

The technique is used for administering isotonic solution of glucose (5%), saline (0.85%) and other electrolytes for a short period. The needle is inserted in the upper limb veins.

Infusion through polythene tube

The technique is used when the intravenous feeding has to be continued for several days or when hypertonic solutions have to be given. The method consists in threading a polythene tube (cannulae) into the deep veins or superior or inferior vena cava. Care should be taken to avoid the danger of infection. This technique has an advantage, i.e. the limbs can be moved freely.

Nutrients Used in Intravenous Feeding

The nutrients used are:

- Water and electrolyte
- Amino acids
- Emulsified fat
- Carbohydrates and alcohol
- Whole blood or plasma
- Vitamins.

Water and electrolytes

The daily minimum water requirement of an adult is about 1.5 liters. Additional water will be required to correct dehydration that might have occurred before the start of therapy. The clinical symptoms of different degrees of dehydration are as follows:

1. Mild symptoms of thirst and oliguria indicating about 2% less of body water (1 L in a 50 kg individual).
2. Moderate symptoms of thirst, oliguria and mental confusion indicating about 6% loss of body water (3 L in a 50 kg man).

3. Severe symptoms of thirst, severe great prostration indicating 8–12% loss of body water. The water loss should be made up in about 24 hours and the urinary excretion restored to about 300–400 mL in every 8 hours.

Carbohydrates and alcohol

The carbohydrates used in intravenous feeding are glucose, fructose and sorbitol. Alcohol can also be given at the rate of 8 g/h as a 3% solution. Glucose is usually administered as a 5% solution. A higher concentration of glucose is likely to result in thrombophlebitis of the infused vein. Fructose is preferable to glucose, as it can be administered at a concentration of 10–15% without causing thrombophlebitis. Sorbitol is also given at 30% concentration without causing any adverse effect.

Both fructose and sorbitol are rapidly metabolized and their metabolism is less dependent on insulin. Alcohol is given as a 3% solution at the rate of 8 g/h. A higher concentration may produce venous thrombosis and intoxication. Alcohol provides 7.1 kcal/kg.

Amino acids

Amino acid solutions available for intravenous feeding are protein hydrolysates, which are usually prepared from acid hydrolysis of casein. The hydrolysate is dialyzed to remove peptides, which may be antigenic or pyrogenic. Tryptophan loss due to acid hydrolysis is made up by the addition of synthetic tryptophan. Synthetic amino acids usually consist of D and L forms.

Since the D form is not utilized by the body, synthetic amino acid mixtures are not commonly used. A solution containing L-amino acid is ideal for use in the intravenous therapy, but is costly. Hence, protein hydrolysates prepared from casein are free from peptides and fortified with tryptophan, and are commonly used in intravenous therapy.

Whole blood and plasma

Up to 1 liter of whole blood provides about 180 g proteins including hemoglobin. Blood is used mainly to combat circulatory failure and loss of blood from the body. A liter of plasma contains about 60–70 g of proteins. Plasma infusion is given as a measure for increasing plasma protein level when it is low.

Emulsified fats

Fat emulsions for intravenous therapy were first introduced in Japan (Nomura, 1928). These are being used at present in some countries. Their keeping qualities are limited and they produce toxic reactions such as dyspnea, urticaria, tachycardia, flushing, vomiting and muscle pain in some patients. In view of the above, fat emulsions for intravenous use have been banned in the USA.

Vitamins

All the vitamins (twice the daily requirements) should be added to the intravenous fluid to meet the daily needs of the patient.

Solution for Parenteral Nutrition

Nutrients solutions for intravenous administrations are given in Tables 35.7 and 35.8. It is evident that it is possible to provide easily the daily requirements of proteins, calories, vitamins, water and electrolytes.

Table 35.7: Solutions for parenteral nutrition for 24 hours

Solutions	No. of bottles	Volume (mL)	Amino acid (g)	Calories (kcal)
Fructose (20%)	2	1,000	–	750
Amino acids (3.3%), fructose (15.0%) and ethanol (2.5%)	5	2,500	80	125
Total	7	3,500	80	875

Table 35.8: Composition of intravenous nutrients solutions used in USA (adult/24 h)

Nutrients	Quantity	Nutrients	Quantity
Water (mL)	2,500–3,000	Vitamin A (IU)	5,000–10,000
Protein hydrolysates (amino acids) (g)	100–140	Vitamin D (IU)	500–1,000
		Vitamin E (IU)	2.5–5.0
Carbohydrate (g) (dextrose)	525–730	Vitamin C (mg)	250–250
Calories (kcal)	2,500–3,500	Thiamine (mg)	25–50
Sodium (mEq)	125–150	Riboflavin (mg)	5–10
Potassium (mEq)	75–120	Pyridoxine (mg)	7.5–15
Magnesium (mEq)	4–8	Niacin (mg) Nicotinic acid (mg)	50–100 12.5–25

HIGH-PROTEIN AND LOW-PROTEIN DIETS

High-Protein Diets

Diets rich in proteins are prescribed for the treatment of PCM and protein deficiency in undernourished patients, before and after surgery, after injury and burns, and in nephritis (type II). The diets are usually based on milk and contain liberal amounts of cheese, eggs, meat and fish (Table 35.9).

Proteins

Diets usually contain about 125–150 g of proteins in case of adult, and 60–100 g for children below 10 years depending on age. The protein intake should be 3–4 g/kg depending on the condition of the patients. The nutritive value of the proteins should be high.

Calories

For the maximum utilization of proteins, the diet should be adequate in calories. Hence, the diets should provide the daily requirements of the calories for the patient.

Table 35.9: High-protein diets in adult (g/caput/day)*

Foodstuffs	Vegetarian	Nonvegetarian
Cereals	200–250	200–250
Legumes	100	100
Milk (cow's)	1,000–1,500	800–1,000
Cheese	80–100	–
Meat and fish	–	100–150
Eggs	–	40–60
Nuts	80–120	80–120
Fats and oils (as vegetable oils)	30–50	30–50
Sugar and jaggery	30–50	30–50
Green leafy vegetables	50–100	50–100
Other vegetables	50–100	50–100
Fruits	100–200	100–200

*Proteins 120–150 g; fat 60–70 g; carbohydrate 250–300 g; calories 3,000–3,500 kcal.

Vitamins and Minerals

Diets containing liberal amounts of milk, egg, meat, fish and green leafy vegetables will also be excellent sources of all essential vitamins and minerals.

Low-protein Diets

Low-protein diets are prescribed for patients suffering from glomerulonephritis, chronic uremia, jaundice and vital hepatitis. Proteins should be mainly derived from milk and other animal foods, and should be of high nutritive value. Since these diets contain only small amounts of protective and protein-rich foods, they will be lacking in several vitamins and minerals (Table 35.10).

Table 35.10: Low-protein diet for adult (g/caput/day)*

Foodstuffs	Vegetarian	Nonvegetarian
Cereals	100–150	100–150
Corn starch or sago	100	100
Legumes	20	20
Milk	300–400	300–400
Meat, fish and egg	–	20–30
Potato	100	100
Green leafy vegetables	100	100
Other vegetables	100	100
Fat and oils	40–60	40–60
Sugar and jaggery	100	100
Fruits	200	200
Multivitamin tablet	1	1

*Proteins 25–30 g; carbohydrate 250–300 g; fat 60–80 g and calories 2,000–2,500 kcal.

HIGH- AND LOW-CALORIE DIETS

High-calorie Diets

High-calorie diets are prescribed for patients who are malnourished and underweight. Weight loss also occurs in many diseases such as tuberculosis, hyperthyroidism, prolong fevers, etc. The composition of high-calorie diets is given in Table 35.11. Hence, the diet should be supplemented with a multivitamin mineral tablet.

Calories

Diets should provide about 500 calories in excess of the daily needs.

Proteins

The protein intake should be 50% more than the requirements. The proteins should be of high quality and derived mostly from milk and other animal foods.

Vitamins and Minerals

High-calorie diets usually contain adequate amounts of different vitamins and minerals. Nevertheless, it is desirable to supplement the diet with a multivitamin mineral diet.

Table 35.11: High-calorie diet for adult (g/caput/day)*

Foodstuffs	Vegetarian	Nonvegetarian
Cereals	300–400	300–400
Legumes	80–100	80–100
Milk (cow's)	1,000–1,500	800–1,000
Meat and fish	–	50
Eggs	–	30
Nuts	100–150	100–150
Fats and oils (half the fat as vegetable oils)	100	100
Sugar and jaggery	100	100
Fruits	200–300	200–300
Green leafy vegetables	100	100
Other vegetables	100	100

*Proteins 80–100 g; fats 60–80 g; carbohydrates 400–500 g; calories 3,000–4,000 kcal.

Low-calorie Diets

Low-calorie diets are prescribed for obese subjects. The aim is to produce calorie deficit in the body, which will result in the fat stored in the adipose tissue being used to meet the calorie needs. It has been observed in obese adults that a diet providing about half the requirement of calories for persons leading sedentary life (1,100 kcal) will help to reduce the body weight by 1–15 kg a week. Consumption of diet providing 1,300 kcal may help to reduce the body weight by 0.5–1.0 kg per week. The composition of diets providing 1,100–1,300 and 1,500 kcal is given in Table 35.12.

Table 35.12: Low-calorie diets for adults (g/caput/day)

Foodstuffs	Diet I		Diet II		Diet III	
	1,100 calories		1,300 calories		1,500 calories	
	V*	NV†	V	NV	V	NV
Cereals	80	80	100	100	130	130
Legumes	60	40	70	50	80	60
Skim milk powder	100	50	100	50	100	50
Skim milk fluid	1,000	500	1,000	500	1,000	500
Cheese	50	–	50	–	50	–
Meet and fish	–	50	–	60	–	70
Egg	–	60	–	80	–	100
Green leafy vegetables	150	150	150	150	150	150
Other vegetables	200	200	200	200	200	200
Roots and tubers	100	100	100	100	100	100
Protein	50	50	50	50	50	50
Fats and oils	15	15	20	20	25	25
Cane sugar	15	15	20	20	25	25
Multivitamin mineral tablet	1	1	1	1	1	1

*V, vegetarian; †NV, nonvegetarian.

LOW- AND HIGH-RESIDUE (FIBER) DIETS

The terms 'fiber' and residue are used interchangeably with respect to the diet, as diets rich in fiber give rise to accumulation of large amounts of undigested residue (bulk) in the large intestines. While diets low in fiber leave only small amounts of residue in the large intestines. The term 'fiber' includes cellulose, hemicelluloses, pentose, etc. They are present in large amounts in bran of cereal grains, the husk of pulses and mature vegetables.

Low-residue Diets

Low-residue diets are recommended for patients suffering from GI disorders, such as peptic ulcer, ulcerative colitis, celiac diseases, diarrhea and dysentery. The composition of low-residue diet is given in Table 35.13.

Table 35.13: Composition of low-residue diets for adults (g/caput/day)*

Foodstuffs	Vegetarian	Nonvegetarian
Milled cereal and cereal product	350	350
Dal	20	20
Milk	1,000	500
Meat and fish	–	40
Egg	–	30
Tender vegetables	50	50
Tender green leafy vegetables	50	50
Potato	100	100
Fleshy fruits	100	100
Fruit juice	200	200
Fats and oils	50	50
Sugar and jaggery	50	50

*Calories 2,400 kcal; proteins 60–70 g.

High-residue Diets

High-residue diets are rich in fiber and recommended for patients suffering from constipation. *Such diets leave large amounts of undigested bulk* in the intestinal tract, which helps to relieve constipation. Recent studies have shown that fiber diets retard the absorption of cholesterol and decreases its level in blood. The composition of high-fiber diet is given in Table 35.14.

Table 35.14: Composition of high-fiber (residue) diets for adults*

Foodstuffs	Vegetarian	Nonvegetarian
Whole cereals	350	350
Whole legume	80	80
Dal	50	50

Contd...

Contd...

Foodstuffs	Vegetarian	Nonvegetarian
Milk	600	400
Meat	–	40
Egg	–	30
Green leafy vegetables	100	100
Other vegetables	200	200
Roots and tubers	100	100
Fruits	100	100
Oils and fats	50	50
Sugar and jaggery	50	50

*Calories 2,400 kcal; proteins 60–70 g.

DIFFERENT TYPES OF THERAPEUTIC DIET (TABLE 35.15)

Table 35.15: Different types of therapeutic diets

Diet	Indication	Foods to be included and avoided
High-fiber diet	Atonic constipation, atherosclerosis, obesity, diabetes	*Foods included:* All long, fiber vegetables such as amaranth greens, cabbage, spinach, etc. Special stress on raw vegetables and salads. All fruits, with skins when tender, whole grain cereals and breads with bran in fine division. Milk, meat, fish, fowl, eggs as desired for normal nutrition *Foods to avoid:* Highly refined and concentrated foods, fried foods, excessive amount of coarse bran, excessive seasonings *Intervals of feeding:* Three meals daily, water and fruit juices between meals before breakfast and before retiring

Contd...

Contd...

Diet	Indication	Foods to be included and avoided
Soft, moderately high-fiber diet	When there is abnormal irritation of the intestines, bulk must be provided in smooth, finely divided form: – Spastic constipation – Mucous colitis – Peptic ulcer	*Foods included:* Modify soft diet to include only pure fruits and vegetables in increased amounts *Food to avoid:* Non-soft diet *Intervals of feeding:* Three to six small meals
Very low-residue diet	Severe diarrhea needs rest to the gastrointestinal (GI) tract Ulcerative colitis during initial stages of treatment preceding and following operations on the colon or rectum when no movement is desired for several days. Partial intestinal obstruction	*Foods included:* Tender meat, fish, clear fat free soups, fruit juices, eggs, refined cereals and breads beverages, coffee, tea, butter and sugar *Foods to avoid:* Coarse bread and cereals, cheese, milk, excessive fat, fried fruits (except juices) and vegetables, tough meats, condiments, excessive sweets *Intervals of feeding:* Usually three meals daily
Bland diet	This diet is used to prevent stimulation of peristalsis and flow of gastric juice by mechanical or chemical irritation and to reduce inflammation: – Gastric and duodenal ulcers – Gastritis (hyperchlorhydria) – Gastric atony – Diarrhea – Ulcerative colitis (refer high-protein diet)	*Foods included:* Milk, cream, butter, milk, cheese, eggs, tender meat, fish, cooked and strained fruits and vegetables, strained citrus juices, white bread, cereals, white potato, rice, etc. *Foods to avoid:* Coarse cereals and breads, rich cheese, though meats, raw and strongly flavored vegetables, raw fruit (except juice), excessive seasonings, pickles, strong coffees, etc. *Intervals of feeding:* Three meals daily with three intermediate feedings

Contd...

Diet	Indication	Foods to be included and avoided
	– Fever (refer high-calorie fluid and soft diet) – Severe jaundice (refer high-CHO and high-protein diets)	
High-calorie diet	When it is desirable to replace lost weight, this diet is used in many conditions, but especially in such diseases as hyperthyroidism, which has a high metabolic rate, fevers and undernutrition in general	*Foods included:* A regular diet with added sugar, cream, butter, eggs, etc. to increase the caloric intake *Foods to avoid:* Fried foods, excessive quantities of bulky low-calorie foods *Intervals of feeding:* Five to six meals daily
High-calorie fluid and soft diet	The diet is used during acute stages of fevers, typhoid, pneumonia, tuberculosis, etc. where there are evidences of malnutrition, but the patient cannot tolerate the full soft or regular diet. Dehydration and weight loss must be combated and corrected	*Foods included:* All foods on the fluid plus eggs in all forms except fried, strained whole grain cereal, white bread, potato, strained vegetables in cream soups and cream *Foods to avoid:* Fried foods, all vegetables except in cream soups, all meat, fish, poultry, breads and cereals, nuts *Intervals of feeding:* Usually every 2 hours, night feeding may be indicated
Low-calorie diet	When body weight exceeds 10% above average weight for height. This is especially important in: – Obesity – Diabetes mellitus	*Foods included:* 1,200 calorie diet, 3 cups milk, meat, 1 egg, 2 bread exchanges, 2 group A vegetables, 1 group B vegetable, 3 fruit exchanges, 1 teaspoon butter *Foods to avoid:* All except those included in exchange list

Contd...

Contd...

Diet	Indication	Foods to be included and avoided
	– Cardiac and kidney disturbances where an extra burden is placed on damaged and overworked organs – Hypertension – Gout – Gallbladder disease	*Intervals of feeding:* Three meals daily, may use six smaller meals
High-carbohydrate (CHO) diet	Toxemias of pregnancy, liver disturbances (refer high-protein diets), preparation for surgery, Addison's disease	*Foods included:* Fruits and vegetables, which are high in CHO, simple starchy puddings, cereals, white and whole wheat bread, fruit desserts and jellies, glucose, sucrose, milk, eggs, meat, fish and butter used as necessary for adequate nutrition *Foods to avoid:* Fried foods, condiments, spices, alcoholic beverages, all rich and fatty foods *Intervals of feeding:* Depends on condition, but usually three meals with three intermediate feedings
High-protein diet	Protein deficiency following inadequate intake, before and after surgery, injury/burns to replace tissue and blood proteins in: – Liver diseases – Hyperthyroidism (refer high-calorie diet) – Pernicious anemia – Diabetes mellitus	*Foods included:* Meat, eggs, milk, fish, pulses, skimmed milk powder, soybeans *Foods to avoid:* If there is restriction of sodium, the diet must be carefully planned *Intervals of feeding:* Usually three meals with three intermediate feeding of high-protein beverage

Contd...

Contd...

Diet	Indication	Foods to be included and avoided
	– Celiac disease, which is characterized by intolerance for CHO and fats	
Moderately low-protein diet	Whenever there is marked retention of nitrogen as in severe nephritis with uremia (refer sodium-restricted diet)	*Foods included:* 2 glasses milk, 1 egg, cereals in combination with milk *Foods to avoid:* In excess of amounts should be avoided, meat, fish, egg, milk, bread, cereal, legumes, nuts and seasoned foods *Intervals of feeding:* Three meals daily, sometimes six small feedings are preferable
Moderate to low-fat diet	– Liver and gallbladder disturbances (refer high-protein diet) – Obesity (low-calorie diet) celiac disease and pancreatic disease (refer high-protein diet) – Intestinal disturbances when membranes show a sensitivity to fatty acids (refer bland diet)	*Foods included:* Milk (whole of skim), egg, meat, cheese, egg white, whole gram, bread, cereals, fruits and vegetables *Foods to avoid:* Fats, depending on disease condition, especially fatty meat, gravy, salad, fried foods, strongly flavored vegetables, nuts and legumes
Low-cholesterol diet	Gallstones atherosclerosis	*Foods included:* Skim milk, meat, poultry or fish, cereal, leafy vegetables, yellow vegetables, other vegetables and fruits

Contd...

Contd...

Diet	Indication	Foods to be included and avoided
		Foods to avoid: Butter, cheese, cream, whole milk, egg yolk, liver, fish. All foods high in fat, oils, fried foods and fatty meats
Sodium-restricted diet	To prevent edema in: – Nephritis – Nephrosis – Cardiac disease – Cirrhosis of liver – Toxemia of pregnancy – ACTH therapy – Hypertension	*Foods in specified amounts:* Milk, meat, eggs, fish, poultry *Unrestricted foods:* Unsalted cereals, breads, fruits, vegetables, unsalted fats, sugars *Foods to avoid:* All salted foods, canned fish, vegetables, pickles, salted butter, bread, nuts. Foods containing baking powder or soda, cakes, prepared mixes, spinach, dry fish
Acid-ash diet	To adjust the reaction of urine, so that salts are held in solution. Kidney stones—calcium and magnesium phosphates, carbonates and oxalates	*Foods included:* Large servings of meat, poultry, fish, eggs, whole grain cereals, bread, cake, rice, noodles and corn *Limit:* Milk, fruits and vegetables *Neutral foods as desired:* Butter, sugar, oils and fat, coffee, tea
Alkaline-ash diet	To adjust the reaction of the urine, so that salts are held in solution—kidney uric acid and cystine calculi	*Foods to avoid:* Legumes, spinach, greens, dried fruits, salty foods such as canned fish and canned vegetables, salted nuts *Intervals of feeding:* Three meals daily *Foods included:* Large amounts of fruits, vegetables, milk *Limited amounts:* Meat, eggs, 1 serving cereal, 1–2 slices bread *As desired:* Butter, sugar, oils and fats

Contd...

Contd...

Diet	Indication	Foods to be included and avoided
		Foods to avoid: Meat, fish fowl, cheese, cereal, rice cakes, cookies
Low-purine diet	Gout	*Foods included:* Milk, eggs, cereals and bread, potato, vegetables, fruits, butter *Foods to avoid:* Meat extracts, meats, especially organic meat, fish—sardines, alcohol beverages *Intervals of feeding:* Three meals daily

Chapter 36

Naturopathic Diet

Naturopathy is an alternative medicinal system that philosophizes on a holistic approach for preventing and curing ailments. This approach includes natural remedies and believes in curing the cause rather than the symptoms. What's more, naturopathy has almost no side effects as it does not require surgery and drugs. Naturopathy gives utmost importance to regular exercise, maintaining the right diet and being mentally stress free. One needs to give up sedentary lifestyle and modify their diet, as it restores the body to good healthy and has long-lasting results.

DEFINITIONS

Naturopathy

1. Naturopathy is the art and science of disease diagnosis, treatment and its prevention using natural therapies including botanic medicine, hydrotherapy, traditional Chinese medicine and lifestyle counseling.
2. Naturopathy is defined as a distinct school of healing, employing nature's forces. It is a system of healing in which diseases are cured by means of natural and rational remedies such as water, sunlight, air, earth power, electricity, magnetism, exercise, rest, proper diet, various kinds of mechanical treatment, mental and moral science. It is also a way of life in which combination of different methods of natural healing are used.

Naturopathic Diet

A system or method of treating disease that employs no surgery or synthetic drugs, but uses special diets, herbs, vitamins, massage, etc. to assist the natural healing processes.

NATUROPATHIC PRINCIPLES APPLIED TO MEAL PLANNING

A naturopathic diet follows the six guiding principles of naturopathic medicine:

1. Trust that the body can heal itself.
2. Identify and treat the cause.
3. Treat the person as an integrative whole.
4. Use non-harming and non-invasive techniques.
5. Focus on overall health, wellness and disease prevention.
6. Use education to allow people to take responsibility for their health.

With this in mind, a typical naturopathic meal includes a combination of approximately 50% organic vegetables, 25% whole grains and 25% protein made up of organic dairy products or free-range meats.

FUNCTIONS OF NATUROPATHY

1. Naturopathic medicine is based on the belief that the diet should not include food that is unnatural or wholesome as it, produces toxins that poison the body.
2. Conditions that are treated and eliminated with a naturopathic diet include digestive issues, food sensitivities and allergies, immune disorders, reproductive imbalances, high cholesterol, insomnia, stress and anxiety.
3. Naturopathy focuses on the body's ability to heal naturally and without external interference.
4. A healthy diet, by naturopathic standards, supports balance and wellness in the body and mind, while stimulating the body's ability to heal.

BASIC GUIDELINES FOR NATUROPATHIC DIET

1. Naturopathic nutrition begins with assessing, which foods cause harmful reactions in the digestive system.
2. Food allergies and intolerances has crucial points of interest in a person's wellness and diet.
3. Once determined, the foods are eliminated and a diet based on whole, natural foods is advised.
4. Naturopathic nutrition encourages eating locally grown organic foods and foods lowest on the food chain, as well as eating slowly to improve digestion.

5. As naturopathy maintains, diet plays an extremely important role in one's health. Our diet has a direct bearing on our health and almost all illnesses are related to our diet.
6. Our diet must include adequate protein, vitamins, calcium, minerals and other nutrients. A well-balanced diet is the key to good health and preventing serious ailments such as heart diseases, increased blood pressure, diabetes, risks of cancer and any other diseases.
7. Avoid consumption of too much sodium, sugary, oily, fried and junk food, processed and refined food. White sugar, white rice and white flour must be substituted by their brown counterparts. One must also consume as little of tea and coffee as possible.
8. Herbal teas such as green tea, ginger root tea, chamomile, mint and holy basil, to name a few are better options, as they are good for health; and avoid consuming alcoholic beverages completely.
9. Consuming the juice of two oranges and an apple in the morning has many health benefits such as easing bowel movements.
10. Start the day with proteins, as it keeps oneself energetic throughout the day and prevents frequent hunger pangs.
11. We must especially consume lots of spinach, broccoli, tomatoes, asparagus, lettuce, cabbage, cauliflower, kale, beetroot and collard greens to name a few, as these are rich sources of vitamin A, C and K, fiber, calcium and vitamins.
12. Also drink coconut water and juices of carrot, spinach, bitter gourd and beetroot as frequently as you can. One must also avoid meats. Oils such as olive and canola are better than hydrogenated vegetable oils.

Intake of Calories in Naturopathic Diet

Naturopathic nutrition does not emphasize caloric intake, though consuming appropriate amounts is important. Roughly 70% of total daily calories should come from grains and legumes, 20% from fruits and vegetables and 10% from concentrated protein, such as meat and eggs.

Optimum Foods

Natural, whole foods are the foundation of a healthy naturopathic diet. Legumes, such as beans, peas, peanuts and lentils, and whole grains such as whole wheat, bulgur, barley, quinoa and spelt, provide rich amounts of vitamins, minerals and dietary fiber. They also provide modest amounts of protein. Fruits and vegetables provide vitamins, minerals, fiber, water and antioxidants, which are disease-fighting nutrients. According to the American Dietetic Association, most people's antioxidants needs can be met by consuming 2 cups of fruit and 2.5 cups of vegetables daily. Organic meat, poultry, fish, dairy products and eggs provide rich amounts of protein, B vitamins, iron and zinc. Fatty fish provide omega-3 fatty acids—healthy fats the body must obtain from food, known to support brain function and heart's health. Refrigerated oils, such as olive oil, also provide healthy fats.

Foods to Avoid

Naturopathic medicine encourages users to avoid foods linked with disease, poor digestion and weight gain. According to Boice, these foods include processed snack foods, fast food, added sugars, saturated fats and trans fats. Saturated fats are found in fatty red meat, dark meat poultry, poultry skin, butter, whole milk, high-fat cheese and cream. Trans fats include shortening, margarine and hydrogenated vegetable oils.

NATUROPATHIC DIET RECIPES

As per naturopathy, a combination of healthy diet along with wheat grass powder shows better health-enhancing results. Following are the recipes for preparing items mentioned in the diet plans:

1. **Brown rice:** This semipolished rice has a reddish brown color and contains more beneficial nutrients than white (polished) rice. It should be washed minimum and soaked for 2–3 hours before cooking it in a pressure cooker using the same water.
2. **Rice soup:** Follow the above method, but add water 8–10 times the quantity of rice. Remove the rice to a side and the thick rice soup that is obtained contains many proteins, amino acids, minerals and vitamins, etc.
3. **Moong dal (green gram) soup:** Add seven to eight times water and boil without stirring, strain out the thick watery soup and add a little salt and pepper for taste. The soup thus obtained contains many proteins, amino acids, minerals, vitamins, etc.
4. **Sprouted pulses:** Pulses such as green moong, matki, harbara dal, etc. are very nutritious when eaten raw after sprouting. For sprouting, first soak the selected pulses in water for 8–12 hours.

Then, drain the water and keep the pulses wrapped in a thick wet cloth for 1 day. Keep the cloth moist by frequent watering. Length of the sprouts increases if kept for another day or two. Longer sprouts are more nutritious. Raw sprouts are recommended to be included in daily diet. The sprouts can also be boiled/stir-fried by adding a little salt, pepper and spices for flavor.

5. **Carrot juice:** Remove the inner whitish stem (as its acidic) and use the outer reddish layer of the carrot for extracting juice by adding water as required.
6. **Vegetable salad:** Use vegetables such as carrot, cucumber, cabbage, radish, beetroot, spinach, lettuce, coriander, etc. by cutting them into small pieces or shredding. Mix them well and add salt and pepper. Another version is to add dry fruits and honey to the previously mixed salad. It has a little sweet taste and is liked by children also.
7. **Basil leaf tea (tulsi kadha):** Take 2 cups of water + 3 or 4 basil (tulsi leaves) + lemon grass (gavati chai) + ginger (2 g) + jaggery as a sweetener. Boil the above ingredients (without adding milk) and pour the tasty drink in a tea cup. Try this tea instead of the regular tea/coffee and you will find it more refreshing.
8. **Jaggery syrup (gud paak):** Use organic jaggery, which is dark brown in color. Break into small pieces. For 1 kg jaggery, add 2 cups water and let it soak for about 10 hours. Then, add a little more water and boil well to form thick syrup. Let it cool naturally, strain the syrup and store it in a glass/ceramic jar. It should be prepared fresh in quantity as required for a week. Jaggery syrup is an excellent sweetener and should be used wherever required instead of sugar. It can be added to milk also or eaten with roti by adding a few drops of lemon juice for taste.
9. **Lime water (nimbu pani):** Take a glass of water (warm or cold water as per the season), squeeze a half/full lemon in it and stir well (do not add any salt or sugar). Having a glass of limewater first thing in the morning has therapeutic value.
10. **Vegetable soup:** Select two/three vegetables from a variety such as bottle gourd (bhopal), ridge gourd (dodka), cabbage (patta gobi), Fenugreek leaves (methi), spinach (palak), cow pea (chowli), etc. Cut them into small pieces, add water twice the quantity of vegetables and steam cook in a cooker. Let it cool a little and then extract its soup by grinding and removing the fiber through a wire-mesh strainer. Give seasoning of cumin

seeds (jeera), garlic, turmeric powder and kari patta. This soup has very high nutritious value.

11. **Baked potatoes:** They are better than the boiled potatoes. Apply a mudpack before baking them over coal amber in a tandoor/barbeque and eat them without removing the skin. In urban areas, they can be baked in an oven/microwave.
12. **Ragi roti (madua/nachni roti):** Ragi is good in minerals and fiber supplement. Rotis are prepared from ragi flour. Another version is to prepare roti by mixing bajra/jowar flour with it.
13. **Ragi (madua/nachni) milk:** Take a bowl of ragi seeds (nachni) and soak for 12 hours. Then grind the sprouted ragi by adding water as required in a mixer. Strain it using a cloth. It is good for diabetes patients.
14. **Khichdi:** Mix two-third part brown rice and one-third part of sprouted green moong + four times the quantity of water + garnishing of turmeric, salt, grinded groundnuts, coriander, jeera, garlic, ginger, etc. Add previously cut vegetables such as bottle gourd, cucumber, carrot, green peas, etc. Mix and steam cook in a cooker.
15. **Vegetable parathas:** Add precut vegetables such as cabbage, potato, cow pea, fenugreek, ginger, garlic, onion, etc. to wheat/jowar dough and roast the parathas over a flat pan by adding a little oil/ghee/butter.
16. **Fruit salad:** Cut and mix sweet fruits such as papaya, chikoo, banana, apple, dates, etc. Add thick buttermilk/sweet whipped curds. Do not add milk with custard powder, as is the general practice. A few mint (pudina) or basil (tulsi) leaves add flavor.
17. **Potato skin soup:** Wash clean 4–5 medium-sized potatoes and scrap off the skin using a scraper. Boil the skin in water and strain out the thick soup. Add a little salt for taste.
18. **Til (sesame seed) chutney:** Dry roast a bowl of til (sesame seeds) on a low flame till they splutter. Add a little dry coconut, roasted garlic 10 flakes, rock salt and red chili powder 1 tsp or dry pepper for taste. Pound or dry grind it in a mixer.
19. **Jawas (flaxseed/linseed) chutney:** Flaxseeds are the best source of essential omega-3 fatty acids and rich in antioxidants. Dry roast a bowl of jawas (flaxseed) on a low flame till they splutter. Add a little dry coconut, roasted garlic 10 flakes, rock salt and red chili powder 1 tsp or dry pepper for taste. Pound or dry grind it in a mixer. One spoonful with every meal is a healthy addition to the diet, It can also be sprinkled over salad sprouts.

DIET THERAPY

Various types of diets are in use all over the world. The names of such diets and the conditions where they are used are as follows:

- Anderson diet: Peptic ulcer
- Lehnartz milk and eggs diet: Peptic ulcer
- Meulengracht diet: Peptic ulcer
- Sippy diet: Peptic ulcer
- Atkins diet: Obesity
- Yo-Yo syndrome diet: Obesity
- Bland diet: Gastrointestinal disturbances and peptic ulcer
- Grollman diet: Hypertension
- Kempner's rice diet: Hypertension
- Karrel milk diet: Myocardial infarction
- Ketogenic diet: Epilepsy
- Pritikin Nathan diet: High performance
- Rowe's diet: Allergy
- Synthetic diets: Allergy.

Convenience Foods

Convenience food items served to patients on regular diets are rarely appropriate for therapeutic diets unless the suppliers of foods prepare them according to rigid specification set by the dieticians or nutritionists.

Dietetic Foods

Foods for special dietary use that are commonly available include fruits canned without the addition of sugar, bread made without salt, vegetables canned without sodium and artificially sweetened pudding mixes, gelatin dessert powder, cookies, jellies, candy, gum and carbonated beverages.

Section VIII

Food Preservation and Hospital Diets

Chapter 37

Cooking

ART OF COOKING

Cooking is an art. It is linked with the dietary habits and cultural pattern of people:

1. Cooking renders the food easy to digest. It makes mastication easier.
2. It lends a new flavor and thereby stimulates digestive juices.
3. It sterilizes food by killing microorganisms, and parasitic ova and eggs.
4. It introduces variety, i.e. many different types of dishes can be prepared with the same ingredients.
5. Good cooking increases the acceptability of food, whereas bad cooking may lead to rejection of even highly nutritious foods.

METHODS OF COOKING

Boiling

Cooking in water at 100°C (212°F) is called boiling. Rice, dal, pulses, roots, tubers and other vegetables are cooked in this way. Boiling in excess of water may result in loss of vitamins and minerals. Therefore, it is a general rule that boiling should be done using minimum amount of water.

Simmering

Cooking below boiling point, i.e. about 84°C is called simmering. Meat and fish are best cooked by simmering, because at high temperature, the fibers of meat are hardened.

Steaming

Steaming is cooking by the heat of direct steam. This principle is employed in pressure cookers. Because of the increased pressure of steam, the temperature attained is higher than 100°C. Pressure cooking is a better method of cooking, since it saves nutrients, fuel and time.

Stewing

Stewing method differs from boiling, in that:

1. Comparatively smaller amounts of liquid is used.
2. Prolonged low degrees of heat is applied; usually 200°F for stewing. The food is half covered with liquid and as soon as it reaches boiling point, the heat is reduced to make it simmer for a prolonged time. For each kilogram of food, approximately 7 liters of fluid is required. For better results, use pan with a well-fitting lid to prevent evaporation. The nutrients, which escape while stewing are not lost, but are present in the liquid, which is served with stew. Stewing is used for cooking meat.

Frying

Frying may be two types, i.e. shallow and deep frying. Shallow frying is suitable for cooking foods such as eggs, savages, dosa and pre-cooked food. In deep frying, food is completely immersed in large-quantity of hot oil. It is suitable for making puri, pakora, vada, cutlets, etc. In deep frying, the oil should be sufficiently hot, otherwise food will absorb lot of oil.

For shallow frying: The fat or oil in the pan needs to be only about one-eighth inch deep. The fat should be hot and quite smooth on the surface when the food is put into it, when browned on one side, the food should be turned and browned on the other side. This method is satisfactory for fish cakes, cutlets and lean cuts of meat, fish and bacon.

Roasting

Food is smeared with a little fat and exposed directly to heat or flame. Chicken or tender mutton may be cooked by this method. It is also called 'barbecue'.

Baking

Baking is cooking food by dry heat. It is done in a hot air oven. Food is enclosed by hot air, so that it gets heat from all sides. The cooking temperature may vary from 250 to 500°F. Baking is an expensive and slow method of cooking.

Broiling or Grilling

Broiling or grilling is cooking by direct dry heat. It can be done either in grill or heavy pan or direct on flame. It is a very quick method of cooking. Only very tender foods can be grilled, viz. kebab, cheese, tomatoes and brinjals.

METHODS OF ENRICHING THE FAMILY DIET

Sprouting Gram

Increasing the vitamin B and C content of the gram. Green gram is best for health. Soak it in water for 24 hours; then spread it out on a damp cloth and keep the cloth damp for 1 or 2 days, until there is a ½ inch sprout. It may be eaten raw or after cooking for a short time. Fermenting cereals and dals increases the vitamin 'B' content. This is done in making the popular South Indian Idly and dosa.

Cereal Millet Mixture

Using a millet such as ragi or bajra or jowar together with the staple cereal, adds extra nutrients to the diet.

Cereal Pulse Mixture

The protein value of a meal is increased by adding dal or groundnuts to rice, roti or chapati.

Milk Porridge

If instead of using water, milk is used to make the porridge out of any cereal flour, an infant gets more protein and calories in the diet.

Powdered Protein Foods

Powdered protein foods can be prepared at home or in a mill. Foods rich in plant proteins such as groundnuts, grams and dals, beans, are pounded or ground into powder. Dried fish can also be powdered. The protein-rich powders can be kept in tins. They need to be cooked and should therefore be added to the cereal flour before cooking. This makes a very nutritious meal for a child.

Pounded Dark Green Leaves

The leaves may be pounded either fresh or dried. Dried leaves makes a green powder, which can also be used to enrich a child's porridge. It can also be added to the dough for making roti or chapati, to enrich the family diet. It is rich in protein and iron.

Chapter 38

Preservation and Storage

HOUSEHOLD/COMMERCIAL METHODS OF PRESERVING AND STORING FOOD

Household Methods

Cold Storage and Freezing

The home refrigerator has now made it possible to store and preserve a variety of foods. Fruits and vegetables should be kept just above the freezing point, i.e. 0°C or 31 to 33°F. Meat and butter are kept at much lower temperatures. There is no growth of food poisoning organisms at this low temperature.

Drying or Dehydration

Drying removes water; and in the absence of water, microorganisms cannot grow. Fruits, fish and meat are preserved by drying. In this method, vitamin 'C' is destroyed, but other nutrients are preserved.

Smoking

Meat may be cured with smoke. Smoke contains phenols, which help in preservation.

Salting and Pickling

Salt is a preservative. By adding certain condiments and spices along with salt, certain foods such as mangoes, vegetables, meat and fish may be preserved.

Canning

Home canning is generally not recommended unless the technique employed is foolproof.

Commercial Methods

Canning

Various foods, e.g. fruit juices, milk and baby foods, soups and fish are preserved by canning. The food is first sterilized at high temperature (275–350°F) for a short time (matter of a few seconds) then cooled and filled in presterilized containers in a sterile atmosphere. There is some loss of heat-labile vitamins during the process of canning.

Freezing

A number of foods, e.g. fruits, vegetables, meat and fish are preserved by the freezing technique. At 0°F, vegetables can be preserved for 8–10 months and meat for about 3 months.

Chemicals

Certain chemicals such as benzoic acid and sodium benzoate may be used for preservation, but their use is strictly limited by government regulations, which prohibit the use of chemicals for preserving food.

Irradiation

Microorganisms are destroyed by gamma rays, wheat, potatoes and onions may be preserved by irradiation.

PRINCIPLES IN METHODS OF COOKING AND SERVING FOR PRESERVATION OF NUTRIENTS

General Principles

1. Plan the daily diet for the family, so that it contains foods from each of the five food groups. The diet should be varied to make it more appetizing.
2. Buy foods, which are in season because they will be cheaper and plenty; try to buy at least one that can be served raw.
3. Select fruits and vegetables, which look fresh; buy just enough for 1 day.
4. Discard any damaged or decayed portions and store in a well-ventilated container or food safe in a cool place from the direct sun. Keep potatoes and onions open in a dry place.
5. Clean and wash the vegetables or fruit before cutting to preserve nutrients; do not soak cut vegetables in water.

6. Well-scrubbed vegetables and fruits do not to be peeled or scraped before cooking or eating. Vegetables such a potatoes cooked with their skins retain more nutrients.
7. Clean and cut vegetables just before cooking or serving raw in order to preserve nutrients.
8. Many kinds of leaves and tops of vegetables, such as beetroot, radish, cauliflower, knol khol, turnip, drumstick and carrot are rich in protective nutrients, and should be used in curries or other dishes.
9. Preserve nutrients in food during cooking by:
   a. Cooking with the minimum amount of water, not throwing any excess water after cooking rice or vegetables and using any water left for making a soup or drink by adding savory or sweet seasonings.
   b. If cereals or dals are soaked before cooking, using the same water for cooking because it contains dissolved nutrients.
   c. Covering root vegetables so as to cook them in their own steam, and also to reduce the cooking time.
   d. Cooking leafy green vegetables quickly in a little boiled salted water.
   e. Not using soda to preserve the color of vegetables or to soften them, because it destroys nutrients.
   f. Avoiding overcooking or refreezing vegetables or keeping them warm on the fire, as these practices destroy the nutrients.

Additional Methods for Increasing the Nutrients in Food

1. **Sprouting pulses:** Bengal gram, black gram or green gram, increases the vitamin B and C content. Such processing also increases the digestibility of pulses, so that they are especially good foods for young children. Sprouted pulses should be prepared and served either raw or lightly cooked in order to preserve the nutrients.
2. **Fermenting cereal and dal:** Increases the vitamin B content of both foods. This is commonly done in South India, e.g. in preparing idly and dosa.
3. **Mixing a pulse with a cereal:** As in khichdi increases the quality of the protein eaten.

FOOD HYGIENE OR PRECAUTIONS IN SELECTION OF FOOD

Food is a potential source of infection. It can be contaminated by bacteria and other microorganisms and parasites at any point during its journey from the producers to the consumer—food hygiene implies hygiene in the production, handling, distribution and serving of all types of food.

Milk

Sources of Infection

The contamination of milk may arise from three sources such as:

1. The dairy animal (tubercle bacilli).
2. The human handler (typhoid bacilli).
3. The environment (through contaminated vessels, polluted water, dust and flies).

Control Measures

Boiling of milk

Boiling is an ancient method of rendering the milk safe for human consumption. In fact, much of the milk produced in India is treated by boiling. The disadvantages of boiling the milk are:

1. Boiling kills all organisms present in the milk, including the useful lactic acid bacteria.
2. It destroys vitamin C and B mostly.
3. Boiling gives 'cooked' taste to milk, due to the burning of lactose during boiling.
4. Proteins in the milk are coagulated.
5. The enzymes are destroyed.

In short, boiling alters the taste, flavor and nutritive value of the milk considerably.

Pasteurization

Pasteurization has been defined by an Expert Committee of WHO (1970) as "the heating of milk to such temperatures and for such period of time as are required to destroy any pathogens that may be present, while causing minimal changes in the composition, flavor and nutritive value". Pasteurization differs from boiling in the following respects:

1. Pasteurization destroys only the harmful pathogenic bacteria, but not the useful lactic acid bacteria.

2. The vitamins are not destroyed by pasteurization.
3. Pasteurization causes only minimal changes in protein and sugar. It is the simplest, safest and the cheapest method rendering milk safe.

Phosphatase test

Phosphatase test is employed to find out if the milk has been properly pasteurized or not. The test is based on the principle that the enzyme phosphatase, which is present in raw milk, is destroyed during pasteurization. If phosphatase enzyme is present after pasteurization, it indicates that the milk has not been properly pasteurized.

Meat

The term 'meat' includes various tissues of animal origin. Meat can be a source of infection, if it is bad or unwholesome.

Meat-borne Diseases and Pathogens

The meat-borne diseases and some causative organisms are:

1. **Tape worms:**
   - *Taenia solium*
   - *Taenia saginata*
   - *Trichinella spiralis*
   - *Fasciola hepatica.*
2. **Bacterial:**
   - Anthrax
   - Actinomycosis
   - Tuberculosis
   - Food poisoning.

Signs of Good Meat

The characteristics of good meat are:

1. **Color:** This should not be pale pink or deep purple.
2. **Touch:** The meat should be firm and elastic to touch; it should not be greasy or slimy.
3. **Smell:** The odor should be agreeable.

Fish

Fish decomposes quickly after death.

Signs of Fresh Fish

The signs of fresh fish are:

1. It must be in a state of stiffness or rigor mortis.
2. The gills must be bright.
3. The eyes must be clear and prominent.

The following diseases are known to be transmitted by fish:

1. A tape worm known as *Diphyllobothrium latum (D. latum).*
2. Fish poisoning—since fish is not eaten raw *D. latum* infestation is a rare disease.

Tinned Fish

More and more people are eating tinned fish and meat these days than ever before. It is necessary to inspect the tin or can before consuming the contents. The following points should be noted when examining tinned fish or meat or any other tinned food:

1. The tin must be from fresh stock, i.e. it must be new and clean.
2. There should be no evidence of having been tampered with, as for example, the presence of sealed openings; such tins should be discarded.
3. On shaking the tin, there should be no sound.
4. On opening the tin, the contents should not be blown out; on the other hand, there should be a hissing noise.

Eggs

Eggs become stale on prolonged storage and storage under unsatisfactory conditions.

Signs/Tests for Freshness

The freshness of the eggs may be tested as follows:

1. **Candling:** When a strong light is projected, the egg must appear transparent. The eggs are rejected, if there are any spots or internal blemishes.
2. **Floating in saline water:** Fresh eggs sink in 10% salt solution; stale eggs will float.

Fruits and Vegetables

Fruits and vegetables, especially those which are eaten raw, e.g. tomatoes, radish can be a source of infection. Those which are grown in sewage irrigated land, are particularly dangerous, if eaten raw and unwashed. They can transmit pathogenic bacteria such as the 'typhoid bacilli' and worm infestations. Vegetables, which are cooked and eaten are free from this danger. Vegetables, which are to be eaten raw, are best treated in a weak solution of potassium permanganate and later washed in running water.

Contamination and its Effect on Health (Food-borne Diseases)

Chapter 39

The term 'food-borne disease' is defined as a disease, usually either infectious or toxic in nature, caused by agents that enter the body through the ingestion of food, with the increase in urbanization, industrialization, tourism and mass catering systems, food-borne diseases are on the increase throughout the world.

TYPES OF FOOD-BORNE DISEASES

Food-borne diseases may be classified as detailed below.

Food-borne Intoxications

1. Due to naturally occurring toxins in some foods:
   a. Lathyrism (beta-oxalyl-amino-alanine).
   b. Endemic ascites (pyrrolizidine alkaloids).
2. Due to toxins produced by certain bacteria:
   a. Botulism.
   b. Staphylococcus poisons.
3. Due to toxins produced by some fungi:
   a. Aflatoxins.
   b. Ergot.
   c. Fusarium toxins.

Food-borne Chemical Poisoning

1. Heavy metals, e.g. mercury (usually in fish), cadmium (in certain shellfish) and lead (in canned food).
2. Oils, petroleum derivatives and solvents, for example, tricresyl phosphate (TCP).
3. Migrant chemicals from package materials.
4. Asbestos.
5. Pesticide residues (DDT, HBC).

Food-borne Infections

1. **Bacterial:** Typhoid, cholera, salmonellosis, shigellosis, etc.
2. **Viral:** Viral hepatitis, gastroenteritis, etc.
3. **Parasitic:** Ascariasis, amebiasis, trichinosis, etc.

Milk-borne Diseases

Milk is an important 'vehicle' or 'medium' for the transmission of disease agents, e.g. tubercle bacilli, typhoid bacilli. The contamination of milk may arise from three sources:

1. The dairy animal, e.g. tubercle bacilli.
2. The human handler, e.g. typhoid bacilli.
3. The environment, e.g. through contaminated vessels, polluted water, dust and flies.

The important milk-borne diseases are:

1. **Directly from the milk animal:**
    - Bovine tuberculosis
    - Brucellosis
    - Streptococcal infections
    - Q fever
    - Cow pox
    - Foot and mouth disease
    - Anthrax
    - Tick-borne encephalitis.
2. **Indirectly from the human handler or environment:**
    - Typhoid and paratyphoid fevers
    - Dysentery
    - Cholera
    - Viral hepatitis
    - Diphtheria.

Nutritional Diseases

1. **Protein-energy malnutrition (PEM):**
    a. Kwashiorkor.
    b. Nutritional marasmus.
    c. Other PEM.

2. **Vitaminosis:**
   a. Vitamin 'A' deficiency.
   b. Thiamine and niacin deficiency states.
   c. Deficiency of B-complex components.
   d. Ascorbic acid deficiency.
   e. Vitamin 'D' deficiency.
   f. Other nutritional deficiencies.
3. **Obesity and other hyperalimentation:**
   a. Obesity.
   b. Hypervitaminosis A.
   c. Hypercarotenemia.
   d. Hypervitaminosis D.
   e. Others.
4. **Diseases of blood and blood-forming organs:**
   a. Iron deficiency anemia.
   b. Other deficiency anemia.

FOOD TOXICITY

Food intoxication refers to food-borne illness caused by the presence of toxin formed in the food. Poison is difficult to define. Many substances present in food would have adverse or toxic effects (Table 39.1), if taken in large doses, but the amounts normally present in foods are harmless.

Toxic factors or toxicants refer to those substances found in foods that produce deleterious effect on health when ingested by man or animals. For example, the contaminants may include dust, dirt, plant material from the same plant or other sources, inedible parts of animal body in case of flesh foods, dirty water in case of milk, chemicals used in feeds that may enter the meat or milk of animals, etc.

CLASSIFICATION OF TOXIC CHEMICALS IN FOODS

1. Natural toxicants in foods.
2. Natural toxicants entering through contaminants:
   a. Plant origin.
   b. Microbial origin.
   c. Biological agents.
3. Chemical toxicants of external origin:
   a. Toxic metals.
   b. Pesticide residues and agrochemicals.

Table 39.1: Some possible toxic effects of foods

Sources	Active agents	Effects
Banana and some other fruits	5-hydroxytryptamine, adrenaline and noradrenaline	Effects on central and peripheral nervous system
Some types of cheese	Tyramine	Raise blood pressure, enhanced by monoamine oxidase inhibitors
Some types of fish, meat or cheese	Nitrosamines	Cancer
Mustard oil	Sanguinarine	Edema
Legumes	Hemagglutinins	Red cell and intestinal cell damage
Some types of beans	Vicine	Hemolytic anemia, toxic effects
	β-aminopropionitrile β-n-oxalyl-amino-alanine	On nervous system
Green potatoes	Solanine	Gastrointestinal upset
Many fish	Various; often confined to certain organs	Mainly toxic effects on nervous system
Many fungi	Various mycotoxins	Mainly toxic effects on nervous system and liver

c. Contaminants from processing practices.
d. Contaminants from packing practices.
e. Accidental contaminants.
f. Contaminants from environment.

Natural Toxicants in Foods

Plants species are often naturally containing chemicals when consumed in large quantities over long period may prove toxic. Such naturally occurring toxicants are also called antinutritional principles. For example, goitrogens that may cause hypothyroidism are found in mustard cabbage and other vegetables. Some vegetables that grow with high levels of nitrogen fertilizers may contain high levels of nitrate, which may prove toxic. It may be necessary to inactivate toxicants by heating or by special treatments.

Toxicants of Natural Origin Entering Through Contaminants

1. **Plant origin:** Toxin-containing seeds such as datura, argemone may enter grains and oil seeds rendering them unsafe for human consumption.
2. **Microbial origin:** Foods with high moisture content are susceptible to contamination by bacteria and mold. High counts of these in foods are necessarily due to poor hygiene and sanitation:
   a. The presence of enteric pathogens in high quantity may cause food-borne diseases such as typhoid, paratyphoid, cholera, gastroenteritis, diarrhea, dysentery and food poisoning.
   b. The infection often comes from persons carrying these contaminants or use of unclean vessels or contaminated vessels multiply speedily as food is a good medium.
   c. Some bacteria grow in the intestines and cause diseases. Some grow in the food and produce toxins.
   d. The bacterial toxins are responsible for food poisoning. Some fungi may grow in foods and produce toxins and are called mycotoxins, some of which may, after chronic consumption, cause cancer of liver or kidney.
3. **Biological agents:** Parasitic worms and flukes that may infect animals and human beings may enter through drinking water or flesh foods, e.g. round worms and liver fluke causing trichinosis.

Chemical Toxicants of External Origin

1. **Toxic metals:** The metals such as lead, antimony, cadmium, arsenic and mercury may enter processed foods through contact with metal containers, pipes, vessels or through chemicals and additives used in processing.
2. **Residues of pesticides and agrochemicals:** Fumigants and pest control chemicals used in storages may enter the grains, nuts, oil seeds and other grain products. Live stock feeds often contain antibiotics and chemicals. The animals may receive drugs to control infections. These may enter their bodies and leave residues in milk, meat and eggs.
3. **Contaminants from processing practices:** Food often undergoes unpermitted processing treatments such as artificial ripening with lime, calcium carbide, methane, artificial coloring with non-permitted synthetic dyes, antimicrobial agents that

may be toxic, pesticides, artificial sweeteners such as saccharine, thickeners such as filter paper. All these practices come under the food adulteration, although they may be practiced due to ignorance. Thermal processing such as roasting and frying may produce polycyclic hydrocarbons. Cyclic polymers of fatty acids may cause toxicity for humans.

4. **Contaminants from packaging materials:** Processed foods are packed in containers of metal, glass, plastic and paper. Acidic foods are known to dissolve metals, e.g. zinc and tin. Levels are known to rise in fruit juices, plastic contain additives such as colors, fillers and chemicals; these may get transferred to the foods. Such contaminants can prove toxic.
5. **Accidental contaminants:** In warehouses where food materials are stored or during transport, these may be accompanied by packs containing toxic materials such as containers of pesticides, paints, etc. If uncleaned containers are used for storing food materials such as edible oils, etc. toxic chemical may contaminate the food products.
6. **Contaminants from environment:** Industrial effluents, automobile exhausts and sewage, drinking water, processed water used for industries and growing crops are likely to get contaminated. Plants exposed to automobile exhausts are known to contain higher lead content. Chemicals from industry, detergents, etc. may contaminate food materials.

COMMON FOOD TOXICANTS

Lathyrus Toxins

The cause of neurolathyrism is a toxin beta-oxalyl-amino-alanine (BOAA), which is found in the seeds of the pulse. Neurolathyrism is a public health problem in certain parts of the country where this pulse is eaten. The pulse is called '*Lathyrus sativus*' is commonly known as 'khesari dal'. It is known by local names such as 'toor dal', 'lak dal', 'batra', 'chura matar', etc.

The seeds of *Lathyrus* have a characteristic triangular shape and gray color. When dehusked, the pulse looks similar to red gram dal or Bengal gram dal. Similar to other pulses, *Lathyrus* is a food source of protein, but for its toxin, which affects the nerves. It is eaten mostly by the poor agricultural laborer, because it is relatively cheap. Students have shown that diets containing over 30% of this dal, if taken over a period of 2–6 months, will results in neurolathyrism. The toxin present in *Lathyrus* seeds has been identified as BOAA. It has been isolated in crystalline form and is water soluble. This property has been made use of in removing the toxin from the pulse by soaking it in hot water and rejecting the soaked water.

Disease

The disease affects mainly young men between the age of 15–45 years and manifest itself in the following stages:

1. **Latent stage:** The individual is apparently healthy, but when subjected to physical stress, exhibits ungainly gait. Neurological examination shows characteristic physical signs. This stage is considered important from the preventive aspect, if the pulse is withdrawn from the diet, it will result in complete remission of the disease.
2. **No-stick stage:** The patient walks with short jerking steps without the aid of a stick. A large number of patients are found in this stage.
3. **One-stick stage:** The patient walks with a crossed gait with a tendency to walk on toes. Muscular stiffness makes it necessary to use a stick to maintain balance.
4. **Two-stick stage:** The symptoms are more severe. Due to excessive bending of knees and cross legs, the patient needs two crutches for support. The gait is slow and clumsy, and the patient gets tired easily after walking a short distance.
5. **Crawler stage:** Finally, the erect posture become impossible as the knee joints cannot support the weight of the body. There is atrophy of the thigh and leg muscles. The patient is reduced to crawling by throwing his/her weight on the hands.

However, it is not possible to avoid consuming khesari dal; it is desirable that the proportion of the dal should never form more than a quarter of the total amount of cereals and pulses eaten per day.

Aflatoxins

Aflatoxins are group of 'mycotoxins' produced by certain fungi, '*Aspergillus flavus*' and '*Aspergillus parasiticus*'. These fungi infest foodgrains such as groundnut, maize, parboiled rice, sorghum, wheat, rice, cotton seed and tapioca under conditions of improper storage, and produce aflatoxins (potent liver carcinogen) of which

B_1 and G_1 are the most potent hepatotoxins, in addition to being carcinogenic. The most important factors affecting the formation of the toxin are moisture and temperature. Aflatoxicosis is quite a public health problem in India.

Control and Preventive Measures

A crucial factor in the prevention of fungal contamination of food-grains is to ensure their proper storage after drying. If food is contaminated, it must not be consumed.

Ergot

Ergot is not a storage fungus, but a field fungus. Foodgrains such as bajra, rye, sorghum and wheat have a tendency to get infested during the flowering stage by the ergot fungus. The fungus grows as a blackish mass and the seeds become black and irregular, and are harvested along with foodgrains. Consumption of ergot-infested grain leads to ergotism.

The symptoms include nausea, repeated vomiting, giddiness and drowsiness extending sometimes for periods up to 24–48 hours after the ingestion of ergot grain. In chronic cases, painful cramps in limbs and peripheral gangrene due to vasoconstriction of capillaries have been reported. Ergot-infested grains can be easily removed by floating them in 20% salt water. They can also be removed by hand picking or air floatation.

Argemone Oil Contamination (Epidemic Dropsy)

From time to time, outbreaks of 'epidemic dropsy' are reported in India. The cause of epidemic dropsy was not known until 1926, when Sarkar ascribed it to the contamination of 'mustard oil' with argemone oil. This toxic substance interferes with the oxidation of pyruvic acid, which accumulates in the blood.

The symptoms of epidemic dropsy consist of sudden, noninflammatory, bilateral swelling of legs, often associated with diarrhea. Dyspnea, cardiac failure and death may follow. Some patients may develop glaucoma; the disease may affect at all ages except breastfed infants. The death rate varies from 5 to 50%.

The contamination of mustard or other oils with argemone oil may be accidental or deliberate. Seeds of *Argemone mexicana* (prickly poppy) closely resemble mustard seeds. The plant grows wild in India. It has prickly leaves and bright yellow flowers. Crops of mustard are gathered during March, and during this period, the seeds of argemone also mature and are likely to be harvested along with mustard seeds. Sometimes unscrupulous dealers mix argemone oil with mustard or other oils.

Argemone oil is orange in color with an acrid odor. The following tests may be applied for the detection of argemone oil—nitric acid test. A simple test is to add nitric acid to the sample of oil in a test tube. The tube is shaken and the development of a brown to orange-red color shows the presence of argemone oil. The accidental contamination of mustard seeds can be prevented at the source by removing the argemone seeds growing among oil seed crops. Unscrupulous dealers may be dealt with by the strict enforcement of the prevention of Food Adulteration Act.

Crotalaria or Weed Seed Contamination (Endemic Ascites)

Studies conducted by the National Institute of Nutrition, Hyderabad showed that the local population subsist on the millet. *Panicum miliare* (locally known as gondi), which gets contaminated with weed seeds of *Crotalaria* (locally known as jhunjhunu). On chemical analysis, jhunjhunu seeds were found to contain pyrrolizidine alkaloids, which are hepatotoxins The symptoms include rapidly developing ascites and jaundice. The preventive measures comprise educating the people in the affected areas about the disease, deweeding of the jhunjhunu plants, which grew along with the staple food crop.

Fluorides

Fluorosis is a disease caused by the consumption of drinking water containing large amounts of fluorides. Toxic effects are seen in the teeth and bone.

Dental Fluorosis (Mottled Enamel)

In many parts of the world where the drinking water contains excessive amounts of fluorine (3–5 ppm), signs and symptoms of dental fluorosis have observed. The enamel of the teeth loses its luster and becomes rough and chalky white patches distributed irregularly over the surface of the teeth, with a secondary infiltration of yellow or brown staining are observed. The enamel is structurally weak and in severe cases, there is marked loss of enamel accompanied by pitting, which gives the tooth surface a corroded appearance.

Skeletal Fluorosis

Chronic fluorosis intoxication through drinking water containing excessive amounts of fluorine (over 10 ppm) or through handling fluoride-containing minerals results in pathological changes in bones. There is sclerosis, i.e. increased density of the bone of the spine, pelvis and limbs due to hypercalcification. In addition, the ligaments of the spine become calcified, producing a 'poker back'. Such persons are crippled and cannot perform simple daily tasks, such as bending, squatting, etc. as the joints are stiff.

Prevention of Toxic Fluorosis

Toxic fluorosis can be prevented only by removing fluorine from the water supplies by treatment with activated carbon or by some other suitable absorbents.

Chapter 40

Safe Food Handling

Food that we serve or eat should be nutritious, pure and safe. When we eat in a restaurant, we expect the surroundings to be clean, the persons who cook or serve the food (food handlers) should maintain hygiene, and the food should be safe and free from any contaminants or harmful disease-causing agents. A food is considered safe when nothing harmful happens after consuming it. Scientists assess food safety in terms of hazard and risk. A hazard is the capacity of a thing to cause harm.

FOOD HANDLING

Food handlers are people who come in contact with food either during cutting, cooking or serving food. Hygiene is the first criterion in terms of handling food. Some steps that are to be followed by food handlers are as follows:

1. It is mandatory for the food handlers to undergo a complete health check at the time of employment. They undergo tests such as chest X-ray, urine and stool routine. They are also physically examined by doctors to ensure that they do not suffer from any communicable diseases.
2. Persons suffering from skin diseases (it could be allergy caused by washing dishes for a long time or any rashes or oozing wounds), diarrhea or dysentery should not be permitted to handle food or utensils till they are completely cured. They should be retested after treatment before resuming duty.
3. Food handlers should be educated in simple terms about personal hygiene (Fig. 40.1) and handwashing technique. Supervisors in food establishments should ensure that proper personal hygiene is implemented and followed with proper training such as:

Keep yourself clean and wear clean protective clothing when working with food
Wash your hands thoroughly
Keep your nails clean and short; do not bite them
No nail varnish or false nails
Keep your hair dean and tidy; cover with a hairnet or hat when working with food; do not scratch your head
Do not smoke or eat when working with food
Do not wear earrings, hairgrips, rings, bracelets or wrist watches
Cover cuts with a waterproof dressing; wear blue one if available
Do not wear strong aftershave or perfume
Do not cough, sneeze or touch your mouth and nose, while working with food

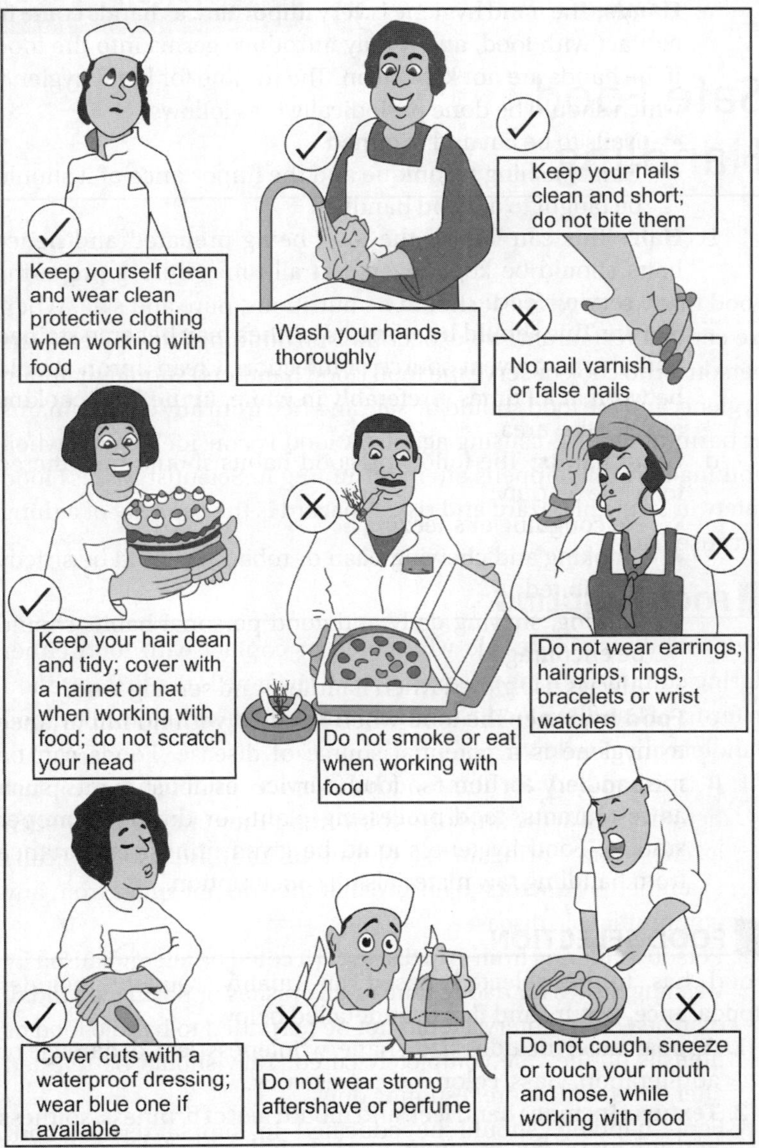

Figure 40.1: Essentials of personal hygiene

a. **Hands:** The hand hygiene is very important, as hands come in contact with food, and it may introduce germs into the food if the hands are not kept clean. The routine for hand hygiene, which should be done periodically is as follows:
   - Nails to be cut and trimmed
   - Handwashing technique and the importance of it should be taught to all food handlers.

b. **Hair:** This can fall on the food being prepared and hence hairs should be kept covered at all times during preparing and serving food.

c. **Apron:** This should be worn, as clothes may become stained and also to prevent source of infection. Clean apron should be worn at all times, preferably in white, in the food cooking and service area.

d. **Good habits:** The following good habits should be adhered to, while on duty:
   - No coughing or sneezing
   - Smoking and chewing paan or tobacco should be strictly prohibited
   - Bathing, shaving daily and good personal habits should be encouraged
   - Always use gloves when handling and serving food.

e. **Food hygiene:** The food when handled with no importance to hygiene is a potential source of disease. Foods can be mishandled at homes, food service establishments such as restaurants, food-processing plants or during improper storage. Food hygiene should be given utmost importance from handling raw materials till consumption.

FOOD SELECTION

Food has to be selected based on quality. Quality includes appearance, texture and flavor, as detailed below:

1. **Appearance:** Includes size, shape, wholeness, lack of damage or adulteration, glass, color and consistency.
2. **Texture:** Includes hand feel, and mouth feel of firmness, softness and juiciness. For example, a crisp apple or a juicy mango is selected for its texture.
3. **Flavor:** Includes sweet, salty, sour or bitter aroma, or smell of a food. Oils such as sesame, groundnut and olive have a distinct flavor. If the oil is rancid, it gives out a bad smell.

PRINCIPLES OF SAFE FOOD PRACTICES

The following rules illustrate the application of the principles of safe food practices.

Personal Hygiene

1. Do not permit individuals with cold or sore throat to handle food until they have recovered.
2. Do not permit anyone with boils, pimples on hands or face to handle food.
3. Avoid sneezing or coughing near food.
4. Always wash hands after using the toilet, scratching the head or other part of the body. Suitable handwashing methods should be followed (warm water, soap, towels).
5. Avoid indiscriminate handling of foods with fingers.
6. Do not return tasting spoon to food without washing it.

Food Processing

1. Select food from plants or markets, which maintain high standards of sanitation.
2. Purchase only pasteurized milk. Buy freshly ground meat and use it within 24 hours after purchase.
3. Protect foods at home or in the market from flies, insects, rodents or contamination by unnecessary handling, sneezing or coughing.
4. Wash all fruits and vegetables before storing in refrigerator.
5. Use a pressure cooker for boiling canned foods such as all non-acidic vegetables, meats and poultry. Boil them for 6–8 minutes before use.
6. Discard without tasting all foods from tin cans, which bulge out from glass jars, which spurt upon being opened.
7. Carefully label insect powders and other chemicals. Do not keep them near foods. Keep them out of the reach of small children.

Refrigeration

1. Keep the refrigerator temperature at 40–45°F.
2. Permit adequate circulation of air around foods in the refrigerator.
3. Protect meats with a loose covering of wax paper, and place vegetables and fruits in the hydrator pan.

4. Refrigerate cooked foods as soon as possible after cooking.
5. Keep cream-filled bakery products, sandwich spreads and salads under constant refrigeration.

Care of Equipment

1. Clean all kitchen equipments thoroughly after use. Meat choppers and mechanical mixers require special attention.
2. Public health regulation require that dishes in public eating places should be washed at least 20 seconds at 140°F in a mechanical washer and then rinsed at 170°F for at least 10 seconds. When handwashing is used, the dishes should remain in rinsed water at 170°F for at least 30 seconds. Detergents or soap powders should be used as directed by the manufacturer and their concentration should be maintained throughout the wash period. Instruct all food handlers for proper use of all equipment.

Other Safe Food Preparation Practices

1. Food comes into contact with human hands during harvestings, storage and service. It is important that food handlers be free from any communicable diseases, i.e. colds, other respiratory ailments, cuts or boils, as they may be responsible for transferring these to the food, thereby spreading the infection to persons consuming the food.
2. Human hair, nasal discharge, skin infections can also be the source of microorganisms. Therefore, persons handling food must wash hands with soap before starting preparation and do not touch hair during preparation.
3. In order to avoid food poisoning, personnel hygiene is very important. The hands of the food handlers must be very clean. Whenever food is handled, use hot water and soap in ample quantities. A person who is ill, should not handle food. Hair should be tied and contact of the hands with hair, mouth and nose should be avoided. Disposable tissues or clean handkerchiefs should be used to cover nose or mouth, while sneezing and coughing. Food should be served using clean serving spoons and not with hands.
4. Kitchen equipments, utensils and appliances should be thoroughly cleaned before contact with any food. Cooked food should not be allowed to stand for more than 2–3 hours at room

temperature. Cooked food should be properly covered, rapidly cooled and then transferred to a refrigerator.

5. Gravies and soups are susceptible to bacterial contamination, especially leftover ones. Such foods should be placed in the refrigerator as soon as possible. They should be reheated and boiled for several minutes before consumption.
6. Milk products should not be stored for more than 2–3 days in the refrigerator.

Commercially Prepared Foods: Food Adulteration/ Food Additives

Chapter 41

FOOD ADDITIVES

Food additives are defined as non-nutritious substances, which are added intentionally to food generally in small quantity, to improve its appearance, flavor, texture or storage properties.

Classification

Food additives may be classified into two categories.

Agents of Various Types

Additives of the first category include:

- Coloring agents, e.g. saffron, turmeric
- Flavoring agents, e.g. vanilla essence
- Sweeteners, e.g. saccharin
- Preservatives, e.g. sorbic acid, sodium benzoate
- Acidity imparting agents, e.g. citric acid, acetic acid, etc.

The various agents mentioned above are generally considered safe for human consumption.

Contaminants

Additives of the 'second category' are, strictly speaking, contaminants incidental through packing, processing steps, farming practices (insecticides) or other environmental conditions. Uncontrolled or indiscriminate use of food additives may pose health hazards among consumers. For example, certain preservatives such as nitrites and nitrates can lead to the production of toxic substances, e.g. nitrosamines that have been implicated in cancer etiology.

Modern science of food technology has revolutionized food processing with the introduction of chemical additives to increase the shelf-life of food, improve its taste and to change its texture or color. Majority of the processed foods such as bread, biscuits, cakes, sweets, confectionary, jams, jellies, soft drinks, ice creams, ketchup and refined oils contain food additives.

Regulations on Food Additives

The use of food additives is subjected to government regulations throughout the world. In India, two regulations, viz. the Prevention of Food Adulteration (PFA) Act and the Fruit Products Order govern the rules and regulations of food additives. Any food that contains food additives that are not permitted, is considered to be adulterated; if the permissible limit exceeds, then also the food is considered adulterated.

The nature and quantity of the additives shall be clearly printed on the label to be affixed to the container. Whenever any extraneous coloring matter has been added to any article of food, the words 'artificially colored' shall be written on the label. At the international level in 1963, a joint Food and Agriculture Organization (FAO)/ World Health Organization (WHO) program on food standards was established, with the FAO/WHO Codex Alimentarius Commission as its principal organ. Protection of the health of consumers is the primary aim of the commission.

FOOD FORTIFICATION

Fortification of food is a public health measure aimed at reinforcing the usual dietary intake of nutrients with additional supplies to prevent/control some nutritional disorders. The WHO has defined 'food fortification' as the process whereby nutrients are added to foods (in relatively small quantities) to maintain or improve the quality of the diet of a group, a community or a population. For example:

1. Foods artificially fortified with vitamin 'D', e.g. milk, margarine, vanaspati and infant foods.
2. Foods fortified with vitamin 'A', e.g. margarine, milk and vanaspati.

ADULTERATION OF FOODS

Adulteration of food is an age-old problem. It is done through a large number of practices such as:

- Mixing
- Substitution
- Abstraction
- Concealing the quality

- Putting up decomposed foods for sale
- Misbranding or giving false labels
- Addition of toxicants.

Food adulteration practices vary from one part of the country to another, and from time to time.

Common Food adulterants (Table 41.1)

The types of adulteration commonly found in India are as follows:

1. **Milk:** Addition of water, removal of fat and addition of starch to make the milk thicker are the common forms of milk adulteration.
2. **Ghee:** This is adulterated with dalda and animal fats such as pig's fat.
3. **Rice and wheat:** These are mixed with stone chips and mud to increase the bulk.

Table 41.1: Food materials and their adulterants

Food materials	Adulteration for foods (adulterants)
Cereals such as wheat, rice, dals	Mud, grits, soap stone bits
Haldi (turmeric powder)	Coal tar dyes, khesari dal
Dhania powder	Lead chromate powder
Black pepper	Starch, cow dung or horse dung powder dried seeds of papaya, saw dust, brick powder
Chili powder	Black gram husk, tamarind seeds powder
Tea dust/leaves	Saw dust, used tea dust
Coffee powder	Date husk, tamarind husk, chicory
Asafetida (hing)	Sand, grit, resins, gums
Mustard seeds	Seeds of prickly poppy—argemone
Edible oils	Mineral oil, argemone oil
Butter	Starch, animal fat
Icecream	Cellulose, starch, non-permitted colors
Sweat meats	Non-permitted colors
Fresh green peas in packing	Green dye
Milk	Extraction of fat, addition of starch and water
Ghee	Vanaspati

4. **Flours:** Wheat flour is mixed with soap stone powder and cheaper flours such as singhara flour.
5. **Pulses:** Chemical substances are added to old stocks to improve the appearance.
6. **Tea and coffee:** Tea leaves are adulterated with old tea leaves, leather and saw dust; coffee is adulterated with chicory.
7. **Honey:** This is adulterated with sugar or jaggery and boiled with empty beehives.
8. **Medicines:** Even drugs are adulterated.

FOOD STANDARDS

The FAO/WHO formulates food standards for international market, Codex Alimentarius Commission, which is the principal organ of the joint FAO/WHO food standards program. The standards in India are based on the standards of the Codex Alimentarius.

PFA Standards

Under the Prevention of Food Adulteration Act, 1954 standards have been established, which are revised from time to time by the 'Central Committee for Food Standards.' The purpose of PFA standards is to obtain a minimum level of quality of foodstuffs attainable under Indian conditions.

Prevention of Food Adulteration Act, 1954

Any food that does not confirm to the minimum standards is said to be of adulterated standards. Provisions have been laid down under this act for various foods. In 1954, the Government of India enacted a Central Prevention of Food Adulteration Act. The act has been amended several times; the latest amendment is that of 1976 and in lately in 1986 to make the act more stringent. Although it is a Central Act; its implementation is largely carried out by the local bodies and state governments.

Agmark Standards

Agmark standards are set by the Directorate of Marketing and Inspection of the Government of India. The Agmark gives the consumer an assurance of quality in accordance with the standards laid down.

Bureau of Indian Standards

The Indian Standards Institute (ISI) mark on any article of food is a guarantee of food quality in accordance with the standards prescribed by the Bureau of Indian Standards (BIS) for that commodity. The Agmark and ISI standards are not mandatory, they are purely voluntary. They express degree of excellence above PFA standards.

Chapter 42

Hospital Diets

TYPES OF DIETS

Generally the diets are of two types (Box 42.1):

- Fluid diets
- Light diets.

Box 42.1: Types of diet

Fluid diets
• Beverages: Tea, coffee, barley water and fruit juice • Milk product preparations: Whey, curd, butter milk, lactic acid milk • Egg preparations: Egg flip, albumin water • Soups: Bones, vegetables, dal (pulses), liver
Light diets
• Toast, poached and boiled eggs, steamed fish • Porridge, soft rice preparations, khichdi, conjee, sago, idlies • Boiled vegetables, salads, jelly and custard • Balanced diet

Fluid Diets

Beverages

Clear tea

Have ready water, which is boiling, but has only just begun to boil. Do not use water that has been boiling for some time, as it spoils the flavor. When it boils, pour a little into the teapot to warm it. Empty out this water and put the tea into pot (one teaspoon of tea for each person). Pour the boiling water over the tea and allow to stand for 3–5 minutes. Strain and pour. Dilute with hot water if desired, and add a few drops of lime or lemon juice and sugar to taste.

Black coffee

One heaped tablespoon of pure coffee powder. Freshly boiled water (300 mL). Heat the coffee jug thoroughly, put the coffee in the jug, pour in the boiling water and allow to stand near the fire for 10 minutes. Strain, reheat and serve as black coffee with sugar if desired.

Barley water (1)

For one tablespoon of barley flour—two tablespoon of cold water, one pint of boiling water and salt to taste. Mix the flour to a smooth paste with cold water and gradually add the boiling water, stirring all the time; boil about 30 minutes and add salt (if permitted), one tablespoon of lime juice, and strain before use.

Barley water (2)

For 50 g of pearl barley, one pint of cold water. Blanch the barley by covering with cold water. Simmer the barley slowly with one pint of water, till it is reduced to two thirds of a pint (about 1½ hour) and strain. A fresh supply should be made at least twice daily. Lime juice may be added to the water before boiling, if desired and sugar added to taste.

Fruit juice (1)

Fruit juice may be prepared from fresh fruit, or by dilution of commercially prepared fruit squashes. Remove the juice from citrus fruit by means of a squeezer, strain, dilute with water and add sugar or glucose to taste.

Fruit juice (2)

Use a fruit squeezer to extract the juice of a lemon or lime. Strain the juice through strainer. Add an equal quantity of drinking water and sugar or glucose to sweeten.

Raw tomato juice

Select ripe, juicy tomatoes, pour boiling water over the tomatoes and let stand for 2 minutes to loosen the skins. Remove skins, mash the tomatoes, and press through the strainer as much of the juice and soft part as possible. Add salt and pepper to taste. Some may prefer little sugar also.

Milk Product Preparation

Whey (1)

Whey is prepared from curds. It contains fats, sugars, salts and vitamins, but no protein. Break up the curds with a fork, then drain off the whey by straining through gauze.

Whey (2) (lime whey)

To one pint of fresh milk, add four tablespoons of lime juice. Boil without stirring until the curd separates. Strain through several thickness of gauze or muslin and add sugar. Cool and serve.

Albumin water (1)

Take the whites of two fresh eggs. Add one cup of water. Put into a wide-necked bottle. Cork it and shake thoroughly. Add little lime juice and sugar. If preferred, orange juice may be substituted for the lime juice.

Albumin water (2)

The white of egg is only used separately from the yolk. Cut with a knife to break up the membrane, then add it to about 150 mL of water, stir well or it may be mixed by shaking gently in a screw-topped jar. Strain before serving and add a little lime juice or glucose if desired. If preferred, orange juice may be substituted for the lime juice. It is especially useful in pyrexia.

Fortified milk

Mix 60 g milk powder (skimmed or whole) with a little cold milk; then add the remainder of the milk, beating thoroughly to ensure complete mixing. This milk may be used when additional food value is required without additional volume. It may be used for all preparations where milk is commonly used.

Curd

Take one cup of lukewarm milk. Add ¼ teaspoon curd as starter and mix well in the milk. Cover it and put it in a hot case or light container. Leave it aside for 6 hours and use it or let it stand at room temperature for 8 hours or more undisturbed. Lime juice can be used for starter, if old curds from the day before is not available.

Butter milk

Add ¼ cup water to one cup curds and whisk or beat, removing the fat if necessary. Add the remainder of the water and mix. Less or more water may be added as desired. If required, a little seasoned oil may be added.

Egg Preparation

Egg flip or egg nog

Beat an egg thoroughly (yolks not used in albumin water may be used) and add 250 mL of milk. Stir well and strain before serving.

This may be flavored with sugar, cinnamon or lemon juice. If desired, it may be added to coffee, tea or cocoa.

Soft cooked egg

1. Lower the egg gently with a spoon into a saucepan of boiling water deep enough to cover it. Put the lid on the pan and allow to stand for 4–5 minutes. Serve immediately after the egg is removed from the hot water. The water should not be allowed to boil after putting in the egg.
2. Place egg in cold water and bring it to boil. Let it boil for about ½ minute. Remove with spoon.

Hard cooked egg

Lower the egg into hot water and keep in simmering temperature for 10–15 minutes according to the size of the egg and how hard is required. If the egg is to be used cold, it should be cooled immediately after cooking by placing in cold water. The shell may then be removed easily.

Poached egg

Use a small pan with water coming about two-thirds up the pan. Add a level teaspoon of salt and a teaspoon of vinegar to each pint of water used. This helps to set the egg. Bring the water almost to boiling point break the egg into cup, taking care to keep it whole, and slide it gently into the water. Tilt the pan, and with a tablespoon gently gather the white round the yolk. Simmer until the white is nicely set (about 3 minute), lift out the egg carefully, draining off the water and serve on hot buttered toast.

Scrambled or buttered egg

Beat the egg well, adding salt, pepper and a tablespoon of milk; melt just enough butter in a saucepan to cover the bottom of the pan. Put the egg and cook slowly over a very gentle heat, stirring lightly to prevent the egg from sticking to the pan. The egg should be soft and creamy when cooked and should be served immediately.

Omelet

Use a perfectly clean, smooth, flat frying pan. Beat two eggs lightly, just enough to mix the whites and yolks, and season with salt and pepper. Add just enough butter to cover the bottom of the pan and when very hot. Pour in the eggs and cook quickly stirring gently with a knife. As the egg sets, tilt the pan slightly to allow the uncooked egg to run down on to the hot pan. As soon as all the egg is set, roll the omelet over, turning in the edges and roll on to a plate; serve hot immediately. If the omelet is to be filled, add the hot cooked filling, e.g. mixed meat, chopped tomato, etc. just before the omelet is rolled over.

Soups

Dal soup

- Dal—½ cup
- Onion—1
- Water—2 cups
- Salt to taste
- Ghee or oil—one teaspoon.

Grind the dal finely, chop and fry the onion, mix all the ingredients and boil for 20–30 minutes.

Vegetable soup

Prepare and dice the vegetables (half cup). Place a saucepan on stove; add melted butter (one teaspoon). After a few minutes, add the boiling meat stock (water in which bones or meat have been simmered slowly for a long time), salt and pepper to taste and boil gently until the vegetables are tender. Mix 45 g flour with a little cold stock, add the boiling stock stirring continually, then return the flour mixture to the soup and boil until thickened. If desired, the vegetables may be rubbed through a strainer before thickening the soup.

Vegetable cream soup

Vegetables are cooked and mashed or forced through a strainer to make pulp, and combined with milk and often their vegetable stock (vegetable stock is the water in which vegetables are cooked). In order to have the vegetable pulp uniformly mixed through the liquid, it is necessary to thicken with a starchy material (flour with butter, mixed and cooked as a white sauce). So cream soups are simple, while in vegetable soup, pulp is added.

General proportions

One part vegetable pulp or puree to two parts of liquid milk, vegetable stock or meat stock (pureed vegetables are mashed and strained vegetables). The proportion of flour to liquid is half tablespoon flour to one cup liquid if starchy vegetable is used; or one tablespoon flour to one cup liquid if a vegetable having little thickening property is used. Different kinds of vegetables are sometimes mixed for a soup or vegetables and meat stock also mixed.

Light Diets

Toast

Cut bread thinly and dry both sides by holding on a fork before fire or placing under grill for a few minutes or use toaster equipment. Toast both sides until golden brown. Cut into neat pieces, and serve hot and crisp.

Poached and Boiled Egg

For poached and boiled egg, refer 'egg preparation' in the same chapter.

Steamed Fish

Clean the piece of fish and drain free from water carefully. Sprinkle a little pepper and salt on the fish, fold in two, lay on a buttered plate and cover with buttered pepper and a lid. Place the plate over a pan of boiling water and steam for 15–20 minutes or until the fish looks quite white, and the flakes separate easily. Serve on a hot dish with the juice poured over it. A small piece of lime or lemon may be served with fish.

Creamed Fish

Prepare a coating sauce as given for creamed vegetables. Prepare and steam 4 ounces of fish as for steamed fish. When the fish is cooked, remove from the bone, if any, and breakup finely. Mix with enough sauce to coat well, and pound thoroughly. If desired, the mixture may be rubbed through a sieve. Add the stiffly beaten white of one egg, turn into a greased tin or mold, cover with greased paper and steam until firm.

Creamed Chicken

Creamed chicken may be prepared as for creamed fish, but the meat must be finely minced before pounding.

Minced Meat

- Cooked meat—250 g
- Heated stock—150 mL
- Pepper and salt
- Small pieces of fried bread.

Method
Remove the fat and skin from the meat and chop or mince nicely. Put into a pan with the heated stock, salt and pepper or other seasonings, and reheat thoroughly. Do not recook. Serve decorated with fried bread.

Minced Liver

- Minced liver—250 g
- Onion—1 (big)
- Water—100 mL
- Oil or fat—2 teaspoons.

Method
Cut the onion into rings and fry in a little hot fat. Add the minced liver and fry very lightly. Add seasonings to the water and bring to the boil. Serve hot.

Light Cereal Preparations

Double boiled rice

- Rice—2 tablespoons
- Milk—240 mL
- Water or milk (water mixed).

Method
Wash the rice and add it to the milk. Simmer gently for 1-1½ hours till it is reduced to pulpy mass. Add sugar, if desired before serving. Cooking in a double boiler or milk cooker is more easily regulated than in an ordinary saucepan.

Ragi congee

- Ragi flour—1 table spoon
- Water or milk
- Salt to taste.

Method
Ragi, after being ground, should be sifted two or three times through muslin. One tablespoon of the ragi flour should be mixed till smooth with a little cold water. Then gradually add 30 mL boiling water with a pinch of salt and boil for 15 minutes. If preferred, half milk and half water may be used.

Arrowroot congee

- Arrowroot—1 tablespoon
- Boiling water—125 mL

- Sugar to taste
- Cold water—2 tablespoons
- Hot milk—125 mL
- Salt—¼ teaspoon.

Method

Mix the arrowroot to a smooth paste with the cold water and add the boiling water gradually. Boil for 10 minutes, stirring constantly. Then add milk, salt and boil for 10 minutes. Add sugar, if desired before serving.

Barley congee

- Prepared barley flour—1 tablespoon
- Cold water—2 tablespoon
- Salt—¼ teaspoon
- Warm milk—150 mL
- Boiling water—150 mL.

Method

Mix barley flour to a smooth paste with the cold water, add it to the boiling water gradually. Stirring constantly, boil for 30 minutes. Add milk and salt or sugar, and bring to the boiling point. Serve it warm.

Sago porridge (1)

- Sago—2 tablespoons
- Milk—150 mL
- Water—150 mL
- Pinch of salt
- Sugar to taste.

Method

Wash the sago, and add milk and water. Bring it to the boiling point, gently stirring in between. After if starts boiling, simmer gently for 15-20 minutes. Add salt and sugar to taste. Serve hot.

Note: If milk and sugar is added to the congee, it is called porridge.

Sago porridge (2)

- Sago rice—50 g
- Milk—200 mL
- Sugar—50 g
- Cardamom powder—1 pinch.

Method

Soak the sago rice in cold water for 1 hour, and drain the water. Heat the milk, add the soaked sago rice and cook it on a low fire till the sago rice become soft. Add sugar and cardamom powder to taste, and serve when it is warm. If desired cold, put in the refrigerator for 1 hour and serve.

Light Puddings

Jelly

1. **Fruit jelly:**
   - Fruit juice—500 mL
   - Powdered gelatin—20 g
   - Sugar—100 g.

   Method: Put all ingredients into a pan and warm gently. Stirring all the time. Turn into a rinsed mold and allow to set, preferably in a refrigerator. Keep cold until served.
2. **Milk jelly:**
   - Milk—500 mL
   - Strip of lime or orange peel
   - Sugar—50 g
   - Powdered gelatin—15 g.

   Method: Put the lime or orange peel in the milk. Bring to boiling point and strain the milk onto the gelatin and sugar. Stirring until all is dissolved. Keep in the basin, stirring from time to time until the mixture is the consistency of thick cream. Pour into rinsed molds and allow to set. Preferably in a refrigerator. Serve cold.

Baked custard

- Egg—1
- Milk—150 mL
- Sugar to taste.

Method

Beat the egg lightly, heat the milk and pour into the egg, stirring all the time. Add sugar to taste and stir well. Pour the mixture into a greased dish and sprinkle a little grated nutmeg on top if desired. Stand the dish in a baking tin with hot water half way up its sides. Bake in a moderate oven until set. If a steamed custard is required, pour the mixtures into individual greased molds, place in a steamer and simmer until set.

Corn flour puddings

- Milk—500 mL
- Sugar—2 tablespoonful
- Custard powder—1 tablespoon

- Corn flour—2 tablespoon
- Thin strip of lime or orange peel or other flavoring.

Method

Pour about three quarters of the milk into a saucepan and add the orange rind or other flavoring sugar; add a pinch of salt and bring to the boil slowly. Mix the corn flour and custard powder together with the remaining cold milk. Pour the boiling milk into the mixed custard and corn flour stirring well. Return to the pan and boil for a few minutes until it thickens. Pour into individual molds and allow to set until cold.

Ice Cream

- Milk—200 mL
- Egg—1
- Sugar—20 g
- Flavoring—vanilla essence.

Method

Beat the egg lightly and mix in the milk and sugar. Heat over a low flame or in a double boiler or milk cooker until the mixture begins to thicken. Remove from the heat and cool quickly. Flavor as desired and freeze.

Idlies

- Parboiled rice or broken raw rice or suji—4 cups
- Black gram dal—1 cup
- Salt to taste
- Baking soda powder—¼ teaspoon.

Method

The following are the methods for the prepare idlies:

1. Soak rice and black gram for 6 hours. Grind separately in a mixer to make a coarse batter. Add salt to batter. Mix well and leave it for overnight to ferment (minimum 10-12 hour).
2. Next morning, take ¼ teaspoon baking soda, mix with—2 tablespoons of water and add in the slightly fermented batter and mix well.
3. Take small six cups idly maker, apply oil inside and fill half of the cups with batter and steam cook in cooker (without weight on it) for 10 minutes serve hot with sugar or any gravy.

Note: If parboiled rice not available, raw rice can be used after making it as suji. Soak the suji for 1 hour. Grind the black gram dal in the mixer as fine batter. Mix the soaked rice, suji and ground black gram dal batter well. Add salt and allow it to ferment for 10 hours. Rest of the procedure is just similar to parboiled rice batter. If raw rice suji not available, rava suji can also be used and prepared in, and served in the same way.

Khichdi

- Fine rice—100 g
- Moong dhal—50 g
- Peeper—1 teaspoon
- Jeera (cumin seed)—1 teaspoon
- Ghee: 2 teaspoons
- Water—4 glasses (800 mL)
- Salt to taste.

Method

Slightly fry the rice and moong dal. Wash and add water, cook on low fire till it becomes soft (dalia). Add salt and cook for few minutes. Keep a frying pan, heat the ghee. When it is hot, put cumin and pepper till it splatters. Put off the fire. Add the splattered cumin (jeera) and peeper with ghee to the soft cooked rice and dal. Serve hot.

Salad

Raw vegetable salad

- Cucumber peeled—¼ kg (cut into round pieces)
- Medium-sized onions—2 (cut into round pieces)
- Spring onions—2 (convenient pieces)
- Tomatoes large size—2 (cut into small pieces or round pieces)
- Small capsicum—1 (thin strip)
- Radishes a few (out into long pieces)
- Black pepper powder and salt to taste.

Method

Decorate all the cut vegetables by keeping each pieces alternatively in circle pattern. Sprinkle salt and pepper powder on them and serve.

Spring salad

- Cooked rice—½ kg
- Orange segments—1 cup
- Diced pineapple, fresh or tinned—1 cup
- Chopped capsicum—½ cup
- Chopped parsley—1 tablespoon

- Peanuts coarsely chopped—½ cup
- Spring onion tops chopped—1 tablespoon
- Peanut oil—4 tablespoons
- Lemon juice—1 tablespoon
- Fresh cottage cheese diced—1 cup
- Cream—2 tablespoons
- Cashew nuts, finely chopped—½ cup
- Ham chopped: 200 g
- Salt and pepper powder to taste
- A pinch sugar.

Method

1. Mix rice, orange, ham, pineapple, capsicum, parsley, onion tops and peanuts in a bowl.
2. Separately mix the oil, lemon juice, salt and pepper and pinch of sugar and blend well.
3. Sprinkle this dressing over the rice mixture and toss lightly. Mix the cheese with cream and cashew nuts, and use as garnish for the salad. Serve chilled.

Note: Chopped ham can be avoided in this recipe, if prepared for vegetarians.

Crushed wheat and chicken salad

- Crushed wheat (dalia)—250 g
- Chicken cooked and shredded—1 cup
- Tomatoes diced—3
- Cucumber diced—1
- Green chilies sliced—2
- Spring onions, chopped—1 bunch
- Parsley chopped—1 bunch
- Mint chopped—1 bunch
- Juice of—3 lemons
- Olive oil—½ cup
- Lettuce chopped—1
- Pepper corns—1 teaspoon (crushed)
- Salt to taste.

Method

Put the wheat in a bowl, cover with cold water and refrigerate for an hour before needed. Remove the parsley leaves from the stems, put in a bowl of water and refrigerate overnight. Prepare a dressing by mixing the lemon juice, olive oil and pepper. Drain the water from the wheat. Mix with all the other ingredients in a bowl, add chicken and salt to taste, pour the dressing over it and mix well. Arrange a bed of lettuce on a platter and pile wheat salad in the center.

Boiled vegetables salad

- Carrot—1 (skin scrapped and diced round)
- Beetroot—1 (skin scrapped and diced round)
- Potato—1 (boiled, peeled and diced)
- Pepper powder and salt to taste.

Method

Pour 100 mL of water—allow it to boil, put diced carrot and beetroot in the boiled water, cover the vessel with heavy lid. Allow it to boil on a low heat for 10 minutes. When tender, remove and strain the remaining water (if it is left out). Decorate all the boiled vegetables attractively, sprinkle salt and pepper to taste and serve.

Note: If prepared, cauliflower shreds can also be boiled in the same way can be served.

Section IX

Nutritional Programs/Education and Role of Nurse

Nutritional Programs/Education and Role of Nurse

- National Programs Related to Nutrition
- National and International Agencies
- Nutrition Education and Role of Nurse

Chapter 43

National Programs Related to Nutrition

Nutritional intervention programs are aimed at provision of food or nutrients directly to people who are at risk of developing malnutrition, pursued by the health and social welfare sectors in many developing countries, including India. This approach aims at supplying the deficient/missing nutrients either through food, which is consumed as a staple (food fortification) or its administration in medicinal form (supplementation) at frequent intervals.

The condition of undernutrition manifests itself among large sections of the poor, particularly amongst the women and the children. Undernutrition is a condition resulting from inadequate intake of food or more essential nutrient(s) resulting in deterioration of physical activity levels, including work levels that are socially necessary. This condition of undernutrition, therefore, reduces work capacity and productivity amongst adults, and enhances mortality and morbidity amongst children. Such reduced productivity translates into reduced earning capacity, leading to further poverty.

The only logical way of overcoming malnutrition on a permanent basis is through economic growth with distributive justice, which ensure people to consume nutritious diet, adequate in quality and quantity, and obtain good health care. But it takes a long time and cannot solve immediate problems of malnutrition affecting low-income groups. Hence, technology is capable of controlling the worst forms of malnutrition and thus preventing the fatal consequences even under low-income conditions have been developed.

Several nutrition intervention programs are currently in operation either singly as vertical programs or as part of health and welfare services in many developing countries. The Government of India have initiated several programs in nutrition on a national scale to control/prevent major nutritional problems. These programs may be classified as:

1. **Programs designed to improve the overall nutritional status:**
   a. Applied Nutrition Program.
   b. Supplementary Feeding Program.
   c. Mid-day Meal Program for School Children.
2. **Program aimed at overcoming specific deficiency diseases:**
   a. National Goiter Control Program.
   b. Vitamin A Prophylaxis Program.
   c. The Iron and Folate Distribution Program.
3. **Others:**
   a. Integrated Child Development Scheme.
   b. India Population Project.

VITAMIN A PROPHYLAXIS PROGRAM

One of the components of the national program for control of blindness is to administer a single massive dose of daily preparation of vitamin A containing 2,000 IU (110 mg of retinyl palmitate) orally to all preschool children in the community every 6 months through peripheral health workers.

This program was launched by the Ministry of Health and Family Welfare in 1970 on the basis of technology developed at the National Institute of Nutrition at Hyderabad. An evaluation of the program has revealed a significant reduction in vitamin 'A' deficiency in children:

1. One of the national health problems in India is blindness due to vitamin A deficiency.
2. According to the recommendation of National Institute of Nutrition, (NIN) Hyderabad, this program was launched by Ministry of Health and Family Welfare in 1970.
3. Under this program, children below 6 years are given every 6 months an oral dose of 200,000 of vitamin A to prevent the nutritional blindness.
4. Vitamin A as the fat-soluble vitamin, will be stored in the liver for as long as 6 months or more.
5. Evaluation of the program shows marked reduction in vitamin A deficiency among children.

Objectives

1. Elimination of blindness due to vitamin A deficiency.
2. Reducing the severe forms of deficiency resulting in blindness and combining it to children below 3 years.

3. Providing adequate diet or vitamin A deficiency and maintaining vitamin A supplementation programs.
4. Targeting diseases such as cataract, refractive error, childhood blindness, corneal blindness, glaucoma and diabetic retinopathy.
5. Developing human resources as well as infrastructure and technology at various levels of health system. The proposed 4-tier structure includes 20 centers of excellence, 200 training centers, 200 service centers and 2,000 vision centers.

NATIONAL IODINE DEFICIENCY DISORDERS PROGRAM (NATIONAL GOITER CONTROL PROGRAM)

Iodized salt is sold at the same price as common salt in goiter endemic areas. Government has aimed to reduce prevalence of goiter under the program of 'Health for All by 2000.' Reduction of 50% of cases by 1985, and 95% by 2000 AD was planned. As a result, a major national program—the iodine deficiency disorders (IDD) control program was mounted in 1986 with the objective to replace the entire edible salt by iodine salt, in a phased manner:

1. The National Goiter Control Program was launched or initiated by the Government of India (GOI) in 1962.
2. Iodine deficiency will be corrected through salt iodization. Banning of entry of common salt.
3. The GOI is implementing universalization of iodized salt. Production of salt is liberalized by inviting and heavily subsidizing to the private salt manufacturers.
4. This program aims at controlling endemic goiter in the Himalayan region.

Objectives

1. To identify and assess the prevalence of goiter in suspected areas through systematic surveys.
2. To prevent and control goiter through production and supply of iodized salt in place of common salt in endemic areas.
3. To assess the impact of the program by undertaking resurvey of the areas after 5 years of continuous supply of iodized salt.
4. Since goiter is known to be due to iodine deficiency, measure has been taken to improve the iodine intake.
5. One method of increasing iodine intake is by adding iodine to common salt.

6. However, surveys show that the iodine deficiency disorders are more widespread than in the earlier period.
7. As a result of major nutritional program, the iodine deficiency disease control program was started in the year 1986 with the objective of replacing the entire edible salt by iodine salt.

Goals

1. The goal of IDD control program in India was to reduce the prevalence of IDD below 10% in the country by 2012.
2. The recent coverage evaluation survey has reported 91% population coverage of iodized salt in India.
3. While 71% population is consuming adequately iodized salt and another 20% is consuming salt with some added iodine.

MID-DAY MEAL PROGRAM

The School Health Committee, 1960 of the GOI recommended a mid-day school meal with the specific objective of providing at least one third of the daily requirement of calories, proteins and other essential nutrients (Table 43.1). For example, in some states, school feeding is an integral part of the applied nutrition program. The mid-day meal program (Table 43.2) has been in operation in many parts of the country since 1962–1963, after it was first organized successfully in Tamil Nadu in 1957. Nearly 12 million children were

Table 43.1: Recommended daily requirement (µg/day)

Target groups	Nutrition
Adult	150
During pregnancy	250

Table 43.2: Model menu for a mid-day meal program

Foodstuffs	g/day
Cereals and millets	75
Pulses	30
Oils and fats	8
Leafy vegetables	30
Other vegetables	30

covered by the program in 1974. The National Institute of Nutrition is of the view of have the desired impact on the children:

1. Mid-day meal program is also known as school lunch program.
2. This program was first introduced in 1925 in Chennai as a part of the people's movements.
3. It has been in operation in many states since 1962.
4. This program seeks to supplement the home diets of children through provision of mid-day meal or school lunch for about 200 days in a year.
5. The beneficiaries of this program are preschool children.

Objectives

1. To attract more children and give admission to schools.
2. To reduce illiteracy and improve education levels of the children.
3. To provide food to meet the gap in nutritional requirements, particularly in poor children.

Principles

In formulating mid-day meals for school children, the following broad principles should be kept in mind:

1. The meal should be a supplement and not substitute to the home diet.
2. The meal should supply at least one third of the total energy requirement and half of the protein requirement.
3. The cost of the meal should be reasonably low.
4. The meal should be prepared easily in schools. No complicated cooking process should be involved.
5. As far as possible, locally available foods should be used. This will reduce the cost of the meal and the menu should be changed frequently to avoid monotony.
6. The meal supplies about 400 calories and 10 g protein for preschool child and about 500 calories and 12 g protein for the older school children. This program introduced other nutritious cooked recipes (rice, pulses, etc.).

Activities

1. The central assistance provided to state under the program is by way of free supply of foodgrains from nearest food corporation of Indian godowns at the rate of 100 g per day and subsidy for transport of foodgrain.

2. To achieve the objective, a cooked mid-day meal with minimum 300 calories and 8–12 g of protein content will be provided to all the children in class I to V.

Goals

- Reorienting eating habits
- Giving nutrition education along with the subjects
- Encouraging the use of local communities
- Improving school attendance and educational performance of the students
- Supplementing nutrition foods for preschool children.

Organizing a School Meal Program

The School Health Committee (1960) recommended that it is desirable to include a protein-rich supplement such as fish (15 g) or skimmed milk reconstituted (120 g) or Indian multipurpose food (15 g) in place of 15 g of pulses.

Indian Multipurpose Food

Indian multipurpose food (IMF) is a cheap supplementary food prepared from groundnut flour and Bengal gram, and fortified with essential minerals and vitamins. The compression of 100 g of the IMF is as follows:

- Proteins: 42.9 g
- Fats: 8.5 g
- Iron: 5.1 g
- Thiamine: 1.3 g
- Niacin: 1.43 g
- Riboflavin: 3.0 g
- Vitamin A: 3,000 IU
- Vitamin D: 300 IU
- Energy value: 387 kcals.

About 1 ounce of this food costs about 4 paise and supplies a fair protein of the daily requirement of proteins, minerals and vitamins. Multipurpose food is finding wide application in school programs.

Balahar

The GOI have taken up the production of a food supplement known as balahar for school feeding programs. It consists of 70% wheat, 25% defatted groundnut meal and 5% t skim milk. A modified version of it contains 75% wheat and 25% defatted groundnut meals.

INTEGRATED CHILD DEVELOPMENT SCHEME

1. As per the national policy for children, the GOI initiated a program called integrated child development scheme (ICDS) on 2nd October, 1975.
2. The beneficiaries are children below 6 years, women with emphasis on pregnant and lactating mothers.
3. This program is operated by the Ministry of Social Welfare in India's response to the challenge of:
   a. Providing preschool education on one hand.
   b. Breaking the vicious cycle of malnutrition, morbidity, reduced learning capacity and mortality on the other.

Objectives

1. To improve the nutritional and health status of children in the age group of 0–6 years through supplementary feeding.
2. To encourage school enrollment as early as possible and five non-formal preschool education.
3. To reduce the incidence of mortality and morbidity rates through coordination with health departments to ensure delivery of the required health inputs.
4. To achieve effective coordination of the policy and implementation levels among the various government departments to promote child development.
5. To bring awareness for mothers to look after the health and well-being of child by providing nutrition and health education.

Activities

1. The ICDS promotes child survival and development through an integrated approach for converging basic services for improved child care.
2. Early stimulation and learning, improved enrolment and retention, health and nutrition, water and environmental sanitation.
3. The ICDS provides increased opportunities for children and their rights.

Achievements

1. New ICDS is effective in 5,659 community development blocks and major urban slums throughout the country.

2. As against 227 crore beneficiaries until March 1997, there were 3.4 crore beneficiaries in April 2001.
3. In 2006, the scheme reached out to about 95 lakh expectants and nursing mothers; and about 244.92 lakh preschool children and 562.18 lakh beneficiaries are getting supplementary nutrition. The package of services available in ICDS is given in Table 43.3.

Table 43.3: Package of services available in ICDS

Beneficiary	Services
Pregnant women	Health check-up Immunization against tetanus Supplementary nutrition Nutrition and health education
Nursing mothers	Health check-up Supplementary nutrition Nutrition and health education
Other women in age group of 15–45 year	Nutrition and health education
Children less than 3 year	Supplementary nutrition Immunization Health check-up Referral services
Children in age group 3–6 year	Supplementary nutrition Immunization Health check-up Referral services Non-formal education

Components of ICDS

In order to achieve these objectives, a package of services is offered. These include the following:

1. Supplementary nutrition.
2. Immunization.
3. Health check-ups/treatment for minor ailments and referral services.
4. Growth monitoring.
5. Non-formal education.

Supplementary Nutrition

1. This is one of the major components of ICDS.
2. At first, identifying the subjects of all families in the community.

3. Field workers are surveyed in the whole community, and then selected poorest children below the age groups of 6 years and pregnant women and lactating, mother for feeding (Table 43.4).
4. The type of supplementary food varies from place to place.

Table 43.4: Energy and protein content of the supplementary food supplied to different target beneficiary groups

Target group	Energy (kcal)	Protein (g)
Infants (6–12 month)	200	8–10
Children (1–6 year)	300	15
Adolescents	500	20
Pregnant women and lactating mother	500	25

Activities

1. Target group identified from community.
2. They are provided supplementary feeding support for 300 days in a year.
3. Weight-for-age growth cards are maintained for all children less than 6 years.
4. Severely malnourished children are given special supplementary feeding and referred to medical services.

Immunization

All infants are immunized against infectious diseases such as diphtheria, measles, whooping cough, tetanus, poliomyelitis and tuberculosis. All pregnant women are immunized against tetanus.

Health Check-up, Treatment for Minor Ailments and Referral Services

1. At anganwadi centers, children, adolescent girls, pregnant and lactating mothers are examined and treated by the local visiting health personnel.
2. In addition, the anganwadi worker diagnoses minor ailments and distributes medicines provided in a medical kit.
3. Women and children who require special investigations and treatment, are referred to doctors at primary health center (PHC).

Growth Monitoring

1. Growth monitoring is done with the help of special growth charts. These are also known as weight/age charts.

2. The charts consist of a card presented in a graphic form and the weight/age curves are drawn across on the charts.
3. For each curve, a different color will be given (i.e. green, yellow, red). Each color indicates the severity of disease. If children were drawn on the yellow curve, it indicates mild; if drawn on the green curve, it indicates moderate and if drawn on the red curve, it indicates severe form.
4. Each curve denotes a particular level of nutrition growth status of the children.

Non-formal Education

Non-formal education of children up to the age of 6 years and pregnant and nursing mothers in rural, urban and tribal areas. It should be given through songs and games.

OTHER NUTRITIONAL PROGRAMS

APPLIED NUTRITION PROGRAM

Applied nutrition program (ANP) is defined as coordinating educational activities among health, agricultural, educational and other interested agencies with active participation of the people of community. The ANP was launched by the GOI in 1963 with aid from UNICEF, FAO and WHO for improving the nutrition of the nursing, and expectant mothers and children.

The chief aim of the program is to stimulate the production of protective foods such as eggs, fish, milk, vegetables and fruits, and by means of health education to promote their consumption by mothers and children who are the vulnerable group from the nutrition standpoint. Health education is an important component of the program; in fact, the program has been developed to teach the village people how they can increase and improve their food supply through their own efforts. An important aspect of the program is to train various categories of personnel such as rural health workers, teachers, doctors, youth and women leaders.

The ANP is one of the largest single programs assisted by United Nations Children's Fund (UNICEF) in many countries in India, it now covers 1,375 community development blocks, and serves 1.7 million women and children. It is connected with the program that has not made the expected impact in terms of stated aims and objectives.

Its demonstration effect has not been felt in most areas. The ANP is demonstrating feeding long-term program.

Aims

1. To provide nutrition education to the community through trained women workers.
2. To create awareness about the dietary requirements, nutritional needs and nutritive value of foods.
3. To raise the nutritional status of mother and children through improved food production.

Objectives

1. Encouraging the rural communities to produce protective foods needed for their family diets.
2. Making people to realize the importance of good health by including the adequate amount of pulses, vegetables and fruits in their diets.
3. Explaining to everyone the need for improving food habits, production, cooking methods, preservation, consumption and utilization of protective foods.
4. Ensuring effective utilization of foods by pregnant, lactating, preschool and school-going children.

Components of ANP

The ANP has three main components. They are:

1. **Production:** To encourage farmers to produce more protective foods such as egg, fish, green leafy vegetables (GLV) rich in vitamin C by organizing a community poultry, fishery unit at host areas, seed samples and equipment were provided by government.
2. **Consumption:** Feeding of protective foods thus produced in the community units through most vulnerable groups:
   - Children below 6 years
   - Pregnant women
   - Lactating mother.

   The ANP distributes one third of production to these people.

Training

1. The training was carried out by government agencies through organization of training programs.

2. The training aspects of this program must be developed in such a manner that it will eventually make an impact at all levels in the community, namely:
   - National level
   - State level
   - District level
   - Village level
   - Block level.
3. Administrative and technical officers associated with this program will organize agriculture, human nutrition, home science and health programs at colleges.
4. They may concern with training of public health workers, teaches, block level officers, village level workers, voluntary organization officials, etc.

Role of Other Agencies

1. **Women's organization:**
   a. They selected women because they are responsible persons in the family.
   b. They have an important role to play as being interested with the feeding of preschool and school children.
2. **Balwadis:**
   a. They have to be applied in each block where the preschool children can gather for recreation and lunch.
   b. They supply lunch for them.
3. **Youth clubs:**
   a. They encourage to take the poultry units and the land for cultivation of vegetables and fruits.
4. **School teachers:**
   a. The success of any program depends on the interest and leadership of teachers.
   b. Teachers have played an important role in encouraging the school children to participate in different community programs arranged by government agencies.

SPECIAL NUTRITION OR SUPPLEMENTARY FEEDING PROGRAM

The special nutritional program (SNP) was started in 1970 for the nutritional benefit of preschool children (6 month to 6 year), pregnant women and nursing mothers, under the overall charge of the Ministry of Social Welfare, GOI. Beneficiaries are selected from the weaker sections of the population. In the initial stages, children in tribal areas and urban slums were covered. Later it was extended to selected backward areas and chronically drought-affected areas.

Objectives

1. To supplement the diet of selected beneficiaries with additional protein and calories to make the deficiency in their daily food intake.
2. The supplementary food supplies 300 calories of energy and 10–12 g of protein/child/day.
3. The beneficiary mothers receive 500 calories and 25 g of protein daily.
4. In addition, vitamin A and D capsules are also supplied for beneficiaries.
5. This supplement is provided to them for about 300 days in a year.

Beneficiary Groups

- Children below 6 years
- Pregnant and lactating women.

Services

- **Preschool children:** 300 kcal and 10–12 g of protein
- **Pregnant and lactating mothers:** 500 kcal and 25 g of protein.

BALWADI NUTRITION PROGRAM

- Balwadi nutrition program was started in the year 1970–1971
- Beneficiaries of this program are preschool children
- Balwadis are established in rural areas for providing preparatory education to the children in the age group of 3–6 years
- This program is under the control of social welfare department
- The food supplement provides 300 kcal and 10 g of protein/day/child.

Beneficiary Group

- Preschool children of 3–5 years of age.

Services

- Provide 300 kcal and protein for 270 days in a year
- They also provide with preschool education

- Balwadis are being phased out because of universalization of ICDS.

TAMIL NADU INTEGRATED NUTRITION PROJECT

1. The Tamil Nadu Integrated Nutrition Project (TINP) covers 9,000 villages in rural Tamil Nadu with a population of over 10 million.
2. This project has a community nutrition center with a community nutrition worker.
3. Beneficiaries of this project are 6–36 months old children. In this project, there are no preschool children.
4. Nutrition and supplementary feeding are given for a limited number of pregnant women and lactating mothers.
5. Under community nutrition center, community nutrition worker is selected by TINP in one village.

Qualities of Community Nutrition Worker

The qualities of community nutrition workers are as follows:

1. She should be married.
2. She should have two healthy children.
3. She should be educated up to class VII.
4. She should belong to Harijan community.

Community nutrition workers focus on the following works:

1. She conducts an initial survey of the village.
2. She weighs and prepares growth charts for children and monitors growth.
3. She also administers ORS, vitamin A solution wherever necessary.
4. She organizes mothers' working groups.
5. She conducts meetings at panchayat offices, houses and schools.
6. She gives nutrition and health education for pregnant women, lactating mothers and preschool children.
7. She distributes medicines wherever needed.
8. She participates in all programs conducted by officials (i.e. medical camps, immunization, etc.).
9. She treats all minor ailments in the community.

RURAL HEALTH PLAN

1. Rural health plan was initiated in the year 1977.
2. The main aim is to prevent diseases and promote good health.

Objectives

1. Encouraging the rural communities to produce protective food needed for their family diets.
2. Determining the food, nutritional and health needs of the population.
3. Assessing the health status of the population.
4. Identifying the health problems in the community.
5. Developing health policies for target group to cope with them.
6. Conducting programs to create awareness about health problems prevailing in the community.
7. Giving health education for people in the community.
8. Improving health levels in the community by available means.
9. Providing safe drinking water for the people.
10. Improving school attendance and educational performance of the students.
11. Providing environmental conditions necessary for proper physical, psychological and social development of the child.
12. Reducing the incidence of mortality and morbidity rates through coordination with health departments to ensure delivery of the required health inputs.
13. Controlling the health problems prevailing in the community, and finding out the factors and causes that are responsible for it.
14. Developing prevention, promotive and curative measure.

ANEMIA CONTROL PROGRAM

1. Nutrition iron deficiency anemia is most prevalent and causing more public health problems in India.
2. Because of the public health importance, a national program for the prevention of nutrition anemia was launched by the government during Fourth- and Fifth Five-year Plans.
3. This program was started in the year 1970–1971.
4. The family welfare program supplies the cost of drugs as granted to the state government.
5. Through this program, pregnant women, young children (1–2 year) are supplied with iron and folic acid tablets. They are distributed through:
   - Maternal child health (MCH) centers in urban areas
   - Primary health centers in rural areas, and even through ICDS projects.

6. This program is implemented in all states.
7. Each beneficiary gets for 100 days:
   - Adults 60 g Iron, 0.5 mg folic acid
   - Children 30 g Iron, 0.1 mg folic acid.
8. New technology for the control of anemia through iron fortification of common salt has also been developed by the NIN, Hyderabad.

Beneficiaries

- Children 1–5 years of age
- Expecting and lactating mothers
- Family planning (IUD) acceptors.

Policy

- **Expecting, lactating mothers and IUD acceptors:** 60 mg of elemental iron + 0.5 mg folate everyday for 100 days
- **Children 1–5 years:** 20 mg of elemental iron + 0.1 mg folate everyday for 100 days.

MONITORING AND EVALUATION OF NUTRITION PROGRAMS

An important advance in this field is the development of the randomized controlled trial for the evaluation of the effectiveness and efficiency of healthcare program. Since health and nutrition of the young child is indivisible from the health and nutrition of the family as a whole. In the long run, we can hope to improve the nutritional status of the children only through improvement in the economic conditions of the community to a level at which families can afford balanced diets. Organized state-sponsored feeding program cannot be the permanent answer to the problem.

National and International Agencies Working Towards Food/ Nutrition

Chapter 44

A number of agencies at national and international level are working towards food and nutrition. Some important agencies are detailed below.

NATIONAL INSTITUTE OF PUBLIC COOPERATION AND CHILD DEVELOPMENT

The National Institute of Public Cooperation and Child Development (NIPCCD) is one of the three organizations working towards food and nutrition, and it is registered under the Society's Registration Act, 1860. The NIPCCD is an autonomous organization with its headquarters in New Delhi. It was sanctioned under the Department of Women and Child Development, and Ministry of Human Resource Development.

Objectives

- Developing and promoting voluntary action in social development
- Taking comprehensive view of child development
- To develop and promote programs in pursuance of the national policy for children
- Developing measures for coordination of governmental and voluntary action in social development
- Evolving framework and perspective for organizing children programs through government and voluntary efforts with a view to achieve the below objectives in the institute:
  - Conducts research and evolution studies
  - Organizes training programs, seminars, workshops and conferences
  - Provides documentation and information services in the field of public cooperation and child development

- It collaborates with regional and international agencies
- The institute is the apex body for training functionaries of the Integrated Child Development Scheme (ICDS).

Structure

The general body and the executive council are the two main constitutional bodies of the NIPCCD. The general body formulates policy for management and administration of the institute. The Union Minister of State for Women and Child Development is the President of the general body and the Chairman of the Executive Council. In addition, there are committees to oversee academic programs and administrative matter. The institute has set up regional centers at Guwahati, Bengaluru, Lucknow and Indore.

Programs and Activities

The programs and activities of the institute may be grouped under following categories:

1. **Regular training programs:** The institute organizes orientation training courses for representatives of voluntary organizations and officials of government departments engaged in implementation of programs of mother care, child development and women's development. The institute also conducts programs in tackling emerging social problems.
2. **Training under Odisha projects:** The NIPCCD is the apex institute for training of functionaries of ICDS program in planning coordination, monitoring the training, building infrastructure, designing syllabi for training of all categories of ICDS functionaries, i.e. anganwadi workers (AWWs), supervisors, child development project officers (CDPOs), etc. In collaboration with WHO, it has undertaken a pilot project on integrated management of childhood illnesses. Under this project, 12 training programs were organized in which 287 AWWs of Haryana were trained.
3. **Documentation and publication:** The resource center of children (RCC) of NIPCCD is a specialized research and reference center for children and women. The RCC database has bibliographic details of documents received and indexed.
4. **New initiatives:** As detailed below:
   - Child rights, policies and legislation
   - Early childhood care and development

- Fund raising and its management
- Gender sensitization of national machinery
- Teleconference between parliamentarians, and women and grass roots
- Reproductive health and human immunodeficiency virus (HIV) or acquired immunodeficiency syndrome (AIDS)
- Gender budgeting and gender indicators.

COOPERATIVE FOR ASSISTANCE AND RELIEF EVERYWHERE

Cooperative for Assistance and Relief Everywhere (CARE) is one of the world's largest, independent, non-profit, non-sectarian, international relief and humanitarian organization. It was founded in 1945 by Wallace Campbell bell to provide relief to supervisors of World War II. It is one of the largest and oldest humanitarian aid organizations focused on fighting global poverty. It helps families in poor communities to improve their lives.

The CARE's programs are developing world to address a broad range of topics including emergency response, food security, water and sanitation, economic development, climate change, agriculture, education and health. CARE also advocates at the local, national and international levels for policy change and the rights of poor people. Within each of these areas, CARE focuses particularly on empowering and meeting the needs of women and girls, and on promoting gender equality. In India, this operation began in 1950. It also helps schools by providing garden tools, pumps and improved seeds to grow more food. CARE has provided mobile medical vans, X-ray machines, diagnosis equipment, eyeglasses, frames, medical books, medicines and vitamins.

Objectives

- To improve basic education
- To prevent the spread of HIV or AIDS
- To increase access to clean water and sanitation
- To expend economic opportunity
- To protect natural resources.

The CARE also delivers emergency aid to supervisors of war and natural disasters, and helps the people to rebuild their lives.

Campaigns

The CARE campaigns in the fight against global poverty, which include the following:

1. **World hunger campaign:** Donation to CARE sponsors' feeding programs, education, sustainable agriculture and other projects designed to reduce world hunger and poverty.
2. **Education:** Partners with government communities and organizations to improve quality and accessibility to basic education.
3. **HIV-AIDS:** The CARE provides educational programs and supports grass root efforts to reduce the spread of disease, and to aid those affected by HIV or AIDS.
4. **Victories over poverty:** The CARE works with communities to provide emergency relief and long-term solution to poverty, i.e.:
   a. In 2003, CARE delivered supplies and equipment including food, water and sanitation kits to pediatric hospitals, health centers and vulnerable families in Southern Iraq.
   b. In 2004, the organization suspended its operations in Iraq in response to kidnapping and apparent death.
   c. In December 2007, CARE announced its sponsorship of the 'Covance CARE'—early childhood development initiative for orphans and vulnerable children in Rwanda.

'CARE' in India

The CARE began its operation in India in 1950. Till the end of 1980s, primary objective of CARE India was to provide food for children in the age group of 6–11 years. From 1980s, CARE India focused its food support in the ICDS program and in development of programs in the areas of health, income and supplementation. It is helping in the following projects:

1. Integrated nutrition and health.
2. Better health and nutrition.
3. Anemia control.
4. Improving women's health.
5. Improved health care for adolescent girls.
6. Child survival.
7. Improving women's reproductive health and family spacing.
8. CARE India works in partnership with Government of India, state governments, non-government organizations (NGOs), etc. Currently, it has projects in Andhra Pradesh, Bihar, Madhya

Pradesh, Maharashtra, Odisha, Rajasthan, Uttar Pradesh and West Bengal.

9. It also advocates for policies that defend human rights and promote the eradication of poverty.
10. It promotes innovative solutions and advocates for global responsibility.
11. Strengthening capacity for self-help.
12. Providing economic opportunity.
13. Delivering relief in emergencies.
14. Influencing policy decisions at all levels.
15. Addressing discrimination in all its forms.

FOOD AND AGRICULTURE ORGANIZATION

The Food and Agriculture Organization (FAO) was founded on 16th October, 1945 in Quebec city, Canada. In 1951 its headquarters were moved from Washington DC, United States to Rome, Italy and regional office in Bangkok. It was the first United Nations Organization's specialized agency, created to look after several areas of world cooperation. India is a founder member of the FAO and has been taking part in all its activities. The FAO was founded in 1945 with a mandate to raise the levels of nutrition and standards of living, to improve agriculture productivity and to better the conditions of rural population to:

- Help nations to raise living standards
- Improve nutrition of the peoples of all countries
- Increase the efficiency of farming, forestry and fisheries
- Better the condition of rural people and through all those means, to widen the opportunity of all people for productive work.

Structure

The FAO is governed by the conference of member nation, which meets every 2 years to review the work carried out by the organization and to approve a program of work and budget for the next biennium. The conference also elects the Director General to head the agency. The FAO is composed of eight departments. They are:

- Administration and finance
- Agriculture
- Economic
- Social
- Fisheries

- Forestry
- General affairs and information
- Sustainable development and technical cooperation.

Budget

The FAO's regular program budget is funded by its members, through contributions set at the FAO conference. This budget covers care, technical work, cooperation and partnerships including technical and cooperation program information and general policy, direction and administrative.

Activities

1. The FAO gives practical help to developing countries through a wide range of technical assistance projects. The organization encourages an integrated approach with environmental, social and economic considerations including the formation of development projects.
2. The FAO collects, analyzes, interprets and disseminates information relating to nutrition, food, agriculture, forestry and fisheries. The organization serves as a clearing house, providing farmers, scientists, traders and government planners with the information they need to make regional decisions on planning, investment, marketing, training or research.
3. The FAO provides independent advice on agricultural policy in planning, and the administrative and legal structures needed for development. It includes national strategies towards rural development, increased food security and the alleviation of poverty.
4. The FAO approves international standards and helps frame international conventions and agreements, and regularly hosts major conferences, technical meetings and consultations of expects.
5. India receives assistance from FAO for time to time in the form of training, consultancy services, equipment and material in the field of agriculture and allied sectors under its technical cooperation program. The various technical cooperation projects in India are:
   a. Transfer on technology for vegetative propogation of walnut in Jammu and Kashmir State.
   b. Assistance to agriculture in Karnataka.

c. Development of integrated plant nutrition system methodology.
d. Training to agriculture in Karnataka.
e. Training in sea safety development programs.
f. Food quality control.

Programs and Achievements

1. **Special program for food security (SPFS):** It is FAO's flagship initiative for reaching the goal of having very less number of hungry people in the world by 2015 through projects in over 100 countries worldwide.
2. **Integrated pest management:** During 1990s, FAO took a leading role in the promotion of integrated pest management for rice production in Asia using an approach known as the farmer field school.
3. **FAO statistics:** The FAO Statistical Division produces FAOSTAT, an online multilingual database on agriculture, nutrition, fisheries, food acid, land use and population from over 210 countries.
4. **Telefood:** In 1997, FAO launched telefood, a campaign of concerns, sporting events and other activities to harness the power of media, celebrities and concerned citizens to help fight hunger.
5. **Right to adequate food:** The FAO's strategic framework (2000–2015) stipulates that the organization is expected to take into full account the progress made in further developing a rights-based approach to food security in carrying out its mission, helping to build a food secure world for present and future generation.
6. **International alliance against hunger (IAAH):** The IAAH was launched on World Food Day, 16th October, 2003. The IAAH works to generate political will, concentrates actions through partnership between inter- and non-governmental organizations, and national alliances.
7. **Goodwill ambassadors:** This program was initiated in 1999. The main purpose of the program is to attract public and media attention to the unacceptable situation that some 800 million people continue to suffer from chronic hunger and malnutrition. The main aim of the goodwill is to make food for all a reality in and beyond 21st century.

NATIONAL INSTITUTE OF NUTRITION

The national institute of nutrition is one of the premier permanent research institutes of the Indian Council of Medical Research (ICMR), an autonomous body under the aegis of the Ministry of Health and Family Welfare, Government of India located at Hyderabad. It was founded in 1918 as part of Coonoor Pasteur Institute.

Objectives

- To identify various dietary and nutrition problems prevalent among different segments of the population
- To continuously monitor diet and nutrition situation of the country
- To evolve effective methods of management, prevention and control of nutritional problems through research, keeping the existing economic, social and administrative set up in view
- To conduct operative research to pave the way for planning and implementation of national nutrition programs
- To investigate nutritional deficiencies, nutrient interactions and food toxicities at basic level for understanding the biochemical mechanism involved
- To provide training and orientation in nutrition to key health professionals
- To disseminate authentic health and nutrition information through appropriate extension activities
- To integrate the institute's research programs with other health, agricultural and economic programs as envisaged by the government
- To advise governments and other organizations on problems of nutrition.

Facilities Available in NIN

Laboratory facilities: These are excellent with all sophisticated instruments needed for modern biomedical research investigations in various laboratories.

Clinical facilities: These include nutritional units for out- and in-patients in three local hospitals to carryout research on clinical aspects of nutrition. A metabolic unit for carrying out metabolic studies on volunteers.

Communication and computation facilities: These are for fast retrieval and efficient communication of information through internet and e-mail facilities.

Education and training program: For planning, implementation and objective evaluation of various community health program needs by trained health personnel. It conducts various programs at undergraduate and postgraduate levels.

Activities

The institute's activities can be broadly categorized under four categories:

1. **Clinical studies:** These are being conducted on the role of intrauterine infections and vitamin nutritional status on the pregnancy outcome. Field studies are being conducted on the impact of women's workload on health. Efficacy of immunization programs in relation to the widely prevalent nutritional disorders such as protein-energy malnutrition (PEM) and vitamin A deficiency have also been investigated.

   Clinical studies in adults include nutritional disorders such as pellagra and degenerative diseases such as diabetes, cancer and cardiovascular diseases. This unit has also been engaged in studies on absorption, metabolism and toxicity of commonly used drugs in various deficiency states in both experimental animals and humans.
2. **Laboratory studies:** The institute has undertaken some laboratory investigations covering a wide range of specialties such as biochemistry, food chemistry, pathology, immunology, hematology, microbiology, endocrinology, physiology and toxicology. Excellent facilities exist for laboratory animal breeding and experimentation.
3. **Community studies:** The institute collaborates with the state and central government, and international agencies in planning and conducting diet and nutrition surveys, evaluating ongoing nutrition programs conducting studies on sociocultural aspects of nutrition.
4. **Teaching programs:** Though primarily a research-oriented institution, teaching and training activities are also given priority. The institute has been recognized by WHO as a center for advanced training in health and nutrition.

CENTRAL FOOD TECHNOLOGY AND RESEARCH INSTITUTE

The Central Food Technology and Research Institute (CFTRI) is the national institute under the Council of Ministry of Scientific and Industrial Research, Government of India and was started in 1950. It deals with the measures of food science and technology.

A local planning advisory committee was constituted in early 1949 under the chairmanship of KC Reddy, the Chief Minister of Mysore, with Dr V Subramanian as its Planning Officer's member. Finally, on Saturday, the 21st October 1950, the CFTRI was declared open by C Rajagopalachari, the Home Minister in the Government of India and Dr V Subramanian became the first Director of the institution. The main scientific disciplines of the institute are as follows:

- Biochemistry and applied nutrition
- Rice and pulse technology
- Flour milling, baking and confectionery
- Food engineering
- Packaging
- Fruits and vegetables technology
- Industrial research, consultancy and extension
- Infestation control and pesticides.

Chapter 45

Nutrition Education and Role of Nurse

DEFINITIONS

1. "Nutrition education as a means of translating nutritional requirements into food and adjusting the food choices to satisfy the nutritional, cultural, psychological and economic needs."
—Albanese, 1971
2. "Nutrition education is a process by which beliefs, attitudes, environmental influences and understanding about food lead to practices that are scientifically sound, practical and consistent with individual needs and available food resources."
—American Dietetic Association, 1973
3. "It is a multidisciplinary process that involves the transfer information, development of motivation and modification of food habits where needed." *—Leviton, 1974*
4. "Nutrition education is the foundation for any program intended for nutritional improvement." *—Devadas, 1970*
5. "It is the process of applying knowledge of nutrition-related scientific information of social and behavioral science in base designed to influence individuals and groups to eat the kinds and amount of foods that we make a maximum contribution to health and social satisfaction." *—Obert, 1978*
6. "It is for making food choices and for the achievement of one's genetic potential, the knowledge of nutrition is perfective."
—White, 1976

NEED OF NUTRITION EDUCATION

India's food and nutrition problems continue to the formidable and malnutrition is still one of the crucial problems in the process of development. Most of the people are suffering from nutritional deficiency diseases such as protein-energy malnutrition (PEM), vitamin A deficiency, iron deficiency anemia and iodine deficiency disorders. Because of lack of awareness about dietary requirements and nutritional values of different foods, illiteracy, ignorance, all the factors directly plays an important role to cause these diseases.

Nearly two third of India's population is a nutritionally deficient. Nutritional surveys conducted and repeated over a number of years indicated that the majority population of every age group (infants, preschooler, school-going children, pregnant women, lactating mother, adolescent girls and old age people) including both the sexes, suffer from malnutrition because both deficiency of protein and calorie or protein starvation and complete lack of food, which is rich in vitamins and minerals [Gopalan 1963, Ranganathan (1968), Devadas (1972), NIN (1982) annual reports].

Malnutrition effects people in general, but adverse effects are more pronounced among the foods of women and children in rural and urban areas. Malnutrition is exclusively due to nonavailability of nutritious food. Failure to use the available rich sources in a meaningful way can be another cause; this is due to lack of knowledge of the value of foods in relation to its individual ignorance; and superstition plays an important role in the detection of chief nutritious foods. The nutritional profile of the Indian women and children focus on the need to take active steps towards prevention of malnutrition. So, for the prevention of nutritional deficiencies prevailing in the community, nutrition education plays a major role to create awareness about nutritional education.

METHODS OF NUTRITION EDUCATION

The important methods of nutritional education are:

1. Lectures and demonstrations.
2. Workshops.
3. Films, still pictures and slides.
4. Posters, charts and exhibitions.
5. Books, pamphlets, bulletins and newspapers.
6. Radio and television.

Lectures and Demonstrations

The lecture should be simple and practical. They should be easily understood by those attending the course. The demonstrations should also be simple and practical, so that they can be adopted by the community.

Workshops

The nutrition workshop should discuss the nutritional problems of the region, and the steps to be taken for solving the problems and for improving the nutrition of the community.

Films, Still Pictures and Slides

The methods are extremely effective education media. They should be practical and illustrative, and easily understood by the people. The narrations should be in the regional language.

Posters, Charts and Exhibitions

Posters should be simple, clear and aesthetic in color and arrangement, written in the regional language. They should stimulate the interests of the people. Charts should be easily visible from a distance. Letters should be big and bar charts should be used to represent the growth of children, and for comparing well-balanced and ill-balanced diets. Exhibitions having posters and charts are a permanent set up for educating the community. Nutrition exhibits should be set up in schools, clubs and other public places, which are readily accessible to the people.

Books, Pamphlets, Bulletins and Newspaper Articles

Printed matter in nutrition and dietetics suitable for educating the students, teacher and other employed in other occupations should be made available in regional languages at low cost price. Popular articles in nutrition and dietetics should be published in newspapers.

Radio and Television

Radio and Television programs reach large number of people at definite times.

OBJECTIVES OF NUTRITION EDUCATION

1. To develop nutrition advisory services and nutrition education of the public.
2. To participate in coordinated community nutrition programs with the cooperation of other disciplines and agencies where necessary.
3. To help for development of supplementary feeding programs wherever necessary and provide continuing consultant services to them.

4. To improve nutrition levels in the community by these and other available means.

SPECIFIC MEANS OF NUTRITION EDUCATION

Specific means include the following:

1. Health or nutrition surveys, for baseline and progress assessment of nutritional status with special reference to vulnerable groups (pregnant and lactating women, infants, preschoolers and school-age children). The nutrition assessment schedule is given in Box 45.1.

Box 45.1: Nutrition assessment schedule

Serial number:	Date: ....
Name:	Age: ....
Address:	Sex: ....
District:	Village: ....

2. Study of food patterns and the socioeconomic factors, beliefs, customs and traditions affecting diets in the area.
3. Nutrition advisory services for individuals and nutrition education programs for vulnerable groups.
4. Participation in the nutrition aspects of other community development, adult education and school education program.
5. Development of nutrition education materials adapted to the local situation.
6. Supplementary feeding programs in MCH activities.
7. Technical advice to school feeding programs on health aspects.
8. Environmental hygiene program, so far, as they influence nutritional status.

TRAINING IN NUTRITION EDUCATION

Training in nutrition can be broadly classified as:

1. Training of professional workers in nutrition and dietetics.
2. Imparting nutrition training for persons engaged in other professions, e.g. teachers, health visitors, nurses, social workers, etc.

Training of Professional Worker in Nutrition and Dietetics

In almost all countries, specialized training facilities are available for the training of nutritionists and dietitians suitable for working as specialists in schools, colleges, hospitals, MCH centers, etc. for imparting nutrition education to the community.

Nutritionists

Nutritionists may be defined as specialists in the field of nutrition who have received both theoretical and practical training in nutrition to qualify them to work in national nutrition programs designed to improve the nutrition of the community. They receive training not only in nutrition and dietetics but also economics and sociology, so that they are aware of the various factors contributing to the wide prevalence of malnutrition in the community.

Dietitians

Dietitians may be defined as workers who have received training in dietetics at the degree level in a university followed by a period of practical training in institutions to qualify them for diet and food management in hospitals, school, lunch rooms and other institutions. During the course of their work, they have the opportunity to impart education in the practical aspects of nutrition and dietetics to nurses, school teachers, social workers, etc.

Training in Nutrition for Workers in other Professions

With suitable instructions in nutrition for short period of 3–4 months, workers in other professions and occupations such as school teachers, welfare workers, public health workers, nurses and community project workers can be given training in nutrition. The course should be practical and should stress on the nutritional deficiencies prevalent in the community and their prevention by the use of local foods.

CHANNELS OF NUTRITION EDUCATION TO THE COMMUNITY

Nutrition education can be conducted through the following channels:

- Health centers
- Women organizations
- Schools and colleges.

Health Centers

The health center is an ideal place for imparting nutrition education to mothers. Nutrition education can be imparted at the centers through:

- Individual consultations
- Lectures and demonstrations
- Distribution of supplementary foods.

Individual Consultations

Pregnant and nursing mothers visit health centers for consultations regarding ailments from which they suffer. The doctor incharge of the center can advise the mothers regarding diets, which they and their children should consume.

Lectures and Demonstrations

The lectures on dietary requirements, deficiency diseases and balanced diets should include practical demonstrations. The use of locally available foods as supplements to the diets of children and mothers should be demonstrated. The effect of supplementary goods on the growth of malnourished children and treatment of PEM and vitamin A deficiency diseases with protein foods and vitamin A concentrates should be explained with the help of charts.

Distribution of Supplementary Foods

Protein-enriched cereal foods should be distributed for feeding children, and processed protein foods and iron tablets for pregnant women and nursing mothers. The value of these foods as supplements to their diet should be explained to the mothers.

Women Organizations

Women organizations can serve as convenient centers for imparting nutrition education and for conducting practical demonstrations of feeding of infants and children with locally available foods. The school teachers and social workers can help in this work.

Schools and Colleges

Nutrition education should be introduced as a compulsory subject in all schools and colleges. This will help the boys and girls who will be future parents to appreciate the role of well-balanced diets in promoting good growth and maintaining good health of infants, children, expectant and lactating mothers.

ROLE OF NURSE IN NUTRITION EDUCATION PROGRAM

Nurse should play a major role for giving nutrition education in the community. The roles of nurse are:

- She should be a communicator
- She should be a demonstrator
- She should be a supervisor
- She should be a organizer
- She should be a teacher
- She should be a educator
- She should be a observer
- She should be a advisor
- She should be a participator
- She should be a evaluator.

The aim of nutrition education is to guide people to choose optimum and balanced diets, remove prejudice and promote good dietary habits. Nutritional problems such as ignorance about the value of breast feeding, traditional food allocation pattern in the families, etc. can be best solved by nutrition education. In recent years, the link between dietary habits and certain chronic diseases such as obesity, diabetes and cardiovascular diseases has been established. Nutrition education is a major intervention in the hands of nurses for the prevention of malnutrition, promotion of health and improving the quality of life.

Today, nutrition is considered as an important aspect of treatment of certain diseases. So, this is the prime responsibility of a nurse to teach about good nutrition to the patients in the hospital and to the families in the community. This teaching helps the people to select right kind of foods to eat, safe methods of cooking, hygienic practices in handling and preservation of food. Nurse is the key person to provide nutrition education to the hospitalized patients and their relatives, and her role is equally important when she works in community. Her main focuses of nutrition education are:

1. **Breastfeeding and weaning:** People should be taught for exclusive breastfeeding at least for 6 months. Breastfeeding should be started during pregnancy period. This information is being provided by clinical nurse and community health nurse.

2. **Preschool and school-going children:** The children have growth spurts at this age period. They require extra protein in their diet. Mothers must be taught regarding the adequate intake of diet by their children. School teacher also need detailed information about nutrition, as they prepare mid-day school meal.
3. **Pregnant and lactating mothers:** This group must be taught by the community health nurse when they come for antenatal and postnatal check-up that they need extra calories, proteins and calcium. This will include a fair amount of milk, GLV, pulses and fruits.
4. **Balanced diet:** People from low income group and rural background have less awareness regarding the balanced diets. Nurse in the community should provide detailed information to the people who want. So, she should have comprehensive knowledge of balanced diet for different age group people.
5. **Malnutrition:** This is a man-made disease. It begins quite commonly in the womb. The main cause of this problem is ignorance, cultural factors and socioeconomic status. Malnutrition can be prevented by providing proper nutrition education and information to the people about cheap and best sources of protein and other nutrients.
6. **Therapeutic diet:** Patients suffering from certain diseases such as diabetes, heart and liver problems can be cured with diet therapy along with medicines, but they need guidance and counseling for therapeutic modifications of diet. Nurse is a team leader in the hospital who provides this information. They should observe either therapeutic diets prepared in the hospital kitchen are provided to the patients properly as per their disease.
7. **Food fads and faulty food habits:** The diet of the people is influenced by local conditions, religious customs and beliefs. The concept of hot and cold food is widely prevalent. There are misconceptions and prejudices, which can be removed by teaching the community. Health education is the main weapon to erase these food fads and habits.

Methods Imparting Nutrition Education (Fig. 45.1)

Community health nurse can use various methods of imparting nutrition education to the people including various audiovisual (AV) aids as follows:

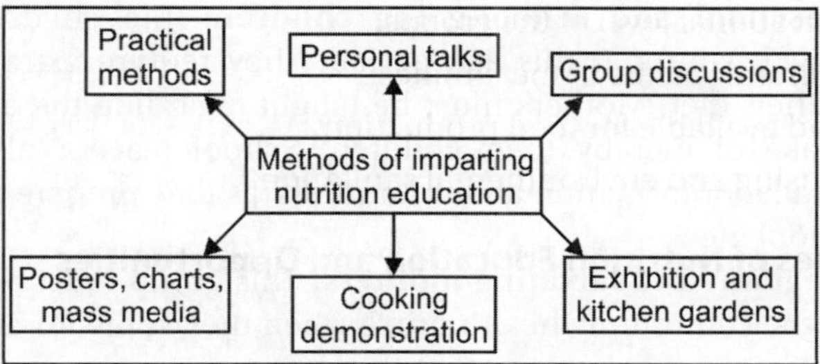

Figure 45.1: Methods of imparting nutrition

1. **Personal talks:** It may be one-to-one casual or formal talks related to any particular topic. It may include menu planning, budgeting the food, etc. People in the rural community are ignorant. They should be provided with detailed knowledge by a nurse.
2. **Group discussion:** It may be organized by a nurse dietician and expert in the field of nutrition. Group should include the person with same characteristics.
3. **Exhibition and kitchen garden:** These are the real aids, which can show the practical means of using fresh vegetables and fruits. Exhibition is also visual demonstration, which helps and motivates people to adopt nutritional preparations.
4. **Cooking demonstration:** This helps the people to change their menu as per their taste. They can learn various methods of cooking.
5. **Posters and charts:** These are visual aids, which can be used to highlight specific features in nutrition. Most of the health professionals display posters to educate people in this field.
6. **Practical methods:** These include short menu planning, food budgeting, etc. During home visits to the families, nurse can guide them as per their family size, income, age group and their food habits.

Factors to be Considered in Nutrition Education

While imparting nutrition education, nurses or other health professional should observe following factors:

1. Culture, religion, food habits and food fads.
2. Food available locally and water supply.

3. Educational level of the groups.
4. Economic status of the families.
5. Land available for food production.
6. Housing and environmental sanitation.

Principles of Nutrition Education and Opportunities

Principles

1. First observe and ask questions to learn about the culture and food habits of the people, and what foods are available?
2. Do not expect people to change food habits easily. New ideas should be introduced gradually and only one thing is taught at a time. Any suggested change should be acceptable and integrated into the present cultural practices.
3. Help people to see that good nutrition is important for them, e.g. if they want their children to grow strong and do well at school, enough of the right kinds of foods must be given to them.
4. Find out the local words for food, so that there will be better communication.
5. In teaching, use actual foods whenever possible, especially home-produced foods, teach also with nutritional posters, flip charts, puppets, role play, etc.
6. Always encourage questions and discussions, to clear doubts. Ask those who have tried out something new to tell others about it.
7. Link the teaching on nutrition with MCH activities and with other health education.
8. Do not teach people the things that is not possible for them to do, nor about foods they cannot afford to buy or cannot get.
9. Follow-up and find out if families are making the needed changes in food practices. Use the information to modify the (own) teaching.

Opportunities

1. Visiting families for any reason may help them in learning better budgeting, selection, storage, preparation and cooking of foods.
2. In the antenatal clinics and at the under-five clinics, there will be opportunities for both group and individual nutrition education.

3. A nutrition education program for mothers, including cooking demonstrations, can be arranged at the outpatient departments and also in the inpatient wards.
4. Nutrition education is an important part of the school health program. It may be linked with a school mid-day meals program.

Clinical Features

1. **General appearance:** Normal built/Thin built/Sickly.
2. **Hair:** Normal/Lack of luster/Dyspigmented/Thin and sparse/Easily pluckable/Flag sign.
3. **Face:** Diffuse depigmentation/Nasolabial dyssebacia/Moon face.
4. **Eyes:** Conjunctiva—normal/Dry on exposure for ½ min/Dry and wrinkled/Bitot's spots/Brown pigmentation/Angular conjunctivitis/Pale conjunctive. Cornea—normal/dryness/hazy or opaque.
5. **Lips:** Normal/Angular stomatitis/Cheilosis.
6. **Tongue:** Normal/Pale and flabby/Red and raw/Fissured/Geographic.
7. **Teeth:** Mottled enamel/Caries/Attrition.
8. **Gums:** Normal/Spongy bleeding.
9. **Glands:** Thyroid enlargement/Parotid enlargement.
10. **Skin:** Normal/Dry and scaly/Follicular hyperkeratosis/Petechiae/Pellagrous dermatosis/Flaky paint dermatosis/Scrotal and vulval dermatosis.
11. **Nails:** Koilonychia.
12. **Edema:** Independent parts.
13. **Rachitic changes:** The knock-knees or bow legs/Epiphyseal enlargement/Beading of the ribs/Pigeon chest.
14. **Internal systems:** Sensory loss/Muscle wasting/Weakness/Loss of position sense/Motor weakness/Loss of vibration sense/Ankle and knee jerks/Calf tenderness/Cardiac enlargement/Tachycardia.

Anthropometric

- Weight (kg)
- Height (cm)
- Mid-upper arm circumference (cm)
- Head circumference (cm)
- Chest circumference (cm)
- Skinfold.

Laboratory findings

- **Hemoglobin:** Specify method)
- **Stool:** Negative ascariasis/Ancylostomiasis/Giardiasis/Amebiasis/ Stongyloides/Others (state)
- **Blood smear:** Negative malaria test/Filaria.

Index

Page numbers followed by *f* and *t* indicate figures and tables, respectively.

C

D

E

G

H

L

M

N